Quality of Life

Jones and Bartlett Series in Oncology

2003 Oncology Nursing Drug Handbook, Wilkes/Ingwersen/Barton-Burke

American Cancer Society Patient Education Guide to Oncology Drugs, Second Edition, Wilkes/Ades/Krakoff

American Cancer Society Consumer's Guide to Cancer Drugs, Second Edition, Wilkes/Ades/Krakoff

Biotherapy: A Comprehensive Overview, Second Edition, Rieger

Blood and Marrow Stem Cell Transplantation, Second Edition, Whedon

Cancer and HIV Clinical Nutrition Pocket Guide, Second Edition, Wilkes

Cancer Chemotherapy: A Nursing Process Approach, Third Edition, Barton-Burke/Wilkes/Ingwersen

Cancer Nursing: Principles and Practice, Fifth Edition, Yarbro/Frogge/Goodman/Groenwald

Cancer Symptom Management, Third Edition, Yarbro/Frogge/Goodman

Chemotherapy Care Plans Handbook, Third Edition, Barton-Burke/Wilkes/Ingwersen

Clinical Guide to Cancer Nursing, Fifth Edition, Yarbro/Frogge/Goodman

Clinical Handbook for Biotherapy, Rieger

Comprehensive Cancer Nursing Review, Fourth Edition, Groenwald/Frogge/Goodman/Yarbro

Contemporary Issues in Breast Cancer: A Nursing Perspective, Second Edition, Hassey Dow

Contemporary Issues in Colorectal Cancer: A Nursing Perspective, Berg

Contemporary Issues in Lung Cancer: A Nursing Perspective, Haas

Contemporary Issues in Prostate Cancer: A Nursing Perspective, Held-Warmkessel

Fatigue in Cancer: A Multidimensional Approach, Winningham/Barton-Burke

Handbook of Breast Cancer Risk-Assessment: Evidence-Based Guidelines for Evaluation, Prevention, Counseling, and Treatment, Vogel/Bevers

Handbook of Oncology Nursing, Third Edition, Johnson/Gross

Health-Care Instruments for Clinical Research, Second Edition, Frank-Stromborg

Homecare Management of the Bone Marrow Transplant Patient, Third Edition, Kelley/McBride/Randolph/Leum/Lonergan

Making the Decision: A Cancer Patient's Guide to Clinical Trials, Mulay

Memory Bank for Chemotherapy, Third Edition, Preston/Wilfinger

Oncology Nursing Review, Second Edition, Yarbro/Frogge/Goodman

Physicians' Cancer Chemotherapy Drug Manual 2003, Chu

Pocket Guide for Women and Cancer, Moore-Higgs/Almadrones/Colvin-Huff/Gossfield/Eriksson

Pocket Guide to Breast Cancer, Second Edition, Hassey Dow

Pocket Guide to Colorectal Cancer, Berg

Pocket Guide to Prostate Cancer, Held-Warmkessel

Progress in Oncology 2002, Devita/Hellman/Rosenberg

Quality of Life: From Nursing and Patient Perspectives, Second Edition, King/Hinds

A Step-by-Step Guide to Clinical Trials, Mulay

Women and Cancer: A Gynecologic Oncology Nursing Perspective, Second Edition, Moore-Higgs/Almadrones/Colvin-Huff/Gossfield/Eriksson

Quality of Life

FROM NURSING AND PATIENT PERSPECTIVES

THEORY • RESEARCH • PRACTICE

SECOND EDITION

CYNTHIA R. KING & PAMELA S. HINDS • EDITORS

JONES AND BARTLETT PUBLISHERS

Sudbury, Massachusetts

BOSTON   TORONTO   LONDON   SINGAPORE

World Headquarters
Jones and Bartlett Publishers
40 Tall Pine Drive
Sudbury, MA 01776
978-443-5000
info@jbpub.com
www.jbpub.com

Jones and Bartlett Publishers
Canada
2406 Nikanna Road
Mississauga, ON L5C 2W6
CANADA

Jones and Bartlett Publishers
International
Barb House, Barb Mews
London W6 7PA
UK

Library of Congress Cataloging-in-Publication Data

Quality of Life : from nursing and patient perspectives / Cynthia R. King and Pamela S.
    Hinds [editors]. – 2nd ed.
        p. ; cm.
    Includes bibliographical references and index.
    ISBN 0-7637-2235-9
    1. Cancer—Nursing. 2. Quality of life. 3. Cancer—Psychological aspects. 4.
Cancer—Social aspects. I. King, Cynthia R. II. Hinds, Pamela S.
    [DNLM: 1. Neoplasms—nursing. 2. Quality of Life. 3. Oncologic Nursing. 4. Patient
Satisfaction. WY 156 Q14 2003]
    RC266.Q35 2003
    610.73'698—dc21

                                                                    2002043336

Acquisitions Editor: Penny M. Glynn
Production Manager: Amy Rose
Associate Production Editor: Karen C. Ferreira
Associate Editor: Karen Zuck
Production Assistant: Jenny L. McIsaac
Senior Marketing Manager: Alisha Weisman
Associate Marketing Manager: Joy Stark-Vancs
Marketing Associate: Jennifer Killam-Zambrano
Manufacturing Buyer: Amy Bacus
Cover Design: Philip Regan
Composition: Chiron, Inc.
Illustrations: Marcia Smith
Printing and Binding: Malloy Inc.
Cover Printing: Malloy Inc.

Printed in the United States of America
07 06 05 04 03   10 9 8 7 6 5 4 3 2 1

We dedicate this special book to our families (Michael, Martha, John, Ron, Ben, and Adam) who have supported us throughout the writing, editing, and publishing process, and to our nursing colleagues, staff, patients, and families (of St. Jude's Children's Research Hospital and many other hospitals and cancer centers) who have taught us to look beyond the outcome of survival to quality of living and to remember the importance of hopefulness, courage, and love.

Contents

Foreword xi
Preface xv
Acknowledgments xvii
Contributors xix

SECTION 1   **OVERVIEW** 1

Chapter 1   Evolution of Quality of Life in Oncology and Oncology Nursing   3
Marcia M. Grant and Grace E. Dean

Chapter 2   Overview of Quality of Life and Controversial Issues   29
Cynthia R. King

SECTION 2   **THEORY** 43

Chapter 3   Theories and Conceptual Models to Guide Quality of Life Related Research   45
April Hazard Vallerand and Judith K. Payne

Chapter 4   Conceptualization and Measurement of Quality of Life and Related Concepts: Guidelines for Clarity   65
Joan E. Haase and Carrie Jo Braden

Chapter 5   Spiritual Quality of Life   93
Elizabeth Johnston Taylor

Chapter 6   Quality of Life and Culture   117
Geraldine V. Padilla

Chapter 7   Quality of Life in Children and Adolescents with Cancer   143
Pamela S. Hinds and Joan E. Haase

SECTION 3   **RESEARCH** 169

Chapter 8   Quality of Life Methodological and Measurement Issues   171
Mel R. Haberman and Nigel Bush

Chapter 9   Quality of Life and Symptoms   199
                 Betty R. Ferrell and Marcia M. Grant

Chapter 10   Quality of Life in Families Experiencing Cancer   219
                 Kathleen M. Stetz

SECTION 4   PRACTICE   239

Chapter 11   Quality of Life Issues in Breast Cancer   241
                 Deanna Kuhn and Karen Hassey Dow

Chapter 12   Clinical Implications of Quality of Life   261
                 Cynthia R. King

Chapter 13   Quality of Life Issues Related to Marrow Transplantation   273
                 June G. Eilers and Cynthia R. King

Chapter 14   A European Perspective on Quality of Life of Stem Cell
                 Transplantation Patients   315
                 Monica C. Fliedner

Chapter 15   Fatigue and Quality of Life A Question of Balance   345
                 Margaret Barton-Burke

SECTION 5   PATIENT PERSPECTIVES   379

Chapter 16   Cancer Survivorship Quality for Life   381
                 Susan A. Leigh and Ellen L. Stovall

Chapter 17   Quality of Life Stories by Patients and Families   397

SECTION 6   CONCLUSION   411

Chapter 18   Nursing and Patient Perspectives on Quality of Life   413
                 Pamela S. Hinds and Cynthia R. King

**APPENDIX 1   Descriptions/Definitions of Quality of Life by Sample (Adult or Youth)
                 and Publication Year   419**

APPENDIX 2   Quality of Life Measurements   427

                 I. Example of the Global Single Item Approach to Measuring
                    Quality of Life   429
                    • Quality of Life Visual Life Analogue Scale (VAS)   429
                      Kate Lorig

II. Examples of Generic Measures of Quality of Life   431
- The McCorkle and Young Symptom Distress Scale   431
  Ruth McCorkle and Kathy Young Graham
- Demands of Illness Inventory   435
  Mel. R. Haberman
- Quality of Life Index   447
  Geraldine V. Padilla and Marcia M. Grant

III. Examples of Cancer-Specific Measures of Quality of Life (Single Measure Approach)   451
- Quality of Life Index: Cancer Version   451
  Carol Ferrans
- Quality of Life Scale: Bone Marrow Transplant   455
  Betty R. Ferrell and Marcia M. Grant

IV. Example of Cancer-Specific Measure of Quality of Life (Battery Approach)   465
- Quality of Life Components for Pediatric Oncology Group (POG) Protocols   465
  Andrew Bradlyn

V. Example of Cancer-Specific Measure of Quality of Life (Modular Approach)   473
- The Bush Bone Marrow Transplant Symptom Inventory   473
  Nigel Bush

VI. Sample Tools for Measuring Quality of Life in Children with Cancer   481
- PedsQL™ Pediatric Quality of Life Inventory for Young Children (ages 5–7)   481
- PedsQL™ Pediatric Quality of Life Inventory for Children (ages 8–12)   495
- PedsQL™ Pediatric Quality of Life Inventory for Teens (ages 13–18)   507

Index   518

Foreword

During my career as an oncology nurse I have been privileged to witness the extraordinary clinical and political changes that have shaped the current treatment and management of cancer care over the past three decades. These changes were initiated in the early 1970s when President Nixon signed the Cancer Act into law. Today, as issues as diverse as access to care, genetic testing, and symptom management routinely employ quality of life (QOL) rhetoric, it is difficult to imagine that in 1979, when the Oncology Nursing Society's president Connie Yarbro asked me to chair the first research committee, QOL was a term unknown to many of us. Drs. Padilla and Grant recognized early on that QOL was an essential part of cancer care and were the first to attempt to capture it as a measure in a nursing context. At the same time, with my colleagues Jeanne Benoliel and Kathy Young, we developed the symptom distress and the enforced social dependency scales to document the impact of cancer and its treatment effects on patients. We knew we needed dependent variables to measure what was happening to patients, especially over time, and these measures seemed to work since they captured the patients' subjective experiences. The major contribution nursing made during those early years was to recognize that patients' perspectives had to be included in order to grasp the full impact of their experiences and plan their care.

The term QOL reached its outcome status when the Food and Drug Administration helped to promote its inclusion in cancer clinical trials in 1985. The federal guidelines were changed to include a favorable effect on either an individual's QOL or survival when new anti-cancer drugs were approved for testing. Subsequently, QOL research has proliferated as a result of this policy change. Although the incidence of many cancers has remained relatively stable over the past century, long-term survival for many types of cancer has improved dramatically. This improvement in overall survival has gradually changed the image of cancer from a disease shrouded in overtones of death to a chronic illness with inherent, episodic, and often long-term needs. Dramatic changes in medical technology and health care delivery continue to impact patient care at every level. New, often toxic, treatments have rendered previously fatal diseases treatable although often with long-term consequences to patients, including varying degrees of symptomatic episodes and functional impairment. When cancer treatments are prescribed, they hopefully have a positive impact on a patient's well-being by controlling or eliminating the cancer and its effects, but treatments often are accompanied by undesirable and lasting side effects. There is a need to weigh the negative and positive effects of a therapy when assessing its value. When put into the context of the patient's life situation, this overall balance is reflected by the concept of QOL. As scientific progress in the fight against cancer continues, QOL issues are increasingly added to the equation when making treatment decisions, including when to halt treatment. King and Hinds are to be commended for expanding the context and increasing our understanding that QOL permeates the total cancer experience for patients and families, making it explicit that it is not just limited to the effects of cancer treatment. In recent years, I have become cautiously optimistic that QOL has finally achieved a position in clinical practice where it can no longer be easily dismissed. This change in position has lasting power because consumer groups have played a critical role in demanding that they have a voice in treatment decision-making and the management of their care. The presence of this book underscores the importance of their voice.

For many of us, the way we view the world and our own personal definition of QOL has been influenced and shaped by the intentional bombings of the World Trade Center in New York City and the Pentagon on September 11, 2001, and the subsequent devastation and loss of life and property that resulted. These senseless acts of violence have given us an opportunity to become introspective about our own mortality, the uncertainty of our future health, and our priorities in life. We can all somehow agree that the quality of our lives was affected by the mass destruction, and we may even be able to achieve agreement on common dimensions. However, consensus is less clear in the context of disease and on an individual level. Our differences are reflected in our values. The experience of cancer holds different meanings and values for each of us and the experience can impact us on a range of dimension. As a group we might have common responses across dimensions, but examination of an individual profile might show that any particular patient could be dramatically different from the overall group. Both perspectives—the individual and the group—are critical to include and this book offers useful strategies for approaching these methodological challenges.

There have been remarkable strides made in the science related to QOL as illustrated by many of the chapters included in the second edition of King and Hinds' book. The ability to publish a second edition reflects the positive reception and success of the first edition and the importance of the content, and provides opportunities to include new advances in the field and to fine tune the previous chapters. The diverse backgrounds of the two editors are reflected in the content, including the state of the science in QOL for both adults and children. They have also expanded their understanding of context by clarifying and adding chapters related to culture and spirituality. The editors have taken an important step in giving educators, students, and clinicians a comprehensive guide of what is known and what can be done about ensuring QOL for our patients and their families. They have enlisted the help of authors, who are experts on studying QOL and its consequences, not only how to measure it, but also what strategies can be used to improve it. The authors are either seasoned researchers or experienced clinicians who are sensitive to the hard realities of trying to translate knowledge into clinical practice. Several authors have focused on the methodological and conceptual issues. Several chapters include issues related to QOL in cancer treatment in general and some in relation to specific diagnoses.

Perhaps the most important accomplishment of this text is its inclusion of all the elements related to QOL into one informative and coherent book that includes both patient and nurses' perspectives. As King and Hinds illustrate, nursing has played an important role in advancing QOL. However, while nursing leadership is critical, it is not by itself sufficient for successful achievement of QOL in cancer care. In addition to the patient's perspective, they recognize the important contributions of professionals from other disciplines, working together in a partnership with patients and families. Many gaps remain between knowledge gained though science and the translation of that information to the actual experience of people who are diagnosed, treated, and surviving cancer. This book helps us look back with pride at all that has been accomplished and the important next steps to continue. King and Hinds' book is a valuable contribution to our ongoing discussion of setting our agenda for research and the implementation of evidence-based practice. Because nurses are present the most frequently and consistently with patients and families in all contexts, we must become the champions for ensuring QOL on all fronts, with our professional colleagues, in our workplace, and in influencing policy to change how care is delivered. I commend King and Hinds for making this valuable contribution to our understanding of QOL that will shape cancer care in the future.

Ruth McCorkle, PhD, FAAN
The Florence S. Wald Professor of Nursing
Director, Center for Excellence in Chronic Illness Care
Chair, Doctoral Program
Yale University, School of Nursing
New Haven, CT

Preface

For many lifetimes, patients have been telling nurses what is of special relevance or meaning to them, particularly during times of threatened health. Nurses have listened earnestly to patients' personal perspectives, realizing that significant information about the quality of these people's lives was being shared. Initially, this information was used to individualize patient care. More recently, nurses have recognized that patients have some similarities in their perspectives on quality of life during health threats, and that they, as nurses, can use these to assist patients in order to have as positive a quality of life as possible. The combined patient and nurse perspectives contribute to an ongoing, enthusiastic effort to identify, describe, measure, and understand quality of life for patients receiving nursing care. The combined perspectives also contribute to the ongoing effort to document the effectiveness of strategies that nurses use to try to contribute to patients' quality of life—providing rich opportunities to examine quality of life from nursing and patient perspectives that currently exist in oncology care.

The purpose of this text is to provide a reference on quality of life that reflects the voice of patients who are receiving or have received care for cancer and the attention (in the form of research, theories, and practice) of their nurses. This text will be useful to oncology nurses from many settings, including inpatient units, outpatient clinics, ambulatory care centers, cancer centers, research centers, home care agencies, hospices, and many others.

The book is divided into six sections. Section 1 provides an overview of the evolution of quality of life in oncology and oncology nursing as well as an overview of the controversial issues related to quality of life. Section 2 highlights theory development related to quality of life. Chapter 3 discusses theories and conceptual models, while Chapter 4 gives guidelines for achieving clarity of concepts related to quality of life. Three additional chapters that describe theory related to quality of life include "Spiritual Quality of Life" (Chapter 5), "Quality of Life and Culture" (Chapter 6) and "Quality of Life for Pediatric and Adolescent Patients" (Chapter 7). The third section focuses on research and begins with an overview of methodological and measurement issues (Chapter 8). This is followed by Chapter 9, which describes the effects of symptoms on quality of life. Chapters 10 and 11 highlight the current research related to families experiencing cancer and patients with breast cancer. Section 4 demonstrates the importance of quality of life in clinical practice. The section opens with a brief overview of the clinical implications of quality of life (Chapter 12) and is followed by two chapters on quality of life issues related to marrow transplantation (Chapters 13 and 14). One of these presents an international perspective. Lastly, Chapter 15 examines fatigue and quality of life for patients with cancer. Section 5 is a unique section with a chapter on cancer survivorship and a chapter with personal perspectives from patients and families. Section 6 concludes the text with a chapter providing recommendations for the future.

Additional resources are located in the appendices. Appendix 1 provides many definitions of quality of life for both adults and youth. Appendix 2 highlights selected examples of quality of life measurement tools. Unique aspects of this book include (1) its presentation of both nursing and patient/family perspectives; (2) quality of life issues related to specific diseases (e.g., breast cancer); (3) quality of life issues related to specific treatments (e.g., marrow transplantation); (4) quality of life issues related to specific populations (e.g., pediatric and adolescent); (5) an international perspective; and (6) discussions of theory, research, and practice throughout the book.

Acknowledgments

Many individuals contribute to the completion of a successful project, including the creation of a book. Different members of our team (patients, families, nursing colleagues, editorial, and production staff) brought different gifts, experiences, and expertise to the completion of this book. We wish to thank all who participated in its development and production. The list of individuals who have provided support, advice, and time is extensive and impressive. Although we are not able to adequately recognize all on that list, we would like to acknowledge a few of these individuals: all of the contributing authors who provided their expertise, time, and special insight into quality of life issues for cancer patients; to Marcia Smith for her sensitive illustrations that portray the important aspects of quality of life and cancer care; to the staff at Jones and Bartlett who guided us in this effort including Jenny McIsaac, Karen Zuck, and Penny Glynn; to John and Martha for their support and encouragement; and to Linda Watts Parker, administrative assistant, for her secretarial talents and good spirits throughout the entire development of the book.

Contributors

Margaret Barton-Burke, PhD, RN

Margaret Barton-Burke is a clinical specialist and nurse resource in Hematology/Oncology at the University of Massachusetts Memorial Medical Center and a Colonel (retired) of the Department of Massachusetts Army National Guard. She has over 25 years of experience in oncology practice, education, and research. Her experience includes working with the Massachusetts Cancer Pain Initiative and the Dana Farber Cancer Institute and teaching, consulting, and holding staff positions. Dr. Barton-Burke is a national leader in the Oncology Nursing Society and the American Cancer Society, and served on the National Advisory Group on Cancer Pain and the editorial committee for the seventh edition of *A Cancer Source Book for Nurses*. Her areas of interest include sexuality, fatigue, pain, and other long-term and palliative care issues. A nationally recognized speaker and author, Dr. Barton-Burke has received the American Journal of Nursing Book of the Year for her book *Cancer Chemotherapy: A Nursing Process Approach* (Jones and Bartlett, 1996).

Carrie Jo Braden, PhD, RN

Carrie Jo Braden is currently the associate dean for research, director of doctoral studies, and Hugh Roy Cullen professor of nursing at the University of Texas Health Science Center, San Antonio School of Nursing. She holds a master's in applied psychology from Winona State University in Winona, Minnesota, a master's in community health nursing, a primary care family nurse practitioner degree, and a PhD in nursing from the University of Arizona in Tuscon. Dr. Braden has published many articles on aspects of chronic illness and has been awarded several research grants from the National Institute of Nursing Research and the National Cancer Institute.

Diane M. Breckenridge, PhD, RN

Diane Breckenridge is a postdoctoral fellow in psychosocial oncology at the University of Pennsylvania School of Nursing. She received her master of science in nursing degree in adult health and illness from the University of Pennsylvania and her PhD in nursing from the University of Maryland. Dr. Breckenridge received the Frensenius USA Research Grant from the American Nephrology Nurses Association to fund her dissertation research on decision making regarding treatment modalities for end stage renal disease patients. Her program of research deals with treatment decision making from the patients' perspective, and her current studies examine decisions regarding treatment for prostate cancer. She is presently funded by Sigma Theta Tau International. Dr. Breckenridge was honored by receiving the 1997–1998 Pennsylvania Nurses' Association Research Award.

Nigel Bush, PhD

Nigel Bush is a staff scientist in the clinical and public health divisions of the Fred Hutchinson Cancer Research Center in Seattle, and a research associate for the National Cancer Institute's Cancer Information Service—Pacific Region. He is a psychologist who has given numerous presentations and media interviews around the country and internationally on health-related quality of life research with marrow and stem cell transplantation, and on the use of the internet and other technologies in health care. He also is the co-founder of the Washington–Alaska Cancer Pain Initiative, a multidisciplinary movement directed toward improving the management of cancer pain. He is a member of the National Cancer Genetics Network Education and Communication working group, the NCI's Cancer Information Service Commmunications working group and the International Society for Quality of Life Research. He holds a bachelor of science from the University of Nottingham, and a PhD from the University of Southampton, both in the United Kingdom.

Grace E. Dean, PhD, RN, MSN

Grace Dean is a research specialist for the nursing research and education department at the City of Hope National Medical Center in Duarte, California. She received her master's in nursing from California State University at Los Angeles and a doctorate in nursing at the School of Nursing, University of California, Los Angeles. She has conducted research on fatigue in patients with cancer and is particularly interested in conducting research on potential physiologic mechanisms that may explain fatigue in patients.

Karen Hassey Dow, PhD, RN, FAAN

Karen Hassey Dow is a professor in the School of Nursing at the University of Central Florida in Orlando. She received her doctorate from Boston College School of Nursing. She has over 25 years experience in oncology nursing and has conducted several funded studies related to quality of life in breast cancer survivors. She is currently the principal investigator of an NIH-funded study examining an individualized psychoeducational intervention for women with early stage breast cancer in the first year after treatment. She has numerous publications and textbooks in the area of cancer survivorship, quality of life, breast cancer, and radiation oncology and was the recipient of the Excellence in Writing Award in Nursing Research from the Oncology Nursing Society in 2000. Dr. Dow was a past recipient of the Oncology Nursing Society's Quality of Life Award in 2000 and 2001. Dr. Dow served on the President's Cancer Panel Special Commission on Breast Cancer, NCI Cancer Education Grant study section, and the Center for Scientific Review Nursing Research Study Section. She recently completed a term on the Oncology Nursing Society Foundation Board of Directors.

June G. Eilers, RN, MSN, PhD, CS

June Eilers is a clinical nurse specialist for the Bone Marrow Transplant Program and a clinical nurse researcher for the Office of Nursing Research at the University of Nebraska Medical Center in Omaha. She has had over 20 years of experience as an advanced practice nurse in cancer care. Her areas of practice and interest have included general oncology/ hematology, hospice and palliative care, bone marrow transplantation, psychological aspects of care, and care of the family. She received her master's and PhD in nursing from the University of Nebraska College of Nursing. Dr. Eilers has been an active member of nursing organizations, including Sigma Theta Research Society, the American Association of Cancer Education, and the Oncology Nursing Society.

Betty R. Ferrell, PhD, RN, FAAN

Dr. Betty Ferrell has been in oncology nursing for 25 years and has focused her clinical expertise and research in pain management, quality of life, and end of life care. Dr. Ferrell is an Associate Research Scientist at the City of Hope National Medical Center. She is a Fellow of the American Academy of Nursing and she has over 250 publications in peer-reviewed journals and texts. Dr. Ferrell received the Oncology Nursing Society Distinguished Nurse Researcher Award in 1996. She is Principal Investigator of a study funded by the American Cancer Society on "Palliative Surgery" and she is also Principal Investigator of the End of Life Nursing Education Consortium (ELNEC) project funded by the Robert Wood Johnson Foundation and several other funded projects related to end of life care in cancer centers and QOL issues in cancer survivors. She is a hospice volunteer and also the chairperson of the Southern California Cancer Pain Initiative. She has authored four books—*Cancer Pain Management* (1995), a text on *Suffering* (1995), *Pain in the Elderly* (1996), and the *Textbook of Palliative Nursing Care* (2001).

Monica Fliedner, RN, CNS, MSN

Monica Fliedner is currently working as research assistant at the Institute for Nursing Science, University of Basel, Switzerland. She holds a bachelor's from the University of Utrecht, the Netherlands and a certificate as a hematology and immunology nurse. She received her master's in nursing from the University of Cardiff in Wales and worked for ten years in the Netherlands, partly as clinical nurse specialist/advanced nurse practitioner on a hematology/SCT unit. Ms. Fliedner is a member of the board of directors of the European Blood and Marrow Transplantation Nurses Group (EBMT-NG) and is a member of the Dutch, American, Swiss, and European Oncology Nursing Society. In 1995 she received the Dutch Glaxo Award for her article on "Sexuality and Intimacy of the Stem Cell Transplant Patient—Nursing Care Issues."

Marcia M. Grant, RN, DNSc, FAAN

Marcia Grant is the director and research scientist for the Nursing Research and Education at the City of Hope National Medical Center in Duarte, California. She received her doctorate from the School of Nursing, University of California, San Francisco. She is a member of the American Academy of Nursing, a recipient of the Distinguished Service Award from the Oncology Nursing Society and the Oncology Nursing Society Award for Excellence of Scholarship and Consistency of Contribution to Oncology Nursing Literature, and the Distinguished Service Award from the Oncology Nursing Society. Dr. Grant has been active in clinical nursing research since the mid-1970s. Her primary program of research focuses on symptom management and quality of life outcomes in cancer patients. She has received local and national funding for her research and has authored over 100 publications. She has conducted research on the development of cancer nursing research and is the principal investigator of an National Cancer Institute training grant that disseminates end of life education to cancer centers.

Margaret Gunther Lee

Margaret Gunther Lee is a graduate of Briarcrest Christian School in Memphis, Tennessee. She grew up in Cordova, Tennessee, with her parents, Jim and Charlotte Lee, her brother, James, and sister, Catherine. Margaret was a patient at St. Jude Children's Research Hospital in Memphis, Tennessee, where she was treated for acute lymphocytic leukemia. Her many years of treatment have given her fresh perspective on patient quality of life. Margaret is currently a senior at Union University where she is studying psychology and family studies. After graduating from college in May 2003, Margaret hopes to pursue a career in mission work.

Joan E. Haase, PhD, RN

Joan Haase is the Emily Holmquist Professor in Pediatric Oncology Nursing in the School of Nursing at the Indiana University, Indianapolis. She received her doctorate from Texas Women's Univerity in 1985. Her area of research is positive health concepts such as resilience and quality of life in children, adolescents, and families experiencing cancer. She has received numerous research awards, including the MNRS Pediatric Section Senior Nurse Researcher Award, Oncology Nursing Society Bristol Myers Research Award, the Oncology Nursing Society Glaxo/Wellcome Research Award, and a Sigma Theta Tau International Faculty Research Award. Dr. Haase has published numerous articles and chapters and was awarded the Oncology Nursing Society Excellence in Writing Award in Nursing Research in 1995. She also has been active in many local, regional, and national nursing organizations, including the Oncology Nursing Society, Association of Pediatric Oncology Nurses, and Sigma Theta Tau International Nursing Honor Society.

Mel R. Haberman, PhD, RN, FAAN

Mel Haberman is the associate dean for research and professor of nursing in the College of Nursing at Washington State University. He received his master's and doctorate from the University of Washington School of Nursing in Seattle. His areas of research interest include quality of life of long-term survivors of marrow transplantaion, psychosocial aspects of cancer survivorship, and instrument development and testing. He has developed questionnaires for research on the demands of illness, cancer survivorship, and recovery from bone marrow transplantation. He co-chaired the State-of-the-Knowledge Conference on Quality of Life and the Cancer Experienced sponsored by the Oncology Nursing Society in 1995. He lives in Spokane with his wife and child.

Pamela S. Hinds, PhD, RN, CS

Pamela Hinds is director of nursing research at St. Jude Children's Research Hospital and is the subcommittee chair on Assent and Research and co-coordinator for the Palliative Care Initiative at the same setting. She is co-chair of the Nursing Research Committee for the Children's Oncology Group and a member of the Institute of Medicine's Committee on Care of the Dying Child and Family. She conducts research on end-of-life decision making by children, their parents, and their health care providers; fatigue and sleep in children and adolescents with cancer; quality of life in children and adolescents across the cancer treatment continuum; and outcomes of nursing care procedures. Her undergraduate degree is in nursing from the University of Vermont, and her graduate degrees in nursing and nursing clinical research are from the University of Arizona.

Nancy A. Hodgson, MSN, RN, CS

Nancy Hodgson is a certified clinical specialist in psychiatric/mental health nursing and is currently a predoctoral fellow in psychosocial oncology at the Center for the Study of Serious Illness at the University of Pennsylvania School of Nursing. She is a clinical instructor in psychiatric nursing and community health nursing for both the University of Pennsylvania and Holy Family College in Philadelphia. She is also a psychiatric liaison consultant to several home care agencies in New Jersey. Ms. Hodgson is a member of the Oncology Nursing Society, Sigma Theta Tau International (Xi Chapter), and the Society of Certified Clinical Specialists in Psychiatric Nursing of the NJSNA. She received her bachelor's degree in nursing from Widener University, her master's degree in psychiatric nursing from the University of Pennsylvania, and is currently pursuing her PhD in Nursing at the University of Pennsylvania.

Marjorie Kagawa-Singer, PhD, RN, MN

Marjorie Kagawa-Singer is an Associate Professor at the University of California—Los Angeles (UCLA) School of Public Health and Asian American Studies Center. She has a master's in Nursing from UCLA School of Nursing and master's and doctorate in anthropology from UCLA. Her clinical work and research has been in oncology, focusing on the disparities in physical and mental health care outcomes of ethnic minority populations with cancer. She serves on multiple local, state, and national committees addressing issues of ethnicity and health care, and has published and lectured extensively on issues in cross-cultural health, cancer, pain, grief and bereavement, end of life decision making, and quality of life. She also serves as consultant to community groups to extend cancer education and services to underserved populations. Presently her research focuses on defining and developing standards of cultural competence in health care. Her current studies related to cancer include intervention studies to promote mammography in Southeast Asian and Pacific Islander women. She is also studying quality of life and doctor–patient communication with Hispanic, African American, and Asian American women post-breast and cervical cancer.

Cynthia R. King, PhD, NP, MSN, RN, FAAN

Cynthia King has experience as owner and nurse consultant with Special Care Consultants, as an advanced practice nurse (CNS and NP), nurse researcher, nurse educator, and administrator. She is a member of the American Academy of Nursing and chair of the Oncology Nursing Society Publishing Council. She has received the ONS/Pharmacia-Upjohn Quality of Life Award, American Journal of Nursing Outstanding Book in Clinical Excellence, Annual Outstanding Alumni Award for School of Nursing, Creighton University, and the Trish Greene Quality of Life Lectureship from the Oncology Nursing Society. She co-chaired the Oncology Nursing Society's State-of-the-Knowledge Conference on Quality of Life and the Cancer Experience. Dr. King has conducted research on quality of life issues for patients with cancer, stress and coping of marrow transplant patients, and nurses' perceptions of quality of life of marrow transplant survivors. She has published numerous articles and chapters in books. Her undergraduate degrees are in biology and psychology from Trinity College and nursing from Creighton University. Her master's in nursing science is from the University of Nebraska Medical Center, her nurse practitioner degree and her PhD are from the University of Rochester.

Deanna Kuhn, RN, MSN, ARNP

Deanna Kuhn is a visiting instructor in the School of Nursing at the University of Central Florida in Orlando. She is the project director of the Breast Cancer Survivor's Study, an National Institutes of Health-funded study designed to test the effectiveness of an individualized, multidimensional, quality of life intervention (the Breast Cancer Educational Intervention) on quality of life for women with newly diagnosed, early stage I or II breast cancer in the first year after initial treatment. She received her bachelor's degree from the University of Cincinnati and her master's from the University of Central Florida.

Susan Leigh, BSN, RN

Susan Leigh is an oncology nurse currently working as a cancer survivorship consultant. She is a founding member and past president of the National Coalition for Cancer Survivorship (NCCS), and is one of the first 15 members selected to the Director's Consumer Liaison Group (DCLG), a new consumer oversight committee at the National Cancer Institute (NCI). Drawing on her experiences as both an oncology nurse and a survivor of Hodgkin's disease, breast cancer, and bladder cancer, she speaks and writes extensively on survivorship issues. Her primary focus is on long-term survival and late effects of treatment. Entering the new millennium, Susan is celebrating 29 years of life after cancer!

Ruth McCorkle, PhD, FAAN

Ruth McCorkle is the Florence Wald Professor of Nursing in the Yale School of Nursing (YSN), the director of the Center for Excellence in Chronic Illness Care, the chair of YSN's Doctoral Program, and a member of Yale Cancer Center's Executive Committee for Cancer Control. Dr. McCorkle has an impressive research career studying patients' responses to cancer at critical points in the cancer illness trajectory: newly diagnosed, undergoing active treatment (acute, stable, and unstable phases), and progressively ill and terminal. Dr. McCorkle is a national and international leader in cancer nursing graduate education and cancer nursing research. She was the first chair of the Oncology Nursing Society, a charter member of the Oncology Nursing Society and the International Society of Nurses in Cancer Care. She has served on the board of directors of both organizations. Dr. McCorkle has served as a member of study sections of the National Cancer Institute (NCI), the National Institute of Nursing Research, and NCI Board of Scientific Counselors. In the early 1980s, she obtained the first nonmedical NCI Institutional Research Training Grant and opened the door for other nonmedical fields to become competitive in securing funding. She has maintained funding for pre- and post-doctoral students since that time. She is presently the program director of an institutional training grant on breast cancer funded by the Department of Defense. In 1993, Dr. McCorkle was recognized by the American Nurses Association as the Nurse Scientist of the Year and in 1994 as the Oncology Nursing Society's Distinguished Nurse Researcher.

Geraldine V. Padilla, PhD

Geraldine Padilla is a professor and associate dean for research at the University of California San Francisco School of Nursing. She was formerly director of nursing research, then Research Scientist at the City of Hope Medical Center in Duarte, California, professor and associate dean at the University of California—Los Angeles (UCLA) School of Nursing and member of the UCLA Jonsson Comprehensive Cancer Center, and vice president for Cancer Control, American Cancer Society California Division. She is internationally known for her work in quality of life. She is associate editor of the journal *Quality of Life Research* and member of the editorial board of the *Journal of Nursing Measurement*. Her own research focuses on quality of life as affected by disease, treatment, and style of care in culturally diverse populations of patients with cancer or arthritis. Dr. Padilla has received intra- and extramural support (e.g., NIH) to examine changes in quality of life in Hispanic and non-Hispanic white women with rheumatoid arthritis; and to develop and test the reliability and validity of Spanish translations of quality of life questionnaires for persons with breast and prostate cancer as well as arthritis. While at UCLA, Dr. Padilla obtained an Institutional National Research Service Award grant from the National Institute for Nursing Research to provide pre- and postdoctoral research training in the area of quality of life. That grant is in its second five-year cycle (current P.I. at UCLA is Dr. L. Sarna).

Judith K. Payne, PhD

Judith Payne is currently an assistant professor of nursing at Wayne State University, and was director of clinical services at the University of New Mexico Cancer Research and Treatment Center. She received her PhD in nursing from the University of Iowa. Her research involves cancer treatment-related fatigue, specifically mechanisms and biomarkers, and new interventions based on evidence-based practice. She is active in the Oncology Nursing Society and Sigma Theta Tau. Dr. Payne is an Advanced Oncology Certified Nurse. She lectures nationally and internationally on fatigue and evidence-based practice.

Lynn M. Rivera, RN, MSN

Lynn Rivera has been a registered nurse for 22 years and an oncology nurse for 15 years. She formerly worked in the Department of Nursing Research and Education at City of Hope National Medical Center in Duarte, California, as a research specialist and is now a school nurse. Ms. Rivera has a master's degree in nursing with a focus in gerontology from California State University, Dominguez Hills in Carson, California. In 1996 she began her doctoral study at the University of California, Los Angeles, School of Nursing.

Kathleen M. Stetz, RN, MN, PhD

Kathleen Stetz is associate professor of nursing in the School of Health Sciences at Seattle Pacific University in Seattle, Washington. She received her master's and doctorate from the University of Washington. She currently teaches undergraduate community health and research courses and graduate courses in research methodology. Dr. Stetz serves as the chair of the Curriculum Committee in the School of Health Sciences, the chair of the University Undergraduate Program Evaluation Committee, and as a member of the University Assessment Task Force.

Michael C. Sullivan

Michael Sullivan had a varied career in service and private industry. He was semiretired from active employment prior to his death from cancer. He was consulting in the areas of sales, marketing, and fund-raising. He also managed the household activities so his wife Lynn Rivera could go to school full time and work. Mr. Sullivan also volunteered as a committeeman-member of the Pasadena Tournament of Roses Association, a member of the Board of Big Brothers of Greater Los Angeles, and a volunteer at the Union Station Foundation, which provides various services for the homeless of the San Gabriel Valley.

Elizabeth Johnston Taylor, PhD, RN

Elizabeth Johnston Taylor is an associate professor at the Loma Linda University School of Nursing. Her clinical experience as an oncology nurse created a deep interest in the relationship between illness and spirituality. In 1992, she earned her doctorate in nursing from the University of Pennsylvania where she focused her studies on the psychosocial and spiritual aspects of living with illness. Her expertisse in researching spirituality and health-related quality of life was further developed during a two-year postdoctoral fellowship at the University of California—Los Angeles School of Nursing. In addition to academic studies, she has obtained two units of Clinical Pastoral Education. Johnston Taylor has received funding for her research and training from the National Cancer Institute (NIH), the Agency for Health Care Policy and Research, the Oncology Nursing Society and ONS Foundation, and the Hospice Nurses Association. She has numerous publications, including articles and book chapters on topics such as quality of life, ethical decision making, pain management, and spiritual responses to illness. Her recent book, published by Prentice Hall, is titled *Spiritual Care: Nursing Theory, Research, and Practice*. Dr. Johnston has also served as Coordinator for the ONS Spiritual Care Special Interest Group. She and her husband, Lyndon, have two daughters, Kathryn (3 years) and Elissa (2 years).

April Hazard Vallerand, PhD, RN

April Hazard Vallerand is currently an assistant professor in the College of Nursing at Wayne State University. Her research involves the improvement and maintenance of functional status in patients with chronic pain. She is currently the principal investigator on a study designed to improve cancer pain management in the home, which is funded by the National Cancer Institute. Dr. Vallerand lectures nationally on the management of pain and has published numerous articles on pain and pain control. She has also written five books on pharmacology for nurses and other health care professionals, including Davis's *Drug Guide for Nurses* (F. A. Davis, 2001), which is in its 7th edition. She is a member of Sigma Theta Tau, the Oncology Nursing Society, the American Pain Society, and the American Society of Pain Management Nurses.

Overview

Evolution of
Quality of Life
in Oncology and Oncology Nursing

MARCIA M. GRANT • GRACE E. DEAN

There is no profit in curing the body if in the process we destroy the soul.
—SAM GOLTER, CITY OF HOPE MEDICAL CENTER, DUARTE, CA

Quality of life (QOL) assessment is an important aspect of the current care provided to cancer patients. This chapter will discuss the theory, research, and practice related to QOL measurement, while addressing the role of oncology nurses in describing and promoting QOL for patients with cancer.

Evolution of Quality of Life as Oncology and Oncology Nursing Outcomes

Traditional medical evaluations of the outcomes of cancer treatments have included disease-free survival, tumor response, and overall survival (U.S. Department of Health and Human Services, 1990). However, clinicians and researchers have come to realize that these outcomes are not adequate in assessing the impact of cancer and its treatment on the patient and daily life, nor in identifying interventions to improve or maintain the patient's QOL. Quality of life measurements provide valuable information to all members of the health care team. Quality of assessment has become an important measure of the outcome of cancer treatment and has been identified as an important nursing outcome variable for well over twenty years (Grant, 2000).

Interest in QOL assessment has continued to increase in recent years. Both national and international activities illustrate the increasing importance of QOL assessment and research. The United States Food and Drug Administration now uses QOL measurements in the process of approving new anti-cancer drugs (Beitz, Gnecco, & Justice, 1996). National and international groups advocating QOL assessment in clinical trials research have recognized its importance (Johnson & Temple, 1985; Nayfield & Hailey, 1991; Osoba, 1992; U.S. Department of Health and Human Services, 1990; World Health Organization, 1993). Interest in QOL research has resulted in a major shift in randomized controlled clinical trials. The Oncologic Drugs Advisory Committee (U.S. Food and Drug Administration) has recommended that a positive effect on QOL and/or survival be the basis for approval of new anti-cancer drugs (Beitz et al., 1996). The importance of a favorable effect on QOL, in the absence of impact on survival, will carry more weight in the approval process than more traditional measures used to assess efficacy, such as objective tumor response. In addition to clinical trials, QOL assessment has evolved into a primary outcome measure in health services research, acute care, and chronic illness (Coleman, Krammer, Johnson, Eilersten, & Hothaus, 1999; Eiser & Morse, 2001; Mandelblatt & Eisenberg, 1995). This evolution has coincided with recent economic changes and pressures forcing health care providers to reconcile quality care and cost effectiveness (Zebrack, 2000).

Inclusion of QOL measurement results to professionals and consumers was recently examined through identifying prescription drugs in the United States that were approved by the FDA and contained information on QOL in the package insert for the drug (Shah, Sesti, Chopra, McLaughlin-Miley, & Copley-Merriman, 2001). The methodology for the study consisted of a search for the terminology "quality of life" or "qol" using an electronic version of the January 2001 *Physicians' Desk Reference*. Eighteen prescription drugs were identified with the most QOL information found in the section Clinical Trials. This study confirms the inclusion of QOL as an outcome and illustrates the dissemination of this information to both professionals and the public.

The World Health Organization (WHO) has a global cancer control program based on knowledge currently available that, if appropriately implemented, can reduce cancer morbidity and mortality worldwide (Stjernswärd & Teoh, 1991). This program includes a focus on palliative care and its impact on the QOL of cancer patients. Since many of the world's cancer patients have no access to effective cancer therapy, only palliative care can be offered. Palliative care programs frequently focus on symptom management and can greatly improve QOL.

Interest in QOL is also reflected in international professional societies. The International Society for Quality of Life Research (ISQOL) was founded in 1994 to promote research in QOL and the scientific study of QOL relevant to health and health care throughout the world. The society promotes the rigorous investigation of health-related QOL measurement from conceptualization to application and

Table 1-1.   **Annual Conferences of International Society for Quality of Life Research**

1994   Inaugural Meeting: Brussels, Belgium
1995   Montreal, Canada
1996   Manila, Philippines
1997   Vienna, Austria
1998   Baltimore, Maryland, USA
1999   Barcelona, Spain
2000   Vancouver, Canada
2001   Amsterdam, The Netherlands
2002   Toronto, Canada

practice. The society's website is located at www.isoqol.org. Annual meetings are held throughout the world (see Table 1-1). A second organization, the International Society for Quality of Life Studies (ISQOLS), has as its mission: to promote and encourage research, discussion, contributions to the research literature and teaching in QOL studies, and provide a liaison among academic, public sector, and private sector researchers, scholars, and teachers in the managerial (policy), behavioral, social, medical, and environment sciences. Their website is located at www.cob.vt.edu/market/isqols. Annual ISQOLS conferences have also been held internationally (Table 1-2).

Other international QOL activities include (*a*) the development of an integrated, modular approach to QOL assessment in oncology patients by the European Organization for Research and Treatment of Cancer (EORTC) (Aaronson et al., 1993); (*b*) the translation of a QOL questionnaire into the eight languages spoken by members of the International Society for Chemo- and Immunotherapy (Tuchler et al., 1992); (*c*) the cultural adaptation of QOL instruments with translations of various cancer and noncancer QOL scales into more than 25 languages ("Cultural Adaptation," 1996); (*d*) the adoption of QOL outcomes in Canadian clinical trials in patients with cancer, including the development of a policy promoting QOL assessment in Phase III trials and the development of written guidelines to assist

Table 1-2.   **Annual Conferences of International Society for Quality of Life Studies**

1997   Charlotte, North Carolina, USA
1998   Williamsburg, Virginia, USA
1999   Girona, Spain
2000   Washington, DC, USA
2001   Williamsburg, Virginia, USA

clinical trials investigators when developing protocols for proposed studies (Osoba, 1992); and (*e*) the adaptation of the Quality of Life Index developed by Padilla and colleagues (1983) for use with colostomy patients by researchers in England and France (Marquis, Marrel, & Blackman, 1996).

Quality of life publications and organizations provide further proof of recent interest in QOL. The first listing of the term *quality of life* appeared in *Index Medicus* in 1972 with 15 citations. In 2002 over 3,280 "quality of life" citations appeared in *Index Medicus*. The first journal focusing specifically on QOL, *Quality of Life Research*, was published in 1992.

Defining Quality of Life

Quality of life assessment is complicated by the fact that there is no universally accepted definition for QOL (see Appendix 1). In the past, many researchers measured only one dimension, such as physical function, economic concern, or sexual function. More recently, researchers have attempted to further define QOL. Spilker (1990) described QOL assessment through three interrelated levels: (*a*) overall assessment of well-being; (*b*) broad domains such as physical, psychological, economic, and social; and (*c*) the components of each domain. This model, shown in Figure 1-1, demonstrates the multidimensional nature of QOL and the importance of assessing all three labels: overall QOL, each domain, and individual items.

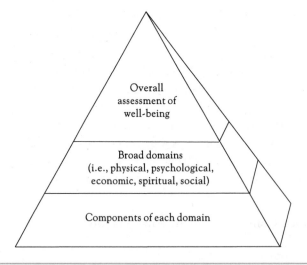

Figure 1-1. **Three levels of quality of life. In their totality, these three levels constitute the scope (and definition) of quality of life.**

Source: Spilker, 1996, pp. 1–10. Used with permission of Lippincott-Raven Publishers.

The World Health Organization defines quality of life as "individuals' perceptions of their position in life in the context of the culture and value system in which they live and in relation to their goals, standards, and concerns" (WHO, 1993). The definition includes six broad domains: physical health, psychological state, levels of independence, social relationships, environmental features, and spiritual concerns.

In the Report of the Workshop on Quality of Life Research in Cancer Clinical Trials cosponsored by the NCI and the Office of Medical Applications of Research, National Institutes of Health, QOL was also identified as a multidimensional concept: "Health-related quality of life is the value assigned to duration of life as modified by impairments, functional states, perceptions, and social opportunities as influenced by disease, injury, treatment, or policy" (U.S. Department of Health and Human Services, 1990). The Workshop recommended that QOL assessment at least include the dimensions generally acknowledged to contribute to QOL (e.g., physical/role functioning, emotional/psychological functioning, social functioning, and somatic/physiological complaints) and a global self-report of QOL.

Within the nursing literature, investigators' definitions of QOL have paralleled those of other disciplines with a focus on the multidimensionality of the concept. Ferrans's (1990) review of QOL literature in relation to conceptual issues identified five broad categories into which QOL definitions could be grouped. These categories focus on the patient's (a) ability to live a normal life, (b) happiness/satisfaction, (c) achievement of personal goals, (d) ability to lead a socially "useful" life, and (e) physical and/or mental capabilities (actual or potential).

Research by Grant, Padilla, and Ferrell has also emphasized the need for a multidimensional definition for QOL, including an existential dimension (Grant, Ferrell, & Sakurai, 1994). These investigators have identified QOL as consisting of four dimensions or domains: physical well-being, psychological well-being, social well-being, and spiritual well-being. Each dimension consists of generic items of concern to all cancer populations, as well as items specific to a type of cancer or treatment. The model has been validated across studies in a number of cancer patient populations (Ferrell et al., 1992b; Ferrell, Grant, Funk, Otis-Green, & Garcia, 1997; Ferrell, Grant, Funk, Otis-Green, & Garcia, 1998a; Ferrell, Grant, Funk, Otis-Green, & Garcia, 1998b; Ferrell, Hassey Dow, Leigh, Ly, & Gulasekaram, 1995; Grant, 1999; Greimel, Padilla, & Grant, 1997; Padilla, Ferrell, & Grant, 1990; Padilla & Grant, 1985; Padilla et al., 1992; Padilla et al., 1983; Padilla, Grant, Ferrell, & Presant, 1996). Figure 1-2 identifies the QOL model as it applies to cancer survivors. This model was identified in investigations involving cancer survivors who were members of the National Coalition of Cancer Survivors and who responded to a mailed QOL questionnaire. The City of Hope Quality of Life model acknowledges that QOL is (a) subjective, (b) based on the patient's self-report, (c) always changing and dynamic, and (d) a multidimensional concept.

Figure 1-2. **Quality of life model applied to cancer survivors.**
Source: Ferrell, Hassey Dow et al., 1995. Used with permission of Oncology Nursing Press.

Measuring Quality of Life

Many questionnaires and surveys have been developed for measuring QOL. Both general and disease-specific approaches have been used, resulting in a multitude of instruments. The Mapi Research Institute in France has approached the challenge of organizing information on the questionnaires by developing a QOL instrument database containing a list of 1,000 instruments, the description of over 300 of them, and copies of 170 original questionnaires. Information on this database is available at www.QOLID.org. Within the context of today's health care environment, the use of QOL as an outcome measure to allocate health care resources has been explored. Distribution of these resources based on expected QOL is tempting. However, because the use of scientific methods to assess QOL is in its infancy and a gold standard for QOL assessment does not exist, caution in applying QOL measures to allocate health care resources is imperative. Research has demonstrated differences between QOL assessments made by health care providers and patients (Fowlie, Berkeley, & Dingwall-Fordyce, 1989; King, Ferrell, Grant, & Sakurai, 1995; Slevin, Plant, Lynch, Drinkwater, & Gregory, 1988). Thus, health care providers are faced with the dilemma of whose QOL it is—society's, the health care provider's, the family's, or the patient's. In assessing QOL, researchers must respond to the following questions: Who should perform QOL assessment? When should QOL be assessed? Are the assessment instruments reliable, valid, and sensitive? and For what purpose is the information being collected (Dean, 1990)?

Relationship of Quality of Life to the Scope of Nursing

Quality of life perspectives are particularly relevant to the scope of nursing practice. Padilla and Grant (1985) state that *quality of life* refers to "that which makes life worth living and connotes the caring aspects of nursing, because nursing is concerned not only with survival and decreased morbidity, but with the whole patient" (p. 45). Nursing is a caring practice in which nurses foster health promotion and maintenance, or restoration of function. Through these nursing activities, nurses promote patient well-being. Since cancer and its treatment impact the entire patient including physical, psychological, social, and spiritual well-being, QOL information gathered by nurses can provide valuable nursing assessment data.

In providing care to patients with cancer, nurses help patients to manage the side effects of therapy and adjust to changes in body image, function, and appearance and to living with a chronic disease. This holistic viewpoint of nursing care delivery can help the patient to maintain or improve life and the quality of that life. The nurse can help the patient to make the changes needed in order to adjust to a life with cancer.

Quality of life is affected by numerous factors including culture, age, and diagnosis. However, many factors may not be amenable to nursing intervention (e.g., diagnosis, family illness history, predisposing characteristics, and medical treatment) (Padilla & Grant, 1985). On the other hand, QOL is also influenced by factors over which nurses have some control, for example, the environment, information provided to patients and family members, personal or social issues, symptom management, and nursing interventions.

In a study of bone marrow transplant survivors, respondents identified ways that nurses and physicians can improve QOL: (*a*) be accessible, (*b*) discover a cure, (*c*) provide support groups, (*d*) reinforce current education, (*e*) provide additional coping strategies, and (*f*) increase patient participation in decision making (Ferrell et al., 1992a). Other researchers have identified similar interventions in other cancer and noncancer patient populations (Davis & Grant, 1994; Felton, Revenson, &

Hinrichsen, 1984; Harrington, Lackey, & Gates, 1996; Karmilovich, 1994; Stetz, McDonald, & Compton, 1996).

Evidence of Nursing Interest in Quality of Life

Nursing as a scientific discipline has been involved in identifying, measuring, promoting, and evaluating QOL in cancer patients for a relatively long period of time. In the 1980s the relevance of QOL as an appropriate outcome to measure the impact of nursing care was identified (Padilla & Grant, 1985). The number of publications related to QOL has steadily increased since the term was first included in the *Cumulative Index of Nursing and Allied Health Literature* (CINAHL) as an indexed topic (Figure 1-3). These references span the various specialities in nursing and include a large portion of nursing contributions to the cancer literature. QOL has also been included as an evaluative component in the cardiac nursing literature (Dracup & Raffin, 1989; Packa, 1989; Packa et al., 1989; Wingate, 1995), nursing care of arthritis patients (Braden, 1990), and nursing care of HIV/AIDS patients (Holzemer & Wilson, 1995; Ragsdale, Kotarba, & Morrow, 1992).

Quality of life, as a concept, fits well with the overall goals of nursing. Nurse researchers are challenged to continue this scientific work and take an active part in the assessment, application, and evaluation of QOL for patients and families. As the focus of health care continues to change, QOL, as an outcome of professional nursing care, may become one of the most important indicators of quality care. Because of this, comparing QOL perceptions among patients, nurses, and family caregivers is

Figure 1-3.   **Citations in CINAHL using quality of life as an index term.**

essential for identifying differences and planning approaches to minimize those differences (King, Ferrell, Grant, & Sakurai, 1995).

Relationship of Nursing QOL Studies with Other Disciplines

The conduct of research on QOL was identified as the second highest priority for research, along with pain management, in the 2000 ONS Research Priorities Survey. This illustrates the continuing importance to the nursing care of oncology patients. Additionally, over the years oncology nurses have been involved in QOL projects in collaboration with other disciplines.

The National Cancer Institute's Clinical Trials Groups have included a QOL measurement in many of the Phase III trials. The Southwest Oncology Group (SWOG), the Gynecologic Oncology Group (GOG), and the National Surgical Adjuvant Project for Breast and Bowel Cancers (NSABP) have all incorporated QOL measures into multiple time periods to determine whether the difference in treatment arms can be described in terms of the impact of QOL. When implementing QOL studies, the medical protocol nurse usually is the one responsible for administering QOL questionnaires. Current approaches to including QOL measurements within these oncology groups may involve development of an interdisciplinary QOL committee responsible for identifying QOL hypotheses, study methods, and analysis approaches. Interpretation of the analysis and writing manuscripts is part of the committee members' responsibilities.

Grant and Ferrell at City of Hope National Medical Center in Duarte, California, have found the interdisciplinary approach valuable. In their research, they have collaborated with physicians, social workers, clergy, and others to explore QOL issues for bone marrow transplant patients (Grant et al., 1992; Grant, 1999b); for colorectal cancer patients (Padilla et al., 1992; Krouse et al., 2000); for nursing home patients (Ferrell, Ferrell, & Rivera, 1995); for women with breast cancer (Ferrell et al., 1996; Ferrell, Grant, Funk, Otis-Green, & Garcia, 1998a&b); in the home care setting (Ferrell & Hassey-Dow, 1997; Ferrell, Taylor, Grant, Fowler, & Corbisiero, 1993; Taylor, Ferrell, Grant, & Cheyney, 1993); and in pediatrics (Ferrell, Rhiner, Shapiro, & Dierkes, 1994).

Interdisciplinary approaches to QOL research have provided data important in expanding the perception of the impact of cancer and cancer treatment on QOL. As a broad outcome of patient care, QOL provides information valuable to physicians, nurses, social workers, psychologists, physical therapists, and pharmacists. As an outcome measure of the impact of health care, QOL will continue to provide valuable information in measuring the impact of health care changes on the lives of cancer patients.

Oncology Nursing Society Research Activities

The Oncology Nursing Society (ONS) and the Oncology Nursing Foundation (ONF) have demonstrated support for QOL research and clinical practice. From 1993 to 1996 the Foundation, in conjunction with corporate sponsors, funded 22 QOL research studies conducted by oncology nurse researchers (Table 1-3). Since 1988 the

Table 1-3. Quality of Life Research Projects Funded by the Oncology Nursing Foundation

Small Grants Program

1989

Quality of Life Perceptions of Bone Marrow Transplant Recipients, Ruth Belec, RN, BSN, CCRN, Marquette University School of Nursing, Milwaukee, WI. Oncology Nursing Foundation/Lederle Research Award.

1990

Testing of a Trait-State Model for Quality of Life, Ann T. Foltz, RN, DNS, Duke University School of Nursing, Raleigh, NC. Oncology Nursing Foundation/Lederle Laboratories Research Grant.

1991

Effect of Pain and Quality of Life in Breast Cancer, Jeri Lynn Ashley, RN, MSN, Baptist Memorial Hospital, Memphis, TN. Oncology Nursing Foundation/Wyeth-Ayerst New Investigator's Research Grant.

1992

Side Effects of Quality of Life in Patients Receiving HDR Brachytherapy, Vickie K. Fieler, RN, MS, University of Rochester Cancer Center, Rochester, NY. Oncology Nursing Foundation/Wyeth-Ayerst New Investigator's Research Grant.

Quality of Life After Autologous Bone Marrow Transplantation, Marie Whedon, RN, MS, OCN, Dartmouth-Hitchcock Medical Center, Hanover, NH. Oncology Nursing Foundation/Wyeth-Ayerst New Investigator's Research Grant.

Quality of Life of Long Term Female Cancer Survivors, Gwen Wyatt, RN, PhD, Michigan State University, East Lansing, MI. Oncology Nursing Foundation/Bristol-Myers Research Grant.

1993

The Experience of Breast Cancer Survivorship, Diane G. Cope, RN, MSN, PhDc, Florida Atlantic University, Boca Raton, FL. Oncology Nursing Foundation/Wyeth Ayerst New Investigator's Research Grant.

Adaptation in Young Breast Cancer Survivors: A Pilot, Karen Hassey Dow, RN, PhD, Beth Israel Hospital, Boston, MA. Oncology Nursing Foundation/Lederle Laboratories Research Grant.

The Impact of Treatment of Endometrial Cancer on Quality of Life, Margaret Anne Lamb, RN, PhD, University of New Hampshire, Durham, NH. Oncology Nursing Foundation/Bristol-Myers Research Grant.

Table 1-3.   **continued**

Development of a Nursing Intervention for Women with Breast Cancer—CMF, Roxanne W. McDaniel, RN, PhD, University of Missouri-Columbia, School of Nursing, Columbia, OH. Oncology Nursing Foundation/Smith Kline Beecham Research Grant.

Pain Relief and Pharmacokinetics of Rectal MS Contin, Cheryl Ann Mummy, RN, BSN, OCN, University of Iowa Hospital and Clinics, Iowa City, IA. Oncology Nursing Foundation/Purdue Frederick Research Grant.

Group Intervention to Home Bound Caregivers of Persons with Cancer and AIDS, Kathleen M. Stetz, RN, PhD, University of Washington, Bothell, WA. Oncology Nursing Foundation/Chiron Therapeutics Research Grant.

1994

The Experience of Being a Family Member of a Breast Cancer Survivor, Diane G. Cope, RN, PhD, OCN, Florida Atlantic University, College of Nursing, Boca Raton, FL. Oncology Nursing Foundation/Bristol-Myers Oncology Division Community Health Research Grant.

Predicting Adjustments in Hispanic Breast Cancer Survivors, Shannon R. Dirksen, RN, PhD, University of New Mexico, Albuquerque, NM. Oncology Nursing Foundation/Immunex Corporation Research Grant.

Black Women's Lived/Caring Experiences with Breast Cancer, Marie F. Gates, RN, PhD, University of Tennessee, College of Nursing, Memphis, TN. Oncology Nursing Foundation Research Grant.

Therapeutic Touch in Breast Cancer: Immune and Quality of Life Effects, Robin A. Meize Grochowski, RN, PhD, University of New Mexico, Albuquerque, NM. Oncology Nursing Foundation/Chiron Therapeutics Research Grant.

Quality of Life: Impact of Head and Neck Cancer, Mary E. Means, RN, BSN, CORLN, University of Iowa Hospital and Clinics, Department of Nursing, Iowa City, IA. Oncology Nursing Foundation Research Grant.

Quality of Life Considerations in Patients with Colon Polyps, Kimberly C. Phillips, RN, MSN, Bowman Gray School of Medicine, Department of Public Health Sciences, Winston-Salem, NC. Oncology Nursing Foundation/Wyeth New Investigator's Research Grant.

Quality of Life in Patients Receiving Monoclonal Antibody Therapy, Lindsey A. Trammell, RN, MSN, OCN, University of Alabama in Birmington, Comprehensive Cancer Center, Birmingham, AL. Oncology Nursing Foundation/Smith Kline Beecham Research Grant.

1995

Risks, Benefits, and Costs of Home and Hospital Care, Linda K. Birenbaum, RN, PhD, Walther Cancer Institute, Indianapolis, IN. Oncology Nursing Foundation/Cerenex Pharmaceuticals Research Grant.

Impact of Silicone Implants on the Lives of Women with Breast Cancer, Ann Coleman, RNP, PhD, OCN, University of Arkansas for Medical Sciences, College of Nursing, Little Rock, AR. Oncology Nursing Foundation/Oncology Nursing Certification Corporation Oncology Nursing Research.

Fear of Cancer Recurrence: A Phenomenological Study, Diane G. Cope, RN, PhD, OCN, University of North Carolina at Charlotte, College of Nursing, Charlotte, NC. Oncology Nursing Foundation Research Grant.

Table 1-3. **continued**

Physiological Fatigue Indicators in Patients with Breast Cancer, Grace E. Dean, RN, MSN, City of Hope National Medical Center, Duarte, CA. Oncology Nursing Foundation/Ortho Biotech Research Grant.

Evaluation of a Hispanic Version of a Pain Education Intervention, Gloria Juarez, RN, MSN, City of Hope National Medical Center, Duarte, CA. Oncology Nursing Foundation Ethnic Minority Researcher and Mentorship Grant.

The Family Experience of Bone Marrow Transplant, Lynne M. Rivera, RN, BSN, City of Hope National Medical Center, Duarte, CA. Oncology Nursing Foundation/New Investigator's Research Grant.

Quality of Life in Persons with Multiple Myeloma, Mary Thomas, RN, MS, OCN, Department of Veteran's Affairs Medical Center, Palo Alto, CA. Oncology Nursing Foundation/Smith Kline Beecham Research Grant.

1996

Quality of Life in Brain Tumor Patients Undergoing Aggressive Therapy, Terri Armstrong, RN, MS, University of Pittsburgh Cancer Institute, Pittsburgh, PA. Oncology Nursing Foundation/ American Brain Tumor Association Grant.

Forgiveness in Terminally Ill Cancer Patients, Jacqueline R. Mickley, RN, PhD, Kent State University, Hudson, OH. Oncology Nursing Foundation/Amgen, Inc. Research Grant.

Conservative Management of Urinary Incontinence Post Radical Prostatectomy: Impact on Urine Loss and Quality of Life, Katherine N. Moore, RN, MN, PhDc, University of Alberta, Edmonton, Alberta, Canada. Oncology Nursing Foundation/Hoechst Marion Roussel Research Grant.

The Relationship of Exercise and Fatigue to Quality of Life in Women with Breast Cancer, Anna L. Schwartz, RN, MS, FNP, University of Utah, College of Nursing, Salt Lake City, UT. Oncology Nursing Foundation/Glaxo Wellcome Research Grant.

Taste Changes of Cancer Patients, Rita Wickman, RN, MS, AOCN, PhDc, Rush Presbyterian St. Lukes Medical Center, Chicago, IL. Oncology Nursing Foundation/Bristol-Myers Oncology Chapter's Grant.

1997

Uncertainty and Watchful Waiting with Prostate Cancer, Donald Bailey, Jr., RN, MN, University of North Carolina, Durham, NC. Oncology Nursing Foundation/Oncology Nursing Certification Corporation Research Grant.

Symptom Management and Successful Outpatient Transplant, Elizabeth Ann Coleman, RN, PhD, AOCN, University of Arkansas for Medical Science, Little Rock, AR. Oncology Nursing Foundation/Smith Kline Beecham Research Grant.

Health Outcomes in Survivors of Breast Cancer, Denise M. Oleske, RN, PhD, Rush University, Chicago, IL. Oncology Nursing Foundation/Amgen, Inc. Research Grant.

Mutual Support Dyads and Quality of Life of Women with Breast Cancer, Laura B. Sutton, RN, MS, CS, University of Pittsburgh, Pittsburgh, PA. Oncology Nursing Foundation/Rhone-Poulence Rorer New Investigator's Research Grant.

Table 1-3.   **continued**

1998

Determination of Preferences and Utilities for the Treatment of Prostate Cancer, Deborah W. Bruner, MSN, RN, Fox Chase Cancer Center, Philadelphia, PA. ONS Foundation/Amgen, Inc. Research Grant.

Evaluation of the Healing Odyssey Program, Nancy J. Raymon, MN, RN, Healing Odyssey, Inc., Irvine, CA. ONS Foundation Nursing Outcomes Research Grant.

1999

Exercise for Patients with Multiple Myeloma, Elizabeth Ann Coleman, PhD, RNP, AOCN®, University of Arkansas for Medical Sciences, College of Nursing, Little Rock, AR. ONS Foundation/Oncology Nursing Society Nursing Outcomes Research Grant.

Effects of Seated Exercise on Fatigue in Breast Cancer, Judith A. Headley, PhD, RN, AOCN®, University of Texas Health Science Center-Houston School of Nursing, Houston, TX. ONS Foundation/Hoechst Marion Roussel Research Grant.

Quality of life and Adjustment for Couples Experiencing Advanced Breast Cancer, Frances Marcus Lewis, PhD, RN, FAAN, University of Washington, School of Nursing, Seattle, WA, ONS Foundation/Amgen, Inc. Research Grant.

The Meaning of Incontinence and Impotence Postprostatectomy, Sally L. Maliski, PhD, RN, University of Pennsylvania, School of Nursing, Philadelphia, PA. ONS Foundation/Ortho Biotech Research Grant.

Prevention of Osteoporosis in Breast Cancer Survivors, Nancy L. Waltman, PhD, RN, University of Nebraska Medical Center, College of Nursing, Omaha, NE. ONS Foundation/Janssen Pharmaceutica Research Grant.

Quality of Life with Photodynamic Therapy vs. Conservative Treatment, Kathy B. Wright, MS, RN, CGRN, CS, Parkland Health and Hospital System, Dallas, TX. ONS Foundation Smith Kline Beecham Research Grant.

2000

Smoking, Alcohol Intake and Depression in Head/Neck Cancer Patients, Sonia Duffy, PhD, RN, HSR&D Field Program, Ann Arbor, MI. ONS Foundation and Sigma Theta Tau International Research Grant.

Symptom Management of Chemotherapy via Telephone Outreach, Janet S. Fulton, PhD, RN, Wright State University, Cincinnati, OH, ONS Foundation/Smith Kline Beecham Research Grant.

African American Women: The Experience of Breast Cancer and Menopause, M. Tish Knobf, PhD, RN, FFAN, Yale University, New Haven, CT. ONS Foundation/Genetech Research Research Grant.

Effects of Symptom Combination on Quality End of Life, Barbara M. Raudonis, PhD, RN, CS, University of Texas at Arlington, Arlington, TX. ONS Foundation/Roxanne Laboratories Research Grant.

Table 1-3.   **continued**

In-Home Pain Education for Cancer Patients–A Pilot Study, Mary Anne Reynolds, PhD, RN, CS, Washington State University Tri-Cities, Richland, WA. ONS Foundation/Knoll Pharmaceutical Research Grant.

2001

Surviving Prostate Cancer and Treatment: Impact on Couples, Michael E. Galbraith, PhD, RN, Loma Linda University School of Nursing, Loma Linda, CA. ONS Foundation/Aventis, Research Grant.

Building a Story: Word Patterns in Writing and Quality of Life, Margaret Saul Laccetti, MSN, RN, AOCN®, Salem State College, Salem, MA. ONS Foundation/Aventis New Investigator Research Grant.

Factors Influencing Quality of Life Following Autologous Bone Marrow Transplantation, Usama S. Saleh, MSN, RN, PhD candidate, University of Kentucky College of Nursing, Lexington, KY. ONS Foundation Ethnic Minority Researcher and Mentorship Grant.

Late Effects and Quality of Life in Long-Term Survivors of Testis Cancer, Linda A. Jacobs, PhD, CRNP, AOCN®, CS, University of Pennsylvania, Philadelphia, PA. ONS Foundation/Bristol-Myers Oncology Research Grant.

2002

Quality of Life in Older Cancer Survivors: Impact of Age and Culture, Kimberly A. Christopher, PhD, RN, OCN®, University of Massachusetts, South Dartmouth, MA. ONS Foundation, Ortho Biotech Research Grant.

Quality of Life in Women Who Carry a BRCA Mutation, Sarah M. McCaffrey, MS, RN, City of Hope National Medical Center, Duarte, CA. ONS Foundation/Genetech Research Grant.

Treatment Decision-Making for the Primary Treatment of Early-Stage Breast Cancer in Chinese American Women, Shiu-yu C. Lee, MSN, RN, Yale University, New Haven, CT. ONS Foundation Ethnic Minority Research Grant.

Major Grants Program
ONS Foundation Center for Leadership, Information, and Research

1999

Living with Lung Cancer: The Women's Perspective, Linda Sarna, DNSc, RN, University of California, Los Angeles, Los Angeles, CA. ONS Foundation/Bristol-Myers Squibb Foundation Inc.

2000

A Behavioral Randomized Trial for Patients on Interferon, Anna L. Schwartz, PhD, ARNP, Oregon Health Sciences University, Portland, OR. ONS Foundation/Schering Oncology Biotherapy Research Grant.

Table 1-3.   **continued**

2001

Telephone Intervention Project: Rural Women with Cancer & Their Partners, Terry A. Badger, PhD, RN, University of Arizona College of Nursing, Tucson, AZ. ONS Foundation/Ortho Biotech, Inc. Symptom Management Phase I Research Grant.

Computerized Cancer Symptom and Quality of Life Assessment, Donna L. Berry, PhD, RN, AOCN®, University of Washington, Seattle, WA. ONS Foundation/Ortho Biotech Inc. Symptom Management Phase I Research Grant.

Upjohn Corporation, in conjunction with ONS, has supported an annual award to recognize nursing excellence in QOL issues (Table 1-4). Manuscripts are requested of ONS members who have submitted an ONS Congress abstract related to QOL and accepted for presentation. If the abstract is accepted for award consideration, the author is required to submit a complete manuscript for review. The manuscripts are evaluated on significance, content, and writing style and address conceptual, research, ethical, or practice issues related to QOL. Established in 1991, a Quality of Life Lectureship has been delivered at ONS's annual Fall Institute and published in

Table 1-4.   **Recipients of the Annual Quality of Life Award Sponsored by the Oncology Nursing Society and Corporations**

1988 *Pregnancy and Parenthood After Treatment for Breast Cancer.* Karen M. Hassey, RN, MS, presented this paper at the 14th Annual Oncology Nursing Society Congress in Pittsburgh, PA. She was the first recipient of the ONS/Upjohn Company QOL Award.

1989 *Effects of Controlled-Release Morphine on Quality of Life for Cancer Pain*, Betty R. Ferrell, RN, PhD; Cheryl Wisdom, RN, MS; Carol Wenzel, RN, MEd; and Judy Brown, RN, MS. Dr. Ferrell presented this paper at the 15th Annual Oncology Nursing Society Congress in San Francisco, CA. The paper was selected for the 1989 ONS/Upjohn Company QOL Award.

1990 *Delirium in Patients with Cancer: Nursing Assessment and Intervention*, Marianne Zimberg, RN, MA, and Susan Berenson, RN, MS. Ms. Zimberg presented this paper at the 16th Annual Oncology Nursing Society Congress in Washington, DC. The paper was selected for the 1990 ONS/Upjohn Company QOL Award.

1991 *Self-Transcendence and Emotional Well-Being in Women with Advanced Cancer.* Doris D. Coward, PhD, RN, presented this paper at the 17th Annual Oncology Nursing Society Congress in San Antonio, TX. The paper was selected for the 1991 ONS/Upjohn Company QOL Award.

Table 1-4. **continued**

1992 *The Oncology Nurse's Role in Patient Advance Directives*. Eileen Parinisi Dimond, MS, RN, OCN, presented this paper at the 17th Annual Oncology Nursing Society Congress in San Diego, CA. The paper was selected for the 1992 ONS/Upjohn Company QOL Award.

1993 *Return-to-Work Experiences of People with Cancer*. Donna L. Berry, RN, PhD, presented this paper at the 18th Annual Oncology Nursing Society Congress in Orlando, FL. The paper was selected for the 1993 ONS/Upjohn Company QOL Award and for the 1993 ONS/Schering Corporation Excellence in Cancer Nursing Research Award.

1994 *Living with Cancer: Children with Extraordinary Courage*, Marilyn Hockenberry-Eaton, RN, PhD, and Ptlene Minick, RN, PhD. Dr. Hockenberry-Eaton presented this paper at the 19th Annual Oncology Nursing Society Congress in Cincinnati, OH. The paper was selected for the 1994 ONS/Upjohn Company QOL Award.

1995 *Quality of Life in Long-Term Cancer Survivors*, Betty R. Ferrell, RN, PhD, RN; Karen Hassey Dow, RN, PhD; Susan Leigh, RN, BSN. Dr. Ferrell presented this paper at the 20th Annual Oncology Nursing Society Congress in Anaheim, CA. The paper was selected for the 1995 ONS/Upjohn Company QOL Award and for the 1995 ONS/Schering Corporation Excellence in Cancer Nursing Research Award.

1996 *Addressing Sexual Dysfunction Following Radiation Therapy for a Gynecologic Malignancy*. Frances Cartwright-Alcarese paper selected at the 21st Annual Oncology Nursing Society Congress in Philadelphia, PA. The paper was selected for the 1996 ONS/Upjohn Company QOL Award.

1997 *Getting Back to Normal: The Family Experience During Early Stage Breast Cancer*. B. Ann Hilton paper selected at the 22nd Annual Oncology Nursing Society Congress in Washington, D.C. The paper was selected for the 1997 ONS/Upjohn Company QOL Award.

1998 *Quality of Life and the Cancer Experience: The State-of-the-Knowledge*. Cynthia R. King paper selected at the 23rd Annual Oncology Nursing Society Congress in Dallas, TX. The paper was selected for the 1998 ONS/Upjohn Company QOL Award.

1999 *End of Life Confusion in Patients*. Deborah A. Boyle paper selected at the 24th Annual Oncology Nursing Society Congress in Atlanta, GA. The paper was selected for the 1999 ONS/Upjohn Company QOL Award.

2000 *The Meaning of Quality of Life in Cancer Survivorship*. Karen Hassey Dow, Betty R. Ferrell, Mel R. Haberman, and Linda Eaton paper selected at the 25th Annual Oncology Nursing Society Congress in San Antonio, TX. The paper was selected for the 2000 ONS/Upjohn Company QOL Award.

2001 *Quality of Life, Survivorship, and Psychosocial Adjustment of Young Women with Breast Cancer After Breast-Conserving Surgery and Radiation Therapy*. Karen Hassey Dow and Patricia Lafferty paper selected at the 26th Annual Oncology Nursing Society Congress in San Diego, CA. The paper was selected for the 2001 ONS/Upjohn Company QOL Award.

2002 *Posttraumatic Stress, Quality of Life, and Psychological Distress in Young Adult Survivors at Childhood Cancer*. Kathleen Meeske paper selected at the 27th Annual Oncology Nursing Society Congress in Washington, D.C. The paper was selected for the 2002 ONS/Upjohn Company QOL Award.

Oncology Nursing Forum (Table 1-5). The purpose of this lectureship is to (*a*) focus ONS membership attention on QOL issues in cancer care; (*b*) describe the contribution of oncology nurse clinicians, educators, administrators, and researchers to QOL in cancer care; (*c*) apply QOL-related information to nursing practice; and (*d*) incorporate QOL philosophy into all aspects of cancer care. In 1988 ONS sponsored a QOL workshop for clinical nurses, which was funded by the Upjohn Corporation. The one-day workshop focused on QOL issues encountered in both acute and ambulatory care settings. In February 1995 AMGEN, U.S.A., and AMGEN, Canada,

---

Table 1-5   **ONS Quality of Life Lectureships**

1991   *The Healthcare Implications of Cancer Rehabilitation in the 21st Century.* Presented by Deborah Mayer, RN, MSN, OCN, at the Second Annual Fall Institute in Atlanta, GA. Sponsored by CIBA-GIEGY Pharmaceuticals.

1992   *Myths, Monsters, and Magic: Personal Perspectives and Professional Challenges of Survival.* Presented by Susan Leigh, RN, BSN, at the Third Annual Fall Institute in Minneapolis, MN. Sponsored by CIBA-GIEGY Pharmaceuticals.

1993   *To Know Suffering.* Presented by Betty R. Ferrell, PhD, RN, at the Fourth Annual Fall Institute in Seattle, WA. Sponsored by CIBA-GIEGY Pharmaceuticals.

1994   *Quality of Life Through the Eyes of Survivors of Breast Cancer.* Presented by Carol Estwing Ferrans, PhD, RN, FAAN, at the Fifth Annual Fall Institute in Pittsburgh, PA. Sponsored by the Purdue Frederick Company.

1995   *Patient-Induced Dehydration: Can It Ever Be Therapeutic?* Presented by Shirley Anne Smith, MSN, RN, OCN, at the Sixth Annual Fall Institute in Nashville, TN. Sponsored by the Purdue Frederick Company.

1996   *Sexuality Issues: Keeping Your Cool.* Presented by Mary K. Hughes, MSN, RN, at the Seventh Annual Fall Institute in Phoenix, AZ. Sponsored by the Purdue Frederick Company.

1997   *Light Your World.* Presented by Rosanne M. Radziewica, RN, MSN, CA, at the 6th Annual Fall Institute in Washington, DC. Sponsored by Purdue Frederick Company.

1998   *Changing Seasons of Care: Harvesting Hope in the Autumn of Life.* Presented by Terri Armstrong, RN, MS, ANP, CS at the 7th Annual Fall Institute in Dallas, TX. Sponsored by Purdue Frederick Company.

1999   *Silence Is Not Golden: Conversations With the Dying.* Presented by Karen J. Stanley, RN, MSN, AOCN at the 8th Annual Fall Institute in Salt Lake City, UT. Sponsored by Purdue Frederick Company.

2000   *The Dance of Life.* Presented by Cynthia R. King, PhD, NP, MSN, RN, FAAN. Presented at the 1st Annual Institutes of Learning in Charlotte, NC. Sponsored by Purdue Pharma L. P.

2001   *Revisiting the Road: Integrating Palliative Care Into Oncology Nursing.* Presented by Marie Bakitas Whedon, ARNP, AOCN®, CHPN, FAAN at the 2nd Annual Institute of Learning in St. Louis, MO. Sponsored by Purdue Pharma L. P.

sponsored the ONS QOL State-of-the-Knowledge Conference in San Diego, California, to address the current knowledge regarding QOL and the cancer experience (King et al., 1997). The conference was attended by oncology nurses and psychologists from the United States and Canada.

Oncology Nursing Society Research Priorities

The ONS Research Committee has periodically surveyed membership over the past 14 years to identify research priorities and provide a focus for nursing education programs and conferences. ONS also uses the findings to advise the Oncology Nursing Foundation and federal agencies about priorities for research funding. Findings from the 2000 ONS Research Priorities Survey have been submitted to the *Oncology Nursing Forum* (Ropka, Guterbock, Krebs, Murphy-Ende, Stetz, Summers, & Given, submitted 2002). Respondents ranked QOL studies as the second most appropriate type of research for nurses.

Quality of Life Research Issues

While progress has been made in defining QOL, developing qualitative and quantitative methodologies to study QOL, and identifying QOL outcomes, many research issues persist, including conceptual and methodological issues.

Authors need to include their definitions of, assumptions about, and conceptual approaches to QOL assessment. To combine findings across studies and synthesize what knowledge has been identified, clarity in defining and measuring QOL is essential. Many quantitative instruments have been developed for measuring QOL, some of which show beginning evidence of reliability, validity, and sensitivity. Future research should focus on the application of these instruments to a variety of patient populations by a variety of researchers. New instruments are unlikely to be needed.

Selection of an appropriate instrument should be related specifically to the questions posed in the research study. One QOL instrument may be valuable in measuring QOL over medical treatment periods, while another may be appropriately suited for evaluating survivors' concerns. Since no gold standard of QOL has been developed, researchers need to select instrumentation based on the nature of the study, the population, and the purpose.

While assumptions are unstated in many research publications, specifying them in QOL research may assist in interpreting findings and building appropriate science. Is it assumed that all items in the selected QOL questionnaire have equal weight? Is it assumed that a baseline value can be gathered anytime before treatment starts? Is it assumed that follow-up evaluation can be obtained anytime after treatment is ended?

These assumptions need to be carefully identified so that studies can be grouped and synthesized.

Missing data in QOL studies is an important issue. In some instances, physicians have been reluctant to collect QOL data when patients are ill, feeling that questions on QOL may be upsetting to them. However, without acute-phase data, follow-up data cannot be compared and the true impact of the disease and treatment on QOL may never be known. To measure QOL during acute treatment periods, it may be necessary to use experienced nurses who are sensitive to the patient's needs but still able to obtain needed information. Qualitative approaches may be very valuable in these situations, as a measure of providing individualized approaches.

Several issues have occurred in the interpretation of QOL study results. One of these is the tension between statistical differences in pre-post QOL scores, and what relationship these differences have to clinical differences. This issue points to the necessity of having a combination of research and clinical expertise available when conducting and interpreting QOL studies. Another issue is the adaptation humans make to changes in health statues, and how this affects their perceptions of QOL. The response-shift concept has been explored and developed to assist in discussing these changes and designing research to demonstrate such shifts. A recent publication provides information on the theoretical underpinnings of the response-shift construct, methodology for assessment in primary and secondary analyses, and application to treatment outcomes research (Schwartz & Sprangers, 2000).

Now that assessment of QOL has become possible, intervention studies and hypothesis-driven studies are needed. We need studies that test interventions directed toward improving the patient's QOL, maintaining QOL during acute treatment periods, and maintaining QOL in cancer survivors and terminally ill patients. Such studies will provide meaningful information for those planning cancer programs, as well as provide sound evidence for appropriating resources for cancer patients in general.

CONCLUSION

Quality of life is a concept relevant to the discipline of nursing. Nurses, and specifically oncology nurses, have actively contributed to the development of the QOL concept through instrument development and population description. Challenges to conducting research on this concept are many, yet research opportunities are abundant and provide a fertile area for continued work.

Nurses have also promoted QOL through clinical nursing activities and by promoting patient well-being. In both research and clinical practice, nurses have collaborated with those in other disciplines to expand the knowledge regarding the impact of cancer and cancer treatment on QOL. Lastly, through the Oncology

Nursing Society and Oncology Nursing Foundation, oncology nurses have demonstrated support for QOL research and clinical practice.

As the interest in quality of life issues continues to increase, nurses will continue to be actively involved locally, regionally, nationally, and internationally. Oncology nurses will continue to assess the impact of cancer and cancer treatment on QOL and implement strategies to decrease adverse physical, psychological, social, and spiritual effects on the lives of patients with cancer.

REFERENCES

Aaronson, N. K., Ahmedzai, S., Bergman, B., Bullinger, M., Cull, A., Duez, N. J., Filiberti, A., Flechtner, H., Fleishman, S. B., de Haes, J. C. J. M., Kaasa, S., Klee, M., Osoba, D., Razavi, D., Rofe, P. B., Schraub, S., Sneeuw, K., Sullivan, M., & Takeda, F. for the European Organization for Research and Treatment of Cancer Study Group on Quality of Life. (1993). The European Organization for Research and Treatment of Cancer QLQ-C30: A quality-of-life instrument for use in international clinical trials in oncology. *Journal of the National Cancer Institute, 85*, 365–376.

Aaronson, N. K., Ahmedzai, S., Bullinger, M., Crabeels, D., Estapè, J., Filiberti, A., Flechtner, H., Frick, U., Hürny, C., Kaasa, S., Klee, M., Mastilica, M., Osoba, D., Pfausler, B., Razavi, D., Rofe, P. B. C., Schraub, S., Sullivan, M., & Takeda, F. (1991). The EORTC core quality of life questionnaire: Interim results of an international field study. In D. Osoba (Ed.), *Effect of cancer on quality of life* (pp. 182–203). Boca Raton, FL: CRC Press.

Beitz, J., Gnecco, C., & Justice, R. (1996). Quality-of-life end points in cancer clinical trials: The U.S. Food and Drug Administration perspective. *Journal of National Cancer Institute Monograph, 20*, 7–9.

Braden, C. J. (1990). A test of the self-help model: Learned response to chronic illness experience. *Nursing Research, 39*, 42–47.

Coleman, E. A., Krammer, A. M., Johnson, M., Eilertsen, T. B., & Holthaus, D. (1999). Quality measure in post-acute care: The need for a unique set of measures. *Abstract Book of Association of Health Service Research, 16*, 78.

Cull, A., Aaronson, N., Ahmedzai, S., Fayers, P., de Haes, H., Kaasa, S., Kiebert, W., Sprangers, M., & Sullivan, M. on behalf of the EORTC Study Group on Quality of Life. (1996, June–January). Instruments. The European Organization for Research and Treatment of Cancer (EORTC) modular approach to quality of life assessment in oncology: An update. *Quality of Life Newsletter*, (13–14), 1-2,8, MAPI Research Institute.

Cultural adaption of quality of life (QOL) instruments. (1996, June–January). *MAPI Research Institute,* (13–14), 5.

Davis, L. L., & Grant, J. S. (1994). Constructing the reality of recovery: Family home care management strategies. *Advances in Nursing Science, 17*(2), 66–76.

Dracup, K., & Raffin, T. (1989). Withholding and withdrawing mechanical ventilation: Assessing quality of life. *American Review of Respiratory Diseases, 140*(Suppl. Part 2), S4–S6.

Eiser, C., & Morse, R. (2001). A review of measures of quality of life for children with chronic illness. *Archives of Disease in Childhood, 84*(3), 205–211.

Felton, B. J., Revenson, T. A., & Hinrichsen, G. A. (1984). Stress and coping in the explanation of psychological adjustment among chronically ill adults. *Social Science and Medicine, 18,* 889–898.

Ferrell, B. A., Ferrell, B. R., & Rivera, L. (1995). Pain in cognitively impaired nursing home patients. *Journal of Pain and Symptom Management, 10*(8), 591–598.

Ferrell, B., Grant, M., Funk, B., Garcia, N., Otis-Green, S., & Schaffner, M. L. J. (1996). Quality of life in breast cancer. *Cancer Practice, 4*(6), 331–340.

Ferrell, B. R., Grant, M., Funk, R., Otis-Green, S., & Garcia, N. (1997). Quality of life in breast cancer, Part I. Physical and social well being. *Cancer Nursing, 20*(6), 398–408.

Ferrell, B. R., Grant, M., Funk, R., Otis-Green, S., & Garcia, N. (1998a). Quality of life in breast cancer, Part II. Psychological and spiritual well being. *Cancer Nursing, 21*(1), 1–9.

Ferrell, B. R., Grant, M. M., Funk, B., Otis-Green, S. A., & Garcia, N. (1998b). Quality of life in breast cancer survivors: Implications for developing support services. *Oncology Nursing Forum, 25*(5), 887–895.

Ferrell, B., Grant, M., Schmidt, G. M., Rhiner, M., Whitehead, C., Fonbuena, P., & Forman, S. J. (1992a). The meaning of quality of life for bone marrow transplant survivors. Part 2: Improving quality of life for bone marrow transplant survivors. *Cancer Nursing, 15*(4), 247–253.

Ferrell, B., Grant, M., Schmidt, G. M., Rhiner, M., Whitehead, C., Fonbuena, P., & Forman, S. J. (1992b). The meaning of quality of life for bone marrow transplant survivors. Part 1: The impact of bone marrow transplant on quality of life. *Cancer Nursing, 15*(3), 153–60.

Ferrell, B. R., & Hassey Dow, K. (1997). Quality of life among long-term cancer survivors. *Oncology, 11*(4), 565–576.

Ferrell, B. R., Hassey Dow, K., Leigh, S., Ly, J., & Gulasekaram, P. (1995). Quality of life in long-term cancer survivors. *Oncology Nursing Forum, 22*(6), 915–922.

Ferrell, B. R., Rhiner, M., Shapiro, B., & Dierkes, M. (1994). The experience of pediatric cancer pain. Part I: Impact of pain on the family. *Journal of Pediatric Nursing, 9*(6), 368–379.

Ferrell, B. R., Taylor, E. J., Grant, M., Fowler, M., & Corbisiero, R. (1993). Pain management at home: Struggle, comfort, and mission. *Cancer Nursing, 16*(3), 169–178.

Fowlie, M., Berkeley, J., & Dingwall-Fordyce, I. (1989). Quality of life in advanced cancer: The benefits of asking the patient. *Palliative Medicine, 3,* 55–59.

Grant, M. (2000). Fatigue and quality of life with cancer. In: M. L. Winningham & M. Barton-Burke (Eds.), *Fatigue in Cancer: A Multidimensional Approach* (pp. 353–364). Sudbury, MA: Jones and Bartlett Publishers.

Grant, M. (1999a). Quality of life issues in colorectal cancer. *Developments in Supportive Cancer Care, 3*(1), 4–9.

Grant, M. (1999b). Assessment of quality of life following hematopoietic cell transplantation. In G. D. Donnell, K. G. Blume, & S. J. Porman (Eds.), *Hematopoietic Cell Transplantation* (2nd ed.) (pp. 407–413) Boston, MA: Blackwell Science, Inc.

Grant, M., Ferrell, B. R., & Sakurai, C. (1994). Defining the spiritual dimension of quality of life assessment in bone marrow transplant survivors. *Oncology Nursing Forum, 21*(2), 376, (Abstract).

Grant, M., Ferrell, B., Schmidt, G. M., Fonbuena, P., Niland, J., & Forman, S. J. (1992). Measurement of quality of life in bone marrow transplantation. *Quality of Life Research, 1*(6), 375–384.

Grant, M., Padilla, G. V., & Ferrell, B. R. (unpublished manuscript). *Manual of the quality of life scale.* Duarte, CA: City of Hope National Medical Center.

Greimel, E. R., Padilla, G. V., & Grant, M. M. (1997). Physical and psychosocial outcomes in cancer patients: A comparison of different age groups. *British Journal of Cancer, 76*(2), 251–255.

Harrington, V., Lackey, N. R., & Gates, M. F. (1996). Needs of caregivers of clinic and hospice cancer patients. *Cancer Nursing, 19*(2), 118–125.

Holzemer, W. L., & Wilson, H. S. (1995). Quality of life and the spectrum of HIV infection. *Annual Review of Nursing Research, 13,* 3–29.

Johnson, D., McGratz, C., Marquis, P., Jambon, B., & Padilla, G. V. (1996, June–January). Determination of QOL as a measure of quality of care in ostomy patients. *Quality of Life Newsletter,* (13–14), 7, MAPI Research Institute.

Johnson, J. R., & Temple, R. (1985). Food and Drug Administration requirements for approval of new anti-cancer drugs. *Cancer Treatment Reports, 69,* 1155–1157.

Karmilovich, S. E. (1994). Burden and stress associated with spousal caregiving for individuals with heart failure. *Progress in Cardiovascular Nursing, 9*(11), 33–38.

King, C. R., Ferrell, B. R., Grant, M., & Sakurai, C. (1995). Nurses' perceptions of the meaning of quality of life for bone marrow transplant survivors. *Cancer Nursing, 18*(2), 118–129.

King, C. R., Haberman, M., Berry, D. L., Bush, N., Butler, L., Dow, K. H., Ferrell, B., Grant, M., Gue, D., Hinds, P., Kruer, J., Padilla, G., & Underwood, S. (1997). Quality of life and the cancer experience: The state-of-the-knowledge. *Oncology Nursing Forum, 24*(1), 27–41.

Krouse, R. S., Grant, M., Nelson, R., Grube, B., Rivera, L., Dean, G., Ferrell, B. R., Wagman, L. D., & Chu, D. Z. J. (2000). Colostomies: A systematic evaluation of quality of life outcomes. *Society of Surgical Oncology*, March 2000, New Orleans, LA.

Mandelblatt, J. S., & Eisenberg, J. M. (1995). Historical and methodological perspectives on cancer outcomes research. *Oncology, 9*(11 Suppl), 23–32.

Marquis, P., Marrel, A., & Blackman, A. (1996, February–May). Quality of care: Management of an international quality of life study in patients with ostomy. *Quality of Life Newsletter*, (15), 12, MAPI Research Institute.

Mooney, K. H., Ferrell, B. R., Nail, L. M., Benedict, S. C., & Haberman, M. R. (1991). 1991 Oncology Nursing Society Research Priorities Survey. *Oncology Nursing Forum, 18*(8), 1381–1388.

Nayfield, S. G., Ganz, P. A., Moinpour, C. M., Cella, D. F., & Hailey, B. J. (1992). Report from a National Cancer Institute (USA) workshop on quality of life assessment in cancer clinical trials. *Quality of Life Research, 1*(3), 203–210.

Osoba, D. (1992). The Quality of Life Committee of the Clinical Trials Group of the National Cancer Institute of Canada: Organization and functions. *Quality of Life Research, 1*, 211–218.

Packa, D. R. (1989). Quality of life of adults after a heart transplant. *Journal of Cardiovascular Nursing, 3*, 12–22.

Packa, D. R., Branyon, M. E., Kenney, M. R., Kahn, S. H., Kelley, R., & Miers, L. J. (1989). Quality of life of elderly patients enrolled in cardiac rehabilitation. *Journal of Cardiovascular Nursing, 3*, 33–42.

Padilla, G. V., Ferrell, B., & Grant, M. M. (1990). Defining the content domain of quality of life for cancer patients with pain. *Cancer Nursing 13*(2), 108–115.

Padilla, G. V., Grant, M., Ferrell, B. F., & Presant, G. A. (1996). Quality of life—cancer. In B. Spilker (Ed.), *Quality of Life and Pharmacoeconomics in Clinical Trials* (2nd ed.) (pp. 301–308). Philadelphia: Lippincott-Raven.

Padilla, G. V., Grant, M., Lipsett, S., Anderson, P., Rhiner, M., & Bogen, C. (1992). Health-related quality of life and colorectal cancer. *Cancer, 70*(5), 1450–1456.

Padilla, G. V., Presant, C., Grant, M., Metter, G., Lipsett, J., & Heide, F. (1983). Quality of life index for patients with cancer. *Research in Nursing and Health, 6*, 117–126.

Ragsdale, D., Kotarba, J. A., & Morrow, J. R. (1992). Quality of life of hospitalized persons with AIDS. *IMAGE: Journal of Nursing Scholarship, 13*, 259–265.

Ropka, M. E., Guterbock, T., Krebs, L., Murphy-Ende, K., Stetz, K., Summers, B., & Given, B. Year 2000 Oncology Nursing Society Research Priorities Survey Summary Report. *Oncology Nursing Forum*, Submitted, 2002.

Schwartz, C. E., & Sprangers, M. A. G. (2000). *Adaptation to Changing Health: Response Shift in Quality-of-Life Research*. Washington, DC: American Psychological Association.

Shah, S., Sesti, A., Chopra, T., McLaughlin-Miley, C., & Copley-Merriman, K. (2001). Quality of life terminology documented in package inserts. *Quality of Life Newsletter, 27*, 1–2.

Slevin, M. L., Plant, H., Lynch, D., Drinkwater, J., & Gregory, W. M. (1988). Who should measure quality of life, the doctor or the patient? *British Journal of Cancer, 57*, 109–112.

Spilker, B. (1990). Introduction. In B. Spilker (Ed.), *Quality of life assessments in clinical trials* (pp. 3–9). New York: Raven Press.

Sprangers, M. A. G., Cull, A., Bjordal, K., Groenvold, M., & Aaronson, N. K. (1993). The European Organization for Research and Treatment of Cancer approach to quality of life assessment: Guidelines for developing questionnaire modules. *Quality of Life Research, 2*, 287–295.

Stetz, K. M., Haberman, M. R., Holcombe, J., & Jones, L. S. (1995). Oncology Nursing Society research priorities survey. *Oncology Nursing Forum, 22*(5), 785–789.

Stetz, K. M., McDonald, J. C., & Compton, K. (1996). Needs and experiences of family caregivers during marrow transplantation. *Oncology Nursing Forum, 23*(9), 1422–1427.

Stjernswärd, J., & Teoh, N. (1991). Perspectives on quality of life and the global cancer problem. In D. Osoba (Ed.), *Effect of cancer on quality of life* (pp. 1–5). Boca Raton, FL: CRC Press.

Taylor, E. J., Ferrell, B. R., Grant, M., & Cheyney, L. (1993). Managing cancer pain at home: The decisions and ethical conflicts of patients, family caregivers, and homecare nurses. *Oncology Nursing Forum, 20*(6), 919–927.

Tuchler, H., Hofmann, S., Bernhart, M., Brugiatelli, M., Chrobak, L., Franke, A., Herold, M., Holowiecki, J., Ihle, R., Jaksic, B., Krc, I., Munteanu, N., Pawlicki, M., Sakalova, A., Schranz, V., Wolf, H., & Lutz, D. (1992). A short multilingual quality of life questionnaire—practicability, reliability, and interlingual homogeneity. *Quality of Life Research, 1*(2), 107–117.

U.S. Department of Health and Human Services, Public Health Service, National Institutes of Health. (1990). *Quality of life assessment in cancer clinical trials. Report of the Workshop on Quality of Life Research in Cancer Clinical Trials.* Bethesda, MD.

Wingate, S. (1995). Quality of life of women after a myocardial infarction. *Heart & Lung, 24*(6), 467–473.

World Health Organization, Division of Mental Health. (1993). WHO-QOL Study protocol: The development of the World Health Organization quality of life assessment instrument (MNG/PSF/93.9). Geneva, Switzerland.

Zebrack, B. (2000). Cancer survivors and quality of life: A critical review of the literature. *Oncology Nursing Forum, 27*(9), 1395–1401.

2

Overview of
Quality of Life
and Controversial Issues

CYNTHIA R. KING

For centuries individuals have been concerned with seeking the "good life." In that search, the prevailing question has been: What is the quality of any specific life? As treatments for cancer become more aggressive and are associated with greater toxicities, and survival time is lengthened significantly by new therapies, there is an increasing need to move beyond the focus of morbidity and mortality and evaluate the nursing and patient perspectives on quality of life (QOL). Both nursing and patient perspectives are important when assessing QOL for individuals with cancer. Oncology nurses, and nurses in general, have been committed to obtaining patients' views on QOL in order to improve nursing care and ultimately the outcomes of care. This chapter highlights the numerous controversies related to QOL and the importance of nursing and patient perspectives.

Many controversies currently exist concerning quality of life and its measurement. How we define and measure the QOL of individuals with cancer reflects much of the ongoing debates related to QOL in general. A more basic question is, Why should we study or use the concept of QOL in cancer care? The answer may be examined at the levels of the individual, the health care provider, or national health care policy. When addressing the question at the level of the patient with cancer, the answer is to improve the quality of the individual's life and treatment. When evaluating a particular therapy, health care providers may evaluate QOL in clinical trials to differentiate between two therapies with similar survival rates. Health care providers are concerned with QOL because it may alter prescribing habits, treatment regimens, and decisions to cease treatment. At the national health care policy level,

QOL is an important concept used to improve the allocation of insufficient health care resources to solve all the health care problems (Spilker, 1990).

Despite the excessive costs of health care, the Census Bureau reported that in 2000 there were 39 million uninsured Americans. This number exceeded the aggregate population of 22 states, plus the District of Columbia. By 2002 there have been reports of 44 million (16%) uninsured Americans. This number is estimated to increase by 1 million each year. Kaplan (1995) describes three major problems with the health care system in the United States: (1) health care costs are excessive, and employers and the government can no longer provide the same level of payment; (2) the system is inequitable, as many individuals are without insurance or adequate resources to cover medical care; and (3) individuals are failing to be good consumers (e.g., individuals may buy unnecessary or ineffective services in an attempt to obtain health). These problems are labeled (1) affordability, (2) access, and (3) accountability. Overall, QOL becomes an important concept when examining health care and cancer care at the levels of the individual, the health care practitioner, and the national health care policy.

The concept of QOL is increasing in importance and growing as a valid indicator of whether a given medical treatment is beneficial. QOL now represents a way to describe the overall results of diagnostic and treatment efforts that makes sense to individuals with cancer and health care professionals (especially nurses). QOL appears to be a relevant goal even in palliative care (Clinch & Schipper, 1993; MacHill et al., 2002).

Definitions

In order to conduct valid QOL studies or adequately describe, assess, or discuss QOL, a clear definition of QOL is required. Unfortunately, many individuals, health care professionals, and researchers have used this term without definition. They may fail to define QOL because they believe that an accepted meaning exists or that the term is too amorphous to be adequately described. For many years there has been a lack of agreement on how to define and describe QOL for patients with cancer (Aaronson, 1990; Clinch & Schipper, 1993; King et al., 1997; Reid & Renwick, 1994; Schipper, Clinch, & Powell, 1990). Numerous authors and researchers have attempted to define QOL, as seen in Appendix 1. These definitions reflect how QOL has been defined for adults, adolescents, and children and how the definitions can vary. Nurses have been actively involved in attempting to define QOL and have found multiple conceptualizations to be helpful.

When discussing QOL, it is important to distinguish it from related, but different, concepts, including well-being, health status, life satisfaction, and hope. In Chapter 4, Haase and Braden discuss the need to clarify the concept of QOL and provide guidelines for obtaining clarity in QOL conceptualization, assessment, and measurement. One method for clarifying this concept is through the use of concept analysis. Whatever method is used, it is crucial to distinguish QOL from other related concepts.

Cella and Tulsky (1991) recommend avoiding the term QOL when discussing or measuring only a single dimension of the concept. Experts in QOL may decide that one definition will not be adequate to describe all the changes in QOL throughout the disease process. Additionally, concept analyses may be needed by various health care disciplines. In fact, the meaning and importance of QOL may be discipline specific or population specific (King et al., 1997). Unfortunately, patients have rarely been involved in defining the concept of QOL; thus, it is not appropriate to assume that patients/survivors and health care professionals share an understanding of the term.

Despite the challenges related to defining QOL, there are areas of conceptual agreement among experts. Most would agree that QOL is comprised of both positive and negative facets of life and is a multidimensional concept. Additionally, many experts agree on the subjectivity and dynamism of the concept (Grant, Padilla, Ferrell, & Rhiner, 1990; Hinds, 1990; Holmes & Dickerson, 1987; Hyland, Kenyon, & Jacobs, 1994; King et al., 1997, Moinpour et al., 1989). The multidimensional aspect of QOL is demonstrated in the numerous dimensions identified as part of the concept (physical, psychological, social, somatic, spiritual). Although some studies include objective measures of QOL, many rely on subjective, self-report measures. The trend toward using patients' self-reports rather than reports of proxies has developed after various studies demonstrated a lack of strong agreement among the ratings of QOL given by patients, family members, and health care providers (Epstein, Hall, Tognetti, Son, & Conant, 1989; King, Ferrell, Grant, & Sakurai, 1995; Osoba, 1994). This is because the QOL assessment by a proxy will be biased by the proxy's own standards of what comprises a desirable QOL (Osoba, 1994). Dynamism reflects the need to measure perceptions of QOL along a continuum, as an individual's QOL may change over time.

Considerable work remains to be done in order to develop consensus definitions of QOL for specific populations or specific disciplines. Until consensus is reached, it is advisable to state the definition of QOL in publications, in research, and in educational or clinical settings.

Dimensions

Despite intensive work by many experts, controversies remain regarding the dimensions of QOL. These controversies are also discussed by Haase and Braden in Chapter 4 and Haberman and Bush in Chapter 8. There has generally been little theoretical basis for the dimensions reflected in the health-related QOL literature (Aaronson, 1991; Padilla, Presant, Grant, Metter, Lipsett, & Heide, 1983). In some instances, researchers developing scales combined factors that were assumed to indicate QOL and then chose items to represent those factors.

Most experts (Aaronson, 1991; Ferrans, 1990, King et al., 1997; Schipper, 1991) would agree that there are four to five generally accepted dimensions to QOL: (1) physical, (2) psychological, (3) social, (4) somatic/disease- and treatment-related symptoms, and (5) spiritual. The physical dimension is the one that most closely approximates the outcome measures traditionally used. Questions asked regarding physical aspects include questions about strength, energy, ability to perform activities of daily living (ADLs), and self-care. These generally correlate with the physicians' estimates of the patient's well-being and functional status (Aaronson, 1991; Padilla, Ferrell, Grant, & Ackley, 1990; Schipper et al., 1990). Psychological well-being is often problematic for health care professionals, who are usually poor estimators of patients' psychological state. Nurses, social workers, and psychologists often are better at estimating the psychological state of patients than are other health care providers. The most frequently studied psychological symptoms are anxiety, depression, and fear. Unfortunately, many of the tests were developed for healthy populations or persons with diagnosed mental or psychological disabilities (Aaronson, 1991; Schipper et al., 1990). Social well-being refers to how individuals carry on relationships with family, friends, colleagues at work, and the general community (Aaronson, 1991; Ferrell et al., 1992a; Ferrell et al., 1992b; Padilla et al., 1990; Schipper et al., 1990). Somatic refers to disease symptoms and treatment side effects (pain, nausea, vomiting), while spiritual well-being refers to the perception that one's life has purpose and meaning (Aaronson, 1991; Ferrell et al., 1992a, Ferrell et al., 1992b; Schipper et al., 1990).

As with the definition of QOL, it is important to specify the domains of QOL when evaluating QOL in education, research, or clinical practice. Additionally, a rationale for the use of these specific dimensions should be included. Some nurses in education, research, or clinical practice include a model that depicts QOL, its dimensions, and associated variables (e.g., Eilers & King, Chapter 13; and Ferrell & Grant, Chapter 9). In the future, nurses should elicit more information from patients/survivors regarding the dimensions of QOL and the associated variables, as work has been limited in this area. Ferrell and colleagues (1992) did evaluate bone marrow transplant recipients' perceptions of QOL and its dimensions and discovered that spiritual well-being was an important separate domain of QOL and not a part of the psychological dimension.

Measurement

Quality of life studies can provide comprehensive and sensitive methods for communicating information on the burden of the disease and effectiveness of treatment if they are designed and implemented well. The impact of cancer and progress in treatment cannot be adequately measured by mortality rates, incidence and prevalence, or average length of stay in the hospital. Cancer affects many dimensions of health and well-being. Ideally, treatment should not only prolong survival and disease-free intervals, but should also decrease symptoms associated with disease, not cause noxious side effects, and improve an individual's ability to return to a normal lifestyle. The use of QOL assessments in clinical trials can help improve clinical practice by suggesting changes in treatment, survivor, and rehabilitation needs (Moinpour, Savage, Hayden, Sayers, & Upchurch, 1995; Schuttiga, 1995). Overall the purpose for assessing QOL is to consider the patient perspective of the disease, identify benefits and risks of treatment choices, and determine the contribution of therapeutic and nursing interventions to QOL (Bowling, 1991; de Haes & van Knippenberg, 1985; Faden & Leplege, 1992).

The potential applications of QOL measures fall into three categories: (1) discrimination, (2) prediction, and (3) evaluation. Discrimination is used to distinguish between individuals or groups with respect to an underlying dimension when no gold standard is available. Prediction is used when the gold standard is available; this method is used to classify individuals into a set of predefined measurement categories. Then a gold standard is used to determine if individuals have been classified correctly (Guyatt & Jaeschke, 1990). An evaluation index is used to measure the magnitude of longitudinal change in an individual or group. These tools have provided the main focus for QOL clinical trials.

Instruments used to measure QOL in patients with cancer need to have reproducibility (reliability), validity, and responsiveness. Reliability is important to ensure that the same results are obtained with repeated measures when the status has not changed. Validity or accuracy is essential for the tool to measure what it is intended to. This is easy if there is a gold standard, but currently no gold standard for QOL measurement exists. Responsiveness or sensitivity to change is the ability to detect clinically important changes. The instrument must register changes in the score when the subject's QOL increases or decreases (Guyatt & Jaeschke, 1990).

Measurement issues are discussed more thoroughly by Haberman and Bush in Chapter 8, yet some QOL controversies deserve mentioning: (1) the use of generic versus specific measurement tools, (2) the use of a single QOL instrument versus a battery of questionnaires, (3) the use of dimension scores versus a total score, (4) the use of self-administered tools versus those of proxies, (5) quantitative versus qualitative tools, (6) measurement at one time point versus measurements on multiple occasions, and (7) whether assessments are culturally sensitive.

Specific versus Generic Measurement Tools

An ongoing controversy exists regarding the use of a generic versus a specific measurement tool. The generic instrument is designed to measure the complete spectrum of dimensions relevant to QOL and can be used to measure QOL for numerous chronic illnesses (e.g., heart disease, pulmonary disease, arthritis, AIDS, and cancer). The two types of generic instruments are health profiles and utility measures. Health profiles are single instruments that measure different aspects of QOL such as the effect of the disease and/or treatment on everyday functioning. These health profiles are designed to be used in a wide variety of conditions and do not reflect a specific disease or treatment. Examples of these instruments are the Sickness Impact Profile (SIP), the Nottingham Health Profile, and the Medical Outcomes Study Short Form-36 (MOS SF-36). Many of these generic tools are lengthy and difficult to use if individuals are seriously ill (Aaronson, 1991; Moinpour et al., 1995; Stewart et al., 1989). Health profile tools are often reliable and valid, but many do not focus adequately on certain aspects of QOL. Utility instruments, on the other hand, are derived from economic decision theory. With these tools QOL is measured as a single number along a continuum of death (0) to full health (10). Some have questioned whether a single measurement can be responsive to small but clinically important changes (Guyatt & Jaeschke, 1990). There is also a problem in using a single overall score for QOL. With this method, different dimensions of QOL may yield different results. For example, treatment 1 may be more effective than treatment 2 in two out of four domains, while treatment 2 may be more effective than treatment 1 in the other two domains (Spilker, 1990). Haberman and Bush provide a list of generic questionnaires in Table 8-3.

Specific instruments focus on problems that are applicable only to certain individuals. These tools may be specific to a disease, a population (individuals with cancer), a certain dimension of QOL (psychological), or a given condition (pain). These instruments are usually more responsive. Unfortunately, specific instruments often are not comprehensive and cannot be used to compare across diseases or conditions (Aaronson, 1991; Guyatt & Jaeschke, 1990). Haberman and Bush provide a list of cancer-specific instruments in Table 8-3.

Single Instrument versus Battery of Tests

Some researchers administer a battery of tests to achieve comprehensiveness. The advantage of this approach is that rich data on multiple dimensions of QOL may be provided. However, this method is problematic if the researcher chooses to use only one section of a tool in the battery of tests (Guyatt & Jaeschke, 1990). When using a battery of tests, it is impossible to combine all the test score results. Also, patients may assign different weights to different dimensions based on their beliefs, which are influenced by the severity of their disease, their cultural background, their religion, and their past experience (Spilker, 1990). Other problems that may be encountered when using a battery of tests include small sample sizes (a large sample size is needed if, for example, researchers are using multiple QOL tests) and the use of univariate statistical techniques to analyze multiple measures of QOL. Also, analyzing change across time is difficult when multiple tools are used (Shumaker, Anderson, & Czajkowski, 1990).

Dimension Scores versus Total Score

Another controversy exists regarding the use of a total score versus the use of dimension scores. Some instruments provide single scores with a total score. Examples include the Cancer Rehabilitation Evaluation System (CARES), the Functional Living Index-Cancer (FLIC), and the Functional Assessment of Cancer Therapy (FACT) (Cella et al., 1993; Ganz, Rofessart, Polinsky, Schag, & Heinrich, 1986; Morrow, Lindke, & Black, 1992). Another method combines several separate tools into a QOL test. In this example each dimension may be measured by a different scale. This was done with the SWOG QOL questionnaire, which combined generic (MOS SF) scales, symptom scales (Symptom Distress Scale), and side effects of treatment (treatment-specific items). The treatment-specific items are revised for each clinical trial depending on the disease site and treatment evaluation in the trial (Moinpour et al., 1995).

Recommendations on Tools

The number of scales that have been used to evaluate QOL issues is enormous, and no consensus has yet been reached as to which are the best tools. It is possible that consensus will be reached on a few widely accepted scales for each domain, or we may be able to better identify specific conditions under which to use certain scales (Spilker, 1990).

Several experts have recently suggested that a "core plus module" be administered to measure QOL. This means that a global QOL index is administered as the core tool that addresses multiple dimensions, and then a smaller additional module is administered that is specific for a particular disease, population, or condition. The European Organization for Research and Treatment of Cancer (EORTC) QOL Core Questionnaire (QLQ-C30) is an example of a core plus module approach (Aaronson et al., 1993; Aaronson et al., 1991; Aaronson et al., 1987; Aaronson, Bullinger, & Ahmedzai, 1988; Schipper et al., 1990). The SWOG Quality of Life Questionnaire is another example of a core plus module (Moinpour et al., 1989; Moinpour, Hayden, Thompson, Feigl, & Metch, 1990). Haberman and Bush in Chapter 8 discuss specific modules that have been developed.

Regardless of other factors, a successful QOL instrument should be brief and easy to read, understand, score, and prepare for analysis. The success of any instrument or series of tests will be related in part to the burden imposed on respondents and their willingness to participate (King et al., 1997).

Self-Report versus Proxies

Most instruments are designed to be self-administered. Frequently, when physicians are used as proxies, they emphasize physiological data. Nurses, social workers, and families place more emphasis on psychosocial measures (Schipper et al., 1990). Other researchers have found that proxy respondents tend to underestimate patients' QOL (King et al., 1995; Sprangers & Aaronson, 1992). While it is generally accepted that QOL information should be directly obtained from the patient/survivor, in some situations data derived from health care professionals or significant others is appropriate to include in the evaluation of QOL (e.g., very young children, very ill patients, comatose patients). It is also important for researchers to consider limitations of self-report data. These limitations can include missing data, language problems, cultural differences, and patient burden.

Quantitative versus Qualitative

A phenomenological approach to QOL may be helpful in that it stresses the importance of individuals' subjective perceptions of their current ability to function as compared to their own internalized standards of what is possible or ideal. Patients may change their expectations and standards throughout treatment and their disease process (Lutgendorf, Antoni, Schneiderman, Ironson, & Fletcher, 1995). A qualitative approach utilizes more open-ended questions and may provide very rich data. However, this approach may be more burdensome for the patient and more time consuming. Quantitative instruments, by contrast, tend to use a closed-question format and categorical scaling and are less time consuming. More recently, nurses in research and clinical settings have begun to combine the two approaches.

Measurements at One versus Multiple Time Points

Previously, much of the QOL research involved measurements at one time point. More recently, experts have recognized the dynamism of QOL and the need for multiple measurement points with the same respondents, or a cross-sectional approach. Unfortunately, measurement of QOL at one time point has not provided a thorough understanding of the nature of QOL or how to improve outcomes through clinical care. As advances continue in the treatment of cancer, multiple measurements are also needed in order to demonstrate improvements over time as a result of new therapies. It must be recognized, however, that the burden for patients/survivors may increase as the number of measurements of their QOL increases. A balance will need to be achieved between not overburdening the patient and providing an opportunity for patients to express their perceptions regarding QOL.

Culture

The question of whether assessments and measurements of QOL are culturally sensitive needs to be raised. It is important to evaluate the relationship of culture and QOL because QOL perceptions of an individual are culture bound, varying from society to society. Padilla and Kagawa-Singer discuss how culture is an important determinant of QOL in Chapter 6. Despite recent research (Phillips & Weekes, 2002), multiculturism has been incorporated more into oncology nursing research between 1999–2000. Little work has been done to address cultural issues in QOL research and the impact of culture on perceptions of QOL. Health care practitioners must be sure they are analyzing QOL beliefs in the context of the patient's culture. Researchers must be careful to avoid ethnocentrism—that is, interpreting the behaviors of patients with cancer in terms of the researchers' own personal feelings and beliefs. Future work should involve translating QOL measures into multiple languages, conducting studies to examine the cross-cultural applicability of theoretical frameworks used to explain QOL, and determining the impact of cultural variables on perceived QOL (Campos & Johnson, 1990; King et al., 1997).

CONCLUSION

Advances in cancer care and increases in survival of patients have caused nurses to take an interest in QOL and its relationship to practice, education, and research. Despite the many ongoing controversies related to QOL, it appears to be an important concept from both a nursing and patient perspective. As the controversies are resolved and our knowledge base increases, both education and clinical practice will improve. If QOL is to be a major outcome variable in nursing research, many of the

---

Table 2-1. **Recommendations for Conducting QOL Research**

Research an aspect of QOL in which you expect a substantial difference in outcome.

Measure QOL and overall survival in addition to other clinical parameters.

You may not need a large sample size as each patient contributes repeated measures over time.

Use tools that are reliable and valid.

Define when the initial measurement of QOL will be performed.

Repeat the measurements at intervals that will allow tracking of the treatment.

Time periods should be 2–4 weeks as this allows for accurate recall.

Follow patients until all influence of treatment is likely to have passed or the endpoint of their disease.

Do not simply average your data; use multivariate ANOVA.

Be modest with extrapolations from the data.

Source: Adapted from Schipper et al., 1990.

---

methodological issues will need to be addressed and resolved. Schipper and colleagues (1990) provide ten recommendations for conducting QOL research (Table 2-1). Additionally, Hinds and King (Chapter 18) provide recommendations for future research or projects to ensure that nursing and patient perspectives are sufficiently reflected. These recommendations are helpful for all nurse researchers. As an outcome of a State-of-the-Knowledge Conference on Quality of Life and the Cancer Experience, King and colleagues (1997) listed recommended topics and questions for future research on QOL. It will be crucial to maintain the nursing and patient perspectives when conducting future research and attempting to influence clinical care and outcomes.

REFERENCES

Aaronson, N. K. (1990). Quality of life research in clinical trials: A need for common rules and language. *Oncology, 4*(5), 59–66.

Aaronson, N. K. (1991). Quality of life research in cancer clinical trials: A need for common rules and language. In N. S. Tchekmedyian & D. F. Cella (Eds.), *Quality of life in oncology practice and research* (pp. 33–42). Williston Park, NY: Dominus Publishing Company.

Aaronson, N. K., Ahmedzai, S., Bergman, B., Bullinger, M., Cull, A., Duez, N. J., Filiberti, A., Fletcher, H., Fleishman, S. B., de Haes, J. C. J. M., Kaasa, S., Klee, M., Osoba, D., Razavi, D., Rofe, P. B., Schraub, S., Sneeuw, K., Sullivan, M., & Takeda, D. for the European Organization for Research and Treatment of Cancer Study Group on Quality of Life. (1993). The European Organization for

Research and Treatment of Cancer QLQ-C30: A quality of life instrument for use in international clinical trials in oncology. *Journal of the National Cancer Institute, 85,* 365–376.

Aaronson, N. K., Ahmedzai, S., Bullinger, M., Crabeels, D., Estape, J., Filiberti, A., Flechtner, H., Frick, U., Hurny, C., Kaasa, S., Klee, M., Mastilica, M., Osoba, D., Pfausler, B., Razavi, D., Rofe, P. B. C., Schraub, S., Sullivan, M., & Takeda, D. for the EORTC Study Group on Quality of Life. (1991). The EORTC Core Quality-of-life Questionnaire: Interim results on an international field study. In D. Osoba (Ed.), *Effect of cancer on quality of life* (pp. 293–305). Boca Raton, FL: CRC Press.

Aaronson, N. K., Bakker, W., Stewart, A. L., van Dam, F. S. A. M., van Zandwijk, N., Yarnold, J. R., & Kirkpatrick, A. (1987). Multidimensional approach to the measurement of quality of life in lung cancer clinical trials. In N. K. Aaronson & J. H. Beckman (Eds.), *Monograph series of the European Organization for Research and Treatment of Cancer* (Vol. 17, pp. 63–82). New York: Raven Press.

Aaronson, N. K., Bullinger, M., & Ahmedzai, S. (1988). A modular approach to quality-of-life assessment in cancer clinical trials. *Recent Results in Cancer Research, 111,* 231–249.

Bowling, A. (1991). Health care research. Measuring health status. *Nursing Practice, 4*(4), 2–8.

Campos, S. S., & Johnson, T. M. (1990). Cultural considerations. In B. Spilker (Ed.), *Quality of life assessments in clinical trials* (pp. 163–170). New York: Raven Press.

Cella, D. F., & Tulsky, D. S. (1991). Measuring quality of life today: Methodological aspects. In N. S. Tchekmedyian & D. F. Cella (Eds.), *Quality of life in oncology practice and research* (pp. 9–18). Williston Park, NY: Dominus Publishing Company.

Cella, D. F., Tulsky, D. S., Gray, G., Sarafian, B., Linn, E., Bonomi, A., Silberman, M., Yellen, S. B., Winicour, P., Brannon, J., Eckberg, K., Lloyd, S., Purl, S., Blendowski, C., Goodman, M., Barnicle, M., Stewart, I., McHale, M., Bonomi, P., Kaplan, E., Taylor, S., IV, Thomas, C. R., Jr., & Harris, J. (1993). The functional assessment of cancer therapy scale: Development and validation of the general measure. *Journal of Clinical Oncology, 11,* 570–579.

Clinch, J. J., & Schipper, H. (1993). Quality of life assessment in palliative care. In D. Doyle, G. W. C. Hanks, & N. MacDonald (Eds.), *Oxford Textbook of Palliative Medicine* (pp. 61–70). Oxford: Oxford University Press.

De Haes, J. C., & Van Knippenberg, F. C. E. (1985). The quality of life instruments for cancer patients. A review of the literature. *Social Science and Medicine, 20*(8), 809–817.

Epstein, A. M., Hall, J. A., Tognetti, J., Son, L. H., & Conant, L. (1989). Using proxies to evaluate quality of life. *Medical Care, 27,* 591–598.

Faden, R., & Leplege, A. (1992). Assessing quality of life. Moral implications for clinical practice. *Medical Care, 30*(5 suppl), MS166–175.

Ferrans, C. C. (1990). Quality of life. Conceptual issues. *Seminars in Oncology Nursing, 6,* 248–254.

Ferrell, B., Grant, M., Schmidt, G. M., Rhiner, M., Whitehead, C., Fonbuena, P., & Forman, S. J. (1992a). The meaning of quality of life for bone marrow transplant survivors. Part 1: The impact of bone marrow transplant on quality of life. *Cancer Nursing, 15*(3), 153–160.

Ferrell, B., Grant, M., Schmidt, G. M., Rhiner, M., Whitehead, C., Fonbuena, P., & Forman, S. J. (1992b). The meaning of quality of life for bone marrow transplant survivors. Part 2: Improving quality of life for bone marrow transplant survivors. *Cancer Nursing, 15*(4), 247–253.

Ganz, P. A., Rofessart, J., Polinsky, M. L., Schag, C. C., & Heinrich, R. L. (1986). A comprehensive approach to the assessment of cancer patient's rehabilitation needs. The cancer inventory of problem situation and a companion interview. *Journal of Psychosocial Oncology, 4,* 27–42.

Grant, M. M., Padilla, G. V., Ferrell, B. R., & Rhiner, M. (1990). Assessment of quality of life with a single instrument. *Seminars in Oncology Nursing, 6,* 260–270.

Guyatt, G. H., & Jaeschke, R. (1990). Measurements in clinical trials: Choosing the appropriate approach. In B. Spilker (Ed.), *Quality of life assessments in clinical trials* (pp. 37–46). New York: Raven Press.

Hinds, P. S. (1990). Quality of life in children and adolescents with cancer. *Seminars in Oncology Nursing, 6,* 285–291.

Holmes, S., & Dickerson, J. (1987). The quality of life: Design and evaluation of a self-assessment instrument for use with cancer patients. *International Journal of Nursing Studies, 24*(1), 15–24.

Hyland, M. E., Kenyon, C. A. P., & Jacobs, P. A. (1994). Sensitivity of quality of life domains and constructs to longitudinal change in a clinical trial comparing almeterol with placebo in asthmatics. *Quality of Life Research 3,* 121–126.

Kaplan, R. M. (1995). Quality of life resource allocation and health-care crisis. In J. E. Dimsdale & A. Baum (Eds.), *Quality of life in behavioral medical research* (pp. 3–30). Hillsdale, NJ: Lawrence Erlbaum Associates.

King, C. R., Ferrell, B. R., Grant, M., & Sakurai, C. (1995). Nurses' perceptions of the meaning of quality of life for bone marrow transplant survivors. *Cancer Nursing, 18,* 118–129.

King, C. R., Haberman, M., Berry, D., Bush, N., Butler, L., Dow, K. H., Ferrell, B., Grant, M., Gue, D., Hinds, P., Kreuer, J., Padilla, G., & Underwood, S. (1997). Quality of life and the cancer experience: The state-of-the knowledge. *Oncology Nursing Forum, 24*(1), 27–41.

Lutgendorf, S., Antoni, M. H., Schneiderman, N., Ironson, G., & Fletcher, M. A. (1995). Psychosocial interventions and quality of life changes across the HIV spectrum. In J. E. Dimsdale & A. Baum (Eds.), *Quality of life in behavioral medical research* (pp. 205–240). Hillsdale, NJ: Lawrence Erlbaum Associates.

McCahill, L. E., Krouse, R., Chu, D., Juarez, G., Uman, G. C., Ferrell, B., & Wagman, L. D. (2002). Indications and use of palliative surgery—results of society of surgical oncology survey. *Annals of Surgical Oncology*, 9(1), 104–112.

Moinpour, C. M., Feigl, P., Metch, B., Hayden, K. A., Meyskens, F. L., Jr., & Crowley, J. (1989). Quality of life endpoints in cancer clinical trials: Review and recommendations. *Journal of the National Cancer Institute*, 81, 485–495.

Moinpour, C. M., Hayden, K. A., Thompson, J. M., Feigl, P., & Metch, B. (1990). Quality of life assessment in southwest oncology group trials. *Oncology 4*, 79–89.

Moinpour, C. M., Savage, M., Hayden, K. A., Sayers, J., & Upchurch, C. (1995). Quality of life assessment in cancer clinical trials. In J. E. Dimsdale & A. Baum (Eds.), *Quality of life in behavioral medical research* (pp. 79–96). Hillsdale, NJ: Lawrence Erlbaum Associates.

Morrow, G. R., Lindke, J., & Black, P. (1992). Measurement of quality of life in patients: Psychometric analyses of the functional living index-cancer (FLIC). *Quality of Life Research*, 1, 287–296.

Osoba, D. (1994). Lessons learned from measuring health-related quality of life in oncology. *Journal of Clinical Oncology*, 12, 608–616.

Padilla, G. V., Ferrell, B., & Grant, M. (1990). Defining the content domain of quality of life for cancer patients with pain. *Cancer Nursing 13*(2), 108–115.

Padilla, G. V., Presant, C., Grant, M. M., Metter, G., Lipsett, J., & Heide, F. (1983). Quality of life index for patients with cancer. *Research in Nursing and Health*, 6(3), 117–126.

Phillips, J., & Weekes, D. (2002). Incorporating multiculturalism into oncology nursing research: The last decade. *Oncology Nursing Forum*, 29(5),807–816.

Reid, D., & Renwick, R. (1994). Preliminary validation of a new instrument to measure life satisfaction in adolescents with neuromuscular disorders. *International Journal of Rehabilitation Research*, 17, 184–188.

Schipper, H. (1991). Guidelines and caveats for quality of life measurement in clinical practice and research. In N. S. Tchekmedyian & D. F. Cella (Eds.), *Quality of life in oncology practice and research* (pp. 25–31). Williston Park, NY: Dominus Publishing Company.

Schipper, H., Clinch, J., & Powell, V. (1990). Definitions and conceptual issues. In B. Spilker (Ed.), *Quality of life assessments in clinical trials* (pp. 11–24). New York: Raven Press.

Schuttiga, J. A. (1995). Quality of life from a federal regulation perspective. In J. E. Dimsdale & A. Baum (Eds.), *Quality of life in behavioral medical research* (pp. 31–42). Hillsdale, NJ: Lawrence Erlbaum Associates.

Shumaker, S. A., Anderson, R. T., & Czajkowski, S. M. (1990). Psychological tests and scales. In B. Spilker (Ed.), *Quality of life assessments in clinical trials* (pp. 95–114). New York: Raven Press.

Spilker, B. (1990). Introduction. In B. Spilker (Ed.), *Quality of life assessments in clinical trials* (pp. 3–9). New York: Raven Press.

Sprangers, M. A. G., & Aaronson, N. K. (1992). The role of health care providers and significant others in evaluating the quality of life of patients with chronic disease: A review. *Journal of Clinical Epidemiology, 45*, 743–760.

Stewart, A. L., Greenfield, S., Hays, R. D., Wells, K., Rogers, W. H., Berry, D. S., McGlynn, E. A., & Ware, J. E., Jr. (1989). Functional status and well-being of patients with chronic conditions: Results from the medical outcomes study. *Journal of the American Medical Association, 262*, 907–913.

Theory

SPIRITUAL

PSYCHOLOGICAL

SOCIAL

PHYSICAL

Theories and Conceptual Models to Guide *Quality of Life* Related Research

APRIL HAZARD VALLERAND • JUDITH K. PAYNE

Over the past two decades, the conception of quality of life (QOL) has evolved from that of a psychosocial concept not given much credence in clinical trials (Aaronson, 1991) to a multidimensional concept used as an outcome variable to determine the efficacy of drugs, treatments, and patients' perceptions of their general health and well-being (Cella & Tulsky, 1990; Ferrell, Wisdom, & Wenzl, 1989; Padilla & Grant, 1985; Ware & Sherbourne, 1992). This rapid evolution of the concept of QOL occurred in a generally atheoretical manner (King et al., 1997). The absence of formal, explicit theoretical models to guide the development of QOL research and the use of study-specific, or ad hoc, approaches to QOL assessment have limited the use and generalizability of QOL assessment in clinical trials in cancer patients (Aaronson, 1991). The difficulty with this study-specific approach is that it does not allow for cross-study comparisons. Also, with few exceptions, study-specific measures are seldom submitted to the rigor of psychometric testing.

This chapter discusses the importance of the conceptual-theoretical relationship, describes the use of theory in nursing- and health-care-related QOL studies, and presents models currently being used to study the QOL of clients with cancer. The task is to explicate the implicit conceptual context and theory-development contributions of QOL research.

The Conceptual and Theoretical Basis in Quality of Life Literature

Research emphasis has evolved from defining the concept of QOL and determining its components or domains to using the concept to ascertain who could benefit from a particular treatment or whether a treatment is effective. This sequence reflects the progression from *theory-generating* research to *theory-testing* research described by Fawcett and Downs (1992). They characterized theory-generating research as that which "seeks to identify a phenomenon, discover its dimensions or characteristics, or specify the relationship between the dimensions" (p. 4). Theory-testing research, in contrast, focuses on testing the ideas developed through theory-generating research in diverse populations (Fawcett & Downs, 1992). Much of the research in QOL to date has been theory-generating. Accordingly, studies have focused on defining the concept and describing the content domains.

A review of many theory-generating QOL studies indicates that although diverse definitions and instruments have been used, researchers tend to agree that the concept is multidimensional (Aaronson et al., 1991; Ferrell, Wisdom, & Wenzl, 1989; Goodinson & Singleton, 1989; Zhan, 1992) and subjective (Aaronson, 1991; Cella, 1994; Cohen, 1982; Donovan, Sanson-Fisher, & Redman, 1989; Goodinson & Singleton, 1989; Ferrans, 1990b; Oleson, 1990; Padilla, Grant, & Martin, 1988). The lack of consensus regarding a definitive definition of QOL may be due to the view that the concept is a "vague and ethereal entity, something that many people talk about, but which nobody very clearly knows what to do about" (Campbell, Converse, & Rodgers, 1976, p. 471).

Agreement on the multidimensional nature of QOL is reflected in three frequently cited domains: physiological, psychological, and sociological (Donovan et al., 1989; Ferrell, Wisdom, & Wenzl, 1989; Padilla, Ferrell, Grant, & Rhiner, 1990; Padilla et al., 1988). A fourth domain—spiritual—has been cited by several investigators (Cella & Tulsky, 1990; Donovan et al., 1989; Ferrell, Grant, Padilla, Vemuri, & Rhiner, 1991).

Due to the subjective nature of QOL, it is now widely accepted that the patient is the most appropriate source to report on his or her QOL. For example, Ferrans and Powers (1985) designed the Quality of Life Index (QLI), "taking into account the life domains noted by the experts, the subjective evaluation of satisfaction with domains, and the unique importance of each domain to the individual" (p. 17).

Theory-testing research has been comprised primarily of studies applying the few models that have been formally explicated to populations other than that from which they were originally developed. Examples of theory-testing studies include that of Ferrell, Grant, Schmidt, Rhiner, Whitehead, Fonbuena, and Forman (1992), who modified the QOL model for cancer patients developed by Ferrell and colleagues (1991), and tested it in a population of patients undergoing bone marrow transplantation. Ferrans (1990a) expanded the testing of the QOL model on patients with cancer from the original population of patients undergoing hemodialysis (Ferrans & Powers, 1985; Ferrans & Powers, 1992). Testing theories with a new population allows for increased generalizability and encourages comparisons of the concept between populations.

Theory-testing research has been hindered by a lack of explicit theories of QOL. In an analysis of nursing research on QOL in the elderly from 1987 to 1991, Moore, Newsome, Payne, and Tiansawad (1993) analyzed 17 studies and found that only 10 of the studies identified theoretical perspectives. Of these 10 studies, 4 studies had minimal linkage of theory and research, 4 used theory or a model as an organizing framework, and 2 tested concepts or relational statements of a model.

Fawcett and Downs (1992) maintained that theory-testing research should be guided not only by an explicit middle-range theory but also by an explicit conceptual model. A prototype of a conceptual-theoretical-empirical structure that could be used as a guideline to depict theoretical linkages for QOL is given in Figure 3-1. The conceptual nursing model used in this depiction is only one example from nursing theory literature. Fawcett (1989) distinguished a conceptual model from a theory by the level of abstraction. She described a conceptual model as "an abstract and general system of concepts and propositions" (p. 26). In contrast, "a theory deals with one or

Figure 3.1.   **Conceptual-theoretical-empirical structure of quality of life.**
Source: Adapted from Fawcett & Downs, 1992.

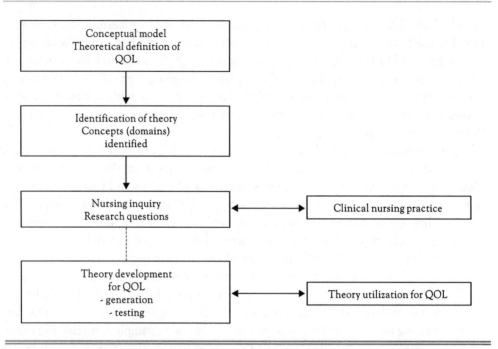

Figure 3-2. **Implications of quality of life theory and research for practice.**
Source: Modified from Fawcett & Downs, 1992.

more relatively specific and concrete concepts and propositions" (p. 26). A conceptual model places concepts in a context and guides the development of new theories (Fawcett & Downs, 1992). To study a concept within a context can allow for a more appropriate interpretation of the meaning of QOL to an individual. Context is particularly relevant with QOL when considering who views the quality of the life situation, for example, the patient, a family member, or the health care provider.

Theories function to describe, explain, and predict phenomena (Fawcett & Downs, 1992). When theory is used to drive research, it provides a structured progression of concept development for its application to a clinical setting (see Figure 3-2). This allows the researcher to determine if the questions being asked fit within the implicit conceptual context and theory development. The use of an explicit conceptual model would help to shape instruments for testing phenomena related to theory and encourages the examination of such instruments for their clinical utility. The abstract nature of QOL, the array of potential indicators, and the lack of conceptual consensus has resulted in nurse researchers focusing their attention to identifying specific, clinically relevant indicators (Mast, 1995). Broad conceptual subcategories, as identified by Ferrans (1996) and Ferrell, Wisdom, and Wenzl

(1989), most notably patients' perceptions of satisfaction with life and level of functioning, have been the result of diverse philosophies and goals of nursing care.

The Theoretical Basis of Quality of Life Measures

Research in the area of QOL and the use of QOL as an outcome in research have increased dramatically in the past decade. However, the rapidity of this growth and the increasing demands for outcome measures in health care have led to measures that are not based in theory. Costain, Hewison, and Howes (1993) suggest that an increasing gap has emerged between the sophistication of statistical analysis used with data obtained from QOL questionnaires and the lack of conceptual sophistication reflected in the operational definitions of the concept. To remedy this weakness, future research should be based on conceptual models and theories that explicate the relationships between the domains of QOL (King et al., 1997). Based on criteria for the evaluation of theories (Fawcett & Downs, 1992), the conceptual-theoretical-empirical linkages of QOL research can be critiqued (see Table 3-1). This critique includes the conceptual basis and theoretical definitions of QOL, as well as the domains identified and the research questions tested.

Models Used in Quality of Life Research for Cancer Patients

Two conceptual models that have most frequently been used to guide research and practice dealing with QOL in clients with cancer are Ferrell and colleagues' (1991) City of Hope Model and Ferrans and Powers' QOL Model (1985). Both of these models were initially developed to generate theory defining the domains of QOL and have since been modified to be used with clients with disorders other than cancer. Both models view QOL from a multidimensional, subjective perspective. The implicit assumptions underlying these models are based on individualistic ideologies and view individuals as complex beings, health as a multidimensional construct, and QOL as dependent on the unique perspective of QOL and reflects the definition of QOL used by the researchers. The way QOL is defined also determines the specific items that must be included in the assessment instrument (Grant, Padilla, Ferrell, & Rhiner, 1990).

The theoretical model developed by Padilla and Grant (1985) that illustrated the relationship between the nursing process and the dimensions of QOL (Figure 3-3) was the conceptual basis initially used by Ferrell and colleagues (1991). QOL was defined as a personal statement of the positivity or negativity of attributes that

Table 3-1. Comparison of Cancer versus Noncancer-Based Quality of Life Theories

Author	Conceptual Basis	Theoretical Definition of Quality of Life	Theory Concepts (Domains) Identified	Research Questions Generated—Concepts Tested
Ferrell, Wisdom, & Wenzl (1989)	Cantril (1965); Lewis (1982); Padilla & Grant (1985); Ware (1984)	Prevent and alleviate physical and mental distress, maintenance of physical/ mental function, and presence of supportive network	Physical well-being Psychological well-being Social well-being Spiritual well-being	The influence of fatigue on the four dimensions of QOL: physical, psychological, social, and spiritual well-being
Ferrans & Powers (1985)	Campbell, Converse, & Rodgers (1976); Cantril (1965); Padilla, Presant, Grant, Lipsett, & Heide (1985)	A person's sense of well-being which stems from satisfaction or dissatisfaction with the areas in life that are important to him/her	Health and function Socioeconomic Psychological/spiritual Family	Patient satisfaction and the importance of experience as seen by survivors of breast cancer
Cella (1994)	None cited except Cella & Cherin (1988)	Patient's appraisal of and satisfaction with his or her current level of functioning compared to what he or she perceives to be possible or ideal	Physical well-being Functional well-being Emotional well-being Social well-being	The relationship of functional status to QOL during and after cancer treatments
Oleson (1990)	Campbell (1981); Cantril (1965); Ferrans & Powers (1985)	A cognitive experience manifested by satisfaction with life domains of importance to the individual and an affective experience manifested by happiness	Health and functioning Socioeconomic Psychological/spiritual Family	Not tested

Author	Theoretical sources	Definition	Concepts	Research question/tested
Zhan (1992)	Campbell, Converse, & Rodgers (1976); Cantril (1965); Ferrans & Powers	The degree to which a person's life experiences are satisfying	Life satisfaction in various domains; Self-concept—psychological well-being; Health functioning—physical well-being; Socioeconomic factors—social well-being	Not tested
Cowan, Graham, & Cochrane (1992)	Burckhardt (1985); Cella & Tulsky (1990); Lewis (1982); McCorkle & Young (1978); Padilla & Grant (1985)	Perceived degree of satisfaction with current life circumstances influenced by functional alterations, symptom distress, and severity of disease	Symptom distress; Cognitive adaptation; Socioeconomic level; Aggressiveness of treatment; Severity of disease; Functional alterations	The relation of symptom distress, cognitive adaptation, and functional alteration to QOL in patients with myocardial infarction and malignant melanoma
Burckhardt (1985)	Campbell, Converse, & Rodgers (1976); Cantril (1965); Cohen & Lazarus (1976)	Not explicitly stated	Perceived support; Negative attitude; Self-esteem; Internal control over health; Severity of pain; Severity of impairment; Social network; Socioeconomic status	What is the impact of pain and functional impairment on the quality of life experienced by persons with arthritis?
Mellon & Northouse (2001)	McCubbin & McCubbin (1991; 1996)	Not explicitly stated	Stressors, family resources, and family meaning	Not tested

characterize one's life and describe an individual's ability to function and the satis-faction in doing so. Padilla and Grant viewed QOL as a multidimensional concept that measured the dimensions of psychological well-being, physical well-being, body image concerns, response to diagnosis or treatment, and social concerns. The model depicted the dimensions of QOL as dependent outcome variables, and nursing process activities manipulated by the investigator as independent variables. Mediating variables that affect QOL are cognitive-emotional changes in the client that enhance self-perceptions and can be affected by nursing care. Because the mediating variable is seen as a necessary antecedent to QOL, the nursing process is viewed as having an indirect impact on QOL. Extraneous variables are those that are not manipulated by the investigator but that may affect the outcomes, such as treatment characteristics, diagnostic characteristics, and personal characteristics. These are usually controlled statistically or directly (Padilla & Grant, 1985). The Padilla and Grant model was then used as a conceptual framework by Ferrell, Wisdom, and Wenzl (1989) in the development and testing of an instrument, the QOL Survey, to measure QOL as an outcome variable in the management of cancer pain. In this study the

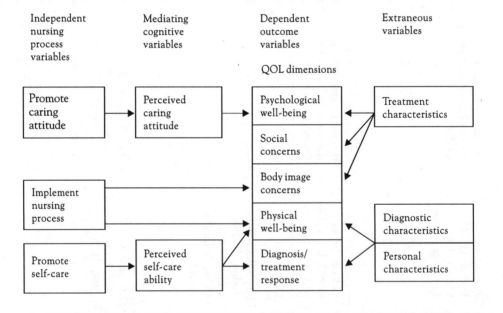

Figure 3.3. **A model of the relationship between the nursing process and the dimensions of quality of life.**

Source: Reprinted with permission from *Advances in Nursing Science*, "Quality of life as a cancer nursing outcome variable," Padilla & Grant, vol. 8, no. 1, p. 53. © 1985 Aspen Publishers, Inc.

conceptual definition of QOL was the prevention and alleviation of physical and psychological distress, the maintenance of physical/mental functioning, and the presence of a supportive network.

After the reliability and validity of the QOL survey were determined (Ferrell, Wisdom, Wenzl, & Brown, 1989), the instrument was revised, and testing continued to gather data about the relationship between pain and QOL (Padilla et al., 1990). From these studies a conceptual model, commonly referred to as the City of Hope Model, was developed to illustrate the influence of pain on the dimensions of QOL (Ferrell et al., 1991; Ferrell, Grant, Rhiner, & Padilla, 1992). The four dimensions included in the model are physical well-being and symptoms, psychological well-being, social well-being, and spiritual well-being. This model demonstrates that pain is an experience that influences all dimensions of QOL (Figure 3-4). Subsequently, fatigue was studied as a variable influencing all four dimensions of QOL (Ferrell, Grant, Dean, Funk, & Ly, 1996).

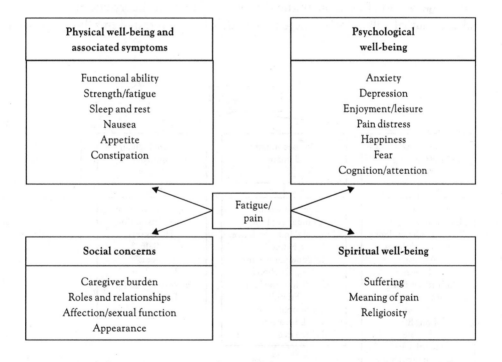

Figure 3-4. **The impact of fatigue and pain on the dimensions of quality of life.**

Source: Modified from Ferrell, Grant, Padilla, Vemuri, & Rhiner, 1991; Ferrell, Grant, Dean, Funk, & Ly, 1996. Used with permission from Oncology Nursing Press.

Ferrans and Powers (1992) defined QOL as "a person's sense of well-being that stems from satisfaction or dissatisfaction with the areas of life that are important to him/her" (p. 29). The conceptual model presented by Ferrans (1990b) described four major domains of QOL: health and functioning, socioeconomic, psychological/spiritual, and family. The four domains encompass 35 aspects of life, conveying the multi-dimensionality of the concept. Ferrans's framework was based on extensive literature review and factor analysis using data from clients on hemodialysis. The Quality of Life Index (QLI) used in these studies was designed to measure QOL, acknowledging the life domains noted by experts, the subjective evaluation of satisfaction with the domains, and the importance of the domains to the individual (Ferrans & Powers, 1985). The initial QLI was modified and tested with a population of clients with cancer. The conceptual model illustrates the hierarchical relationships between the global construct of QOL, the four major domains, and specific aspects of the domains (Figure 3-5; Ferrans, 1990b; Ferrans, 1996). Ferrans's model, which links satisfaction and QOL, has a strong conceptual basis, clearly distinguishes between the domains, and provides a solid example of the connection between theory and research. External and mutual validation of these two models has been tested in subsequent studies

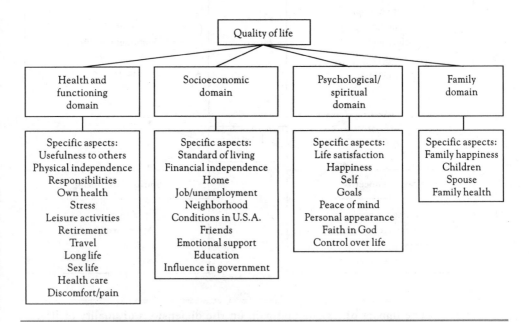

Figure 3-5. **Hierarchical relationship between the global construct of quality of life, four major domains, and specific aspects of the domains.**

Source: Ferrans, 1990b. Used with permission from Dr. Carol Estwing Ferrans.

by these researchers. Although developed independently and simultaneously in diverse samples, both Ferrell's and Ferrans's models identify four common domains or dimensions.

Cella (1994) contended that while there are many diverse areas of the concept of QOL, "most can be grouped into one of four correlated but distinct areas: physical, functional, emotional and social" (p. 188). The two fundamental components of the definition of QOL are multidimensionality and subjectivity. Multidimensionality of QOL refers to a broad range of content that includes physical, functional, emotional, and social well-being. The assumption is that by combining measures of these aspects one can approximate a single index of QOL. Subjectivity refers to the fact that QOL can only be understood from the patient's perspective. The underlying processes include perception of illness, perception of treatment, expectation of self, and appraisal of risk/harm. A complex relationship exists between treatment and effects. The two distinct aspects of the relationship between symptoms and overall QOL are symptom intensity and symptom duration.

End of life care is an emerging component of QOL theoretical development. Presently there is no identified QOL palliative care model. Mainly, care is based on the whole person concept.

Noncancer QOL Models in Nursing

Two QOL models reported in the nursing literature, which were developed conceptually but have not yet been tested clinically, are those of Oleson (1990) and Zhan (1992). Oleson (1990) used a concept analysis procedure to develop a model of subjectively perceived QOL (Figure 3-6). She identified the critical attributes of satisfaction and happiness and applied the life domain categories of health and functioning, socioeconomic, psychological/spiritual, and family, which were identified by Ferrans and Powers (1985) as causes of a client's satisfaction or happiness. Finally, she identified the consequences of a positively perceived QOL as the development of potential and self-actualization. QOL was conceptually defined as a cognitive experience, manifested by satisfaction with life domains of importance to the individual, and an affective experience, manifested by happiness. True to the assumptions of a phenomenological research approach, the individual's own perceptions of levels of satisfaction and happiness in relation to life domains influence how he or she will experience QOL.

Zhan (1992) also developed a model of QOL citing the works of Campbell, Cantril, Ferrans, Ferrell, Padilla, and others. Based on the definition of QOL as "the degree to which a person's life experiences are satisfying" (p. 796), Zhan described QOL as a multidimensional concept that cannot be completely measured by either a

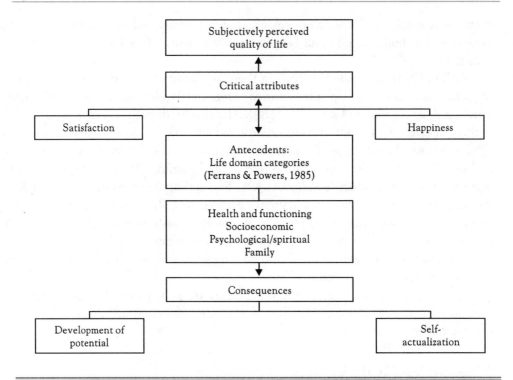

Figure 3-6. **Model of subjectively perceived quality of life.**
Source: Oleson, 1990. Copyrighted material of Sigma Theta Tau International, used with permission.

subjective or an objective approach. She identified dimensions of QOL as life satisfaction, self-concept, health and functioning, and socioeconomic factors. According to this model, QOL is also influenced by one's personal background, health, social situation, culture, environment, and age (Figure 3-7). The perceived meaning of QOL comes from the interaction between the person and his or her environment. Both Oleson's and Zhan's models require testing in clinical settings to determine their applicability to various client populations, including cancer populations.

An example of the testing necessary to determine the clinical usefulness of a model was demonstrated by Cowan, Young-Graham, and Cochrane (1992). In their theoretical model of QOL for chronic illness, the concepts of symptom distress, functional alterations, and cognitive adaptation were identified as mediating variables (Figure 3-8). The authors noted that in many studies, functional alterations and/or symptom distress are used as definitions of QOL instead of as factors influencing it (McCorkle & Young, 1978; Young & Longman, 1983). Perceived QOL is viewed as the outcome variable and defined as "the extent to which the person's assessed level

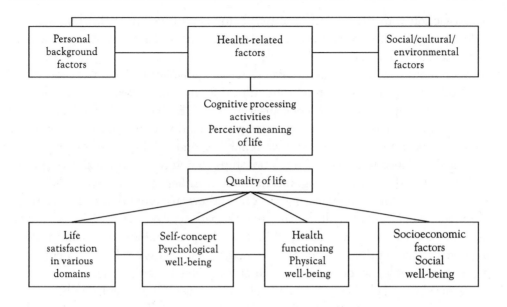

Figure 3-7. **Conceptual model of quality of life.**

Source: Zhan, 1992. Used with permission from Blackwell Science Ltd.

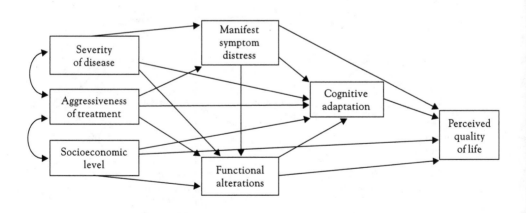

Figure 3-8. **Theoretical model of quality of life for chronic illness.**

Source: Cowan, Young-Graham, & Cochrane 1992. Copyright © 1990. Used with permission of Katherine Young-Graham and Marie J. Cowan.

of satisfaction with life and sense of well-being is positive" (p. 19), while the antecedent variables are severity of disease, aggressiveness of treatment, and socioeconomic level. Initial testing of the model was accomplished by comparing the results between subjects with myocardial infarction and malignant melanoma, to ascertain if the model was generalizable to chronic illness, rather than disease specific. In addition, relationships between the concepts were tested. Each of the theoretical concepts was measured two to four times to gain empirical clarity regarding the dimensions of the concepts and to test for sensitivity, reliability, and validity. The results provided empirical evidence to support the relationships among the theoretical concepts and indicated that there were no significant differences between the myocardial infarction and malignant melanoma subjects. The authors suggested that further testing of the model would entail multivariate analysis, path analysis, or LISREL on a larger sample size with greater variability of illness. The potential for developing and testing nursing interventions aimed toward specific components or all components of the mediating variables affecting QOL based on this model is promising.

Another example of the use of models in nursing QOL research can be seen in a study by Burckhardt (1985) which explored the impact of pain and functional impairment on the QOL of persons with arthritis (Figure 3-9). She used a cognitive framework to develop a causal model in which the disease-related variables interact-

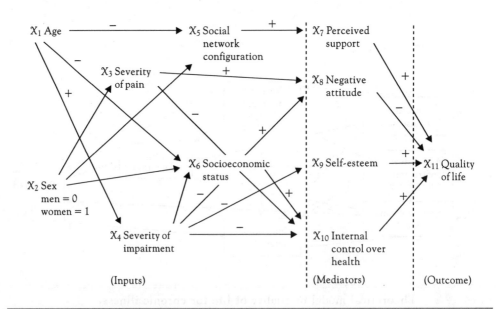

Figure 3-9. **The hypothesized causal model.**
Source: Burckhardt, 1985. Used with permission from Lippincott-Raven Publishers.

ing with demographic and social factors were hypothesized to indirectly affect quality of life through psychological mediators (Figure 3-9). The definition of QOL used in this study was not stated explicitly. Definitions focusing on satisfaction and subjectivity, however, are presented in the review of the literature. The model explained 46 percent of the variance in QOL. In addition, the psychological mediators of positive self-esteem, internal control over health, perceived support, and low negative attitude toward the illness were found to contribute directly to a higher QOL. Severity of arthritis-related impairment was also seen to indirectly affect QOL through the mediating variables. The findings suggested that manipulating input variables such as pain or impairment may not directly affect QOL but may instead affect cognitive mediating variables such as self-esteem and perceived control over health, which are directly related to changes in QOL (Padilla & Grant, 1985). Burckhardt (1985) further suggested that nursing strategies that decrease pain and functional impairment should be tested in experimental designs for their impact on both the mediating variables and QOL. Burckhardt's 1985 study is an excellent example of how a model may direct nursing practice. Although these models were not developed with cancer patients, they may be used to generate research questions to be tested in cancer populations.

Recent attention has been given to the Medical Outcomes Study's (MOS) conceptual framework and evolving MOS SF-36 instrument (Figure 3-10). The purpose of the MOS was to relate variations in patient outcomes to differences in systems and to develop a practical tool to measure outcomes (Tarlov et al., 1989).

CONCLUSION

A universally accepted definition of QOL has not been developed; in fact, over 30 different definitions for proposed dimensions of QOL in persons with cancer have been used (Cella & Tulsky, 1990). Nevertheless, the majority of researchers have agreed that QOL is a multidimensional, subjective concept. The variability of the definition of the concept is reflected by the models used in QOL research. A number of studies do not identify a theoretical basis for the concept. This theoretical insufficiency becomes a problem when QOL is used to guide study design or as an outcome variable. Only a few nursing studies were found with a strong theoretical basis (King et al., 1997). These studies demonstrated the use of a conceptual model to guide nursing practice.

Most of the researchers who cited a theoretical basis used Campbell and colleagues' (1976) subjective definition of QOL as their conceptual basis for instrument development and for testing the phenomenon of QOL. An exception is the Medical Outcomes Study conceptual framework (Tarlov et al., 1989), which emphasizes the patient's perspective across systems of care. An issue remains that we still do not have

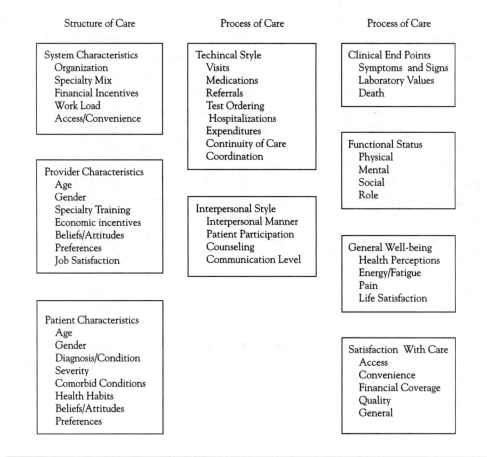

Structure of Care

System Characteristics
  Organization
  Specialty Mix
  Financial Incentives
  Work Load
  Access/Convenience

Provider Characteristics
  Age
  Gender
  Specialty Training
  Economic incentives
  Beliefs/Attitudes
  Preferences
  Job Satisfaction

Patient Characteristics
  Age
  Gender
  Diagnosis/Condition
  Severity
  Comorbid Conditions
  Health Habits
  Beliefs/Attitudes
  Preferences

Process of Care

Techincal Style
  Visits
  Medications
  Referrals
  Test Ordering
  Hospitalizations
  Expenditures
  Continuity of Care
  Coordination

Interpersonal Style
  Interpersonal Manner
  Patient Participation
  Counseling
  Communication Level

Process of Care

Clinical End Points
  Symptoms and Signs
  Laboratory Values
  Death

Functional Status
  Physical
  Mental
  Social
  Role

General Well-being
  Health Perceptions
  Energy/Fatigue
  Pain
  Life Satisfaction

Satisfaction With Care
  Access
  Convenience
  Financial Coverage
  Quality
  General

igure 3-10. **The Medical Outcomes Study's conceptual framework.**
Source: Tarlov et al., Medical Outcomes Study. JAMA, August 1, 1989.

a universally accepted definition of quality of life. Therefore, a future recommendation is for a more realistic theoretical definition that reflects quality of life from the patient's perspective today.

Another important recommendation for the future is to base research on conceptual models of QOL that incorporate the multidimensionality of the concept and that attempt to explicate the interrelationships among QOL domains (Aaronson et al., 1991). Future research based on conceptual models that explicate the interrelationships among QOL domains is needed. In order to be tested, a theory must have concepts that can be observed empirically; that is, the concepts must be connected to empirical indicators by operational definitions. Hypotheses must be stated and must be testable (Fawcett & Downs, 1992). Once the operational definition used to measure QOL is based on theoretical notions of the construct, the linkage between theory and research will be strengthened by allowing the development of instruments consistent with the theory that can be tested for clinical utility. The use of theoretically based conceptual models will enhance the applicability of the concept as a reliable and valid outcome measure. Future QOL studies should attempt to provide a definition of the concept, describe the theory from which the research questions were developed, and explicate the conceptual model illustrating the relationship among the concepts. The provision of this information will allow the concept to be tested and encourage the use and further testing of instruments to measure QOL.

REFERENCES

Aaronson, N. K. (1991). Methodologic issues in assessing the quality of life of cancer patients. *Cancer, 67,* 844–850.

Aaronson, N. K., Meyerowitz, B. E., Bard, M., Bloom, J. R., Fawzy, F. I., Feldstein, M., Fink, D., Holland, J. C., Johnson, J. E., Lowman, J. T., Patterson, W. B., & Ware, J. E. (1991). Quality of life research in oncology: Past achievements and future priorities. *Cancer, 67,* 839–843.

Burckhardt, C. S. (1985). The impact of arthritis on quality of life. *Nursing Research, 34*(1), 11–16.

Campbell, A. (1981). *The sense of well-being in America.* New York: McGraw-Hill.

Campbell, A., Converse, P., & Rodgers, W. (1976). *The quality of American life.* New York: Russell Sage Foundation. Rutgers University Press.

Cantril, H. (1965). *The pattern of human concerns.* New Jersey: Rutgers University Press.

Cella, D. F. (1994). Quality of life: Concepts and definitions. *Journal of Pain and Symptom Management, 9,* 186–192.

Cella, D. F., & Cherin, E. A. (1988). Quality of life during and after cancer treatment. *Comprehensive Therapy, 14,* 69–75.

Cella, D. F., & Tulsky, D. S. (1990). Measuring quality of life today: Methodological Aspects. *Oncology, 4*(5), 29–38.

Cohen, C. (1982). On the quality of life: Some philosophical reflections. *Circulation, 66*(Suppl. III), III-29–III-33.

Costain, K., Hewison, J., & Howes, M. (1993). Comparison of a function-based model and a meaning-based model of quality of life in oncology: Multidimensionality examined. *Journal of Psychosocial Oncology, 11*(4), 17–37.

Cowan, M. J., Young-Graham, K., & Cochrane, B. L. (1992). Comparison of a theory of quality of life between myocardial infarction and malignant melanoma: A pilot study. *Progress in Cardiovascular Nursing, 7*(1), 18–28.

Donovan, K., Sanson-Fisher, R. W., & Redman, S. (1989). Measuring quality of life in cancer patients. *Journal of Clinical Oncology, 7*(7), 959–968.

Fawcett, J. (1989). *Analysis and evaluation of conceptual models of nursing* (2nd ed.). Philadelphia: F. A. Davis.

Fawcett, J., & Downs, F. S. (1992). *The relationship of theory and research* (2nd ed.). Philadelphia: F. A. Davis.

Ferrans, C. E. (1990a). Development of a quality of life index for patients with cancer. *Oncology Nursing Forum, 17*(3, Suppl), 15–21.

Ferrans, C. E. (1990b). Quality of life: Conceptual issues. *Seminars in Oncology Nursing, 6*(4), 248–254.

Ferrans, C. E. (1996). Development of a conceptual model of quality of life. *Scholarly Inquiry for Nursing Practice: An International Journal, 10*(3), 293–304.

Ferrans, C. E., & Powers, M. J. (1985). Quality of life index: Development and psychometric properties. *Advance in Nursing Science, 8*(1), 15–24.

Ferrans, C. E., & Powers, M. J. (1992). Psychometric assessment of the quality of life index. *Research in Nursing and Health, 15*, 29–38.

Ferrell, B., Grant, M., Padilla, G., Vemuri, S., & Rhiner, M. (1991). The experiences of pain and perceptions of quality of life: Validation of a conceptual model. *The Hospice Journal, 7*(3), 9–24.

Ferrell, B. R., Grant, M. M., Rhiner, M., & Padilla, G. V. (1992). Home care: Maintaining quality of life for patient and family. *Oncology, 6*(2), 136–140.

Ferrell, B., Grant, M., Schmidt, G. M., Rhiner, M., Whitehead, C., Fonbuena, P., & Forman, S. J. (1992). The meaning of quality of life for bone marrow transplant survivors. Part 1: The impact of bone marrow transplant on quality of life. *Cancer Nursing, 15*(3), 153–160.

Ferrell, B., Grant, M., Dean, G., Funk, B., & Ly, J. (1996). "Bone tired": The experience of fatigue and its impact on quality of life. *Oncology Nursing Forum, 23*(10), 1539–1547.

Ferrell, B. R., Wisdom, C., & Wenzl, C. (1989). Quality of life as an outcome variable in the management of cancer pain. *Cancer, 63*, 2321–2327.

Ferrell, B., Wisdom, C., Wenzl, C., & Brown, J. (1989). Effects of controlled-release morphine on quality of life for cancer pain. *Oncology Nursing Forum, 16*, 521–526.

Goodinson, S. M., & Singleton, J. (1989). Quality of life: A critical review of current concepts, measures and their clinical implications. *International Journal of Nursing Studies, 26*(4), 327–341.

Grant, M., Padilla, G. V., Ferrell, B. R., & Rhiner, M. (1990). Assessment of quality of life with a single instrument. *Seminars in Oncology Nursing, 6*(4), 260–270.

King, C., Haberman, M., Berry, D., Bush, N., Butler, L., Dow, K., Ferrell, B., Grant, M., Gue, D., Hinds, P., Kreuer, J., Padilla, G., & Underwood, S. (1997). Quality of life and the cancer experience: The state-of-the-knowledge. *Oncology Nursing Forum, 24*(1), 27–41.

Lazarus, R. S., Cohen, J. B. (June, 1976). Study of stress and coping in aging. Paper presented at the 5th WHO Conference on Society, Stress, and Disease: Aging and Old Age, Stockholm: Sweden.

Lewis, F. M. (1982). Experienced personal control and quality of life in late-stage cancer patients. *Nursing Research, 31*, 113–119.

Mast, M. (1995). Definition and measurement of quality of life in oncology nursing research: Review and theoretical implications. *Oncology Nursing Forum, 22*(6), 957–964.

McCorkle, R., & Young, K. (1978). Development of a symptom distress scale. *Cancer Nursing, 1*, 373–378.

McCubbin, M. A., & McCubbin, H. I. (1991). Family stress theory and assessment: The resiliency model of family stress, adjustment, and adaptation. In H. I. McCubbin and A. I. Thompson (Eds.), *Family assessment: Inventories for research and practice* (pp. 3–32). Madison, WI: University of Wisconsin.

McCubbin, M. A., & McCubbin, H. I. (1996). Resiliency in families: A conceptual model of family adjustment and adaptation in response to stress and crisis. In H. I. McCubbin, A. I. Thompson, & M. A. McCubbin (Eds.), *Family assessment: Resiliency, coping and adaptation—Inventories for research and practice* (pp. 1–64). Madison, WI: University of Wisconsin System.

Mellon, S., & Northouse, L. (2001). Family survivorship and quality of life following a diagnosis. *Research in Nursing and Health, 24*, 446–459.

Moore, B. S., Newsome, J. A., Payne, P. L., & Tiansawad, S. (1993, November). Nursing research: Quality of life and perceived health in the elderly. *Journal of Gerontological Nursing*, 7–14.

Oleson, M. (1990). Subjectively perceived quality of life. *Image: Journal of Nursing Scholarship, 22*(3), 187–190.

Padilla, G. V., Ferrell, B., Grant, M. M., & Rhiner, M. (1990). Defining the content domain of quality of life for cancer patients with pain. *Cancer Nursing, 13*(2), 108–115.

Padilla, G. V., & Grant, M. M. (1985). Quality of life as a cancer nursing outcome variable. *Advances in Nursing Sciences, 8*(1), 45–60.

Padilla, G. V., Grant, M. M., & Martin, L. (1988). Rehabilitation and quality of life measurement issues. *Head & Neck Surgery, 10* (Suppl. 11), S156–S160.

Padilla, G. V., Presant, C., Grant, M., Lipsett, J., & Heide, F. (1983). Quality of life index for patients with cancer. *Research in Nursing and Health, 3*, 117–126.

Tarlov, A., Ware, J., Greenfield, S., Nelson, E., Perrin, E., & Zubkoff, M. (1989). The medical outcomes study: An application of methods for monitoring the results of medical care. *JAMA, 262,* 925–930.

Ware, J. (1984). Conceptualizing disease impact and treatment outcomes. *Cancer,* 53(Suppl.), 316–323.

Young, K. J., & Longman, A. J. (1983). Quality of life and persons with malignant melanoma: A pilot study. *Cancer Nursing, 6,* 219–235.

Zhan, L. (1992). Quality of life: Conceptual and measurement issues. *Journal of Advanced Nursing, 17,* 795–800.

Chapter

4

Conceptualization and Measurement of
Quality of Life
and Related Concepts:
Guidelines for Clarity

JOAN E. HAASE • CARRIE JO BRADEN

The purposes of this chapter are to: (1) clarify quality of life (QOL) conceptualization and measurement issues that make it difficult to distinguish concepts *related* to QOL from concepts that are *indicators* of QOL, and (2) provide guidelines for achieving conceptual clarity, illustrating the use of the guidelines to specify and define concepts related to QOL. The introductions in much of the literature about QOL begin with a discussion of the complex and elusive nature of the term and the subsequent difficulties with adequate definition or measurement (Aaronson et al., 1991; Ballatori, 2001; Calman, 1987; Cella & Tulsky, 1990; Costain, Hewison, & Howes, 1993; de Haes & van Knippenberg, 1989; Donovan, Sanson-Fisher, & Redman, 1989; Fallowfield, 1990; Ganz, Schag, & Cheng, 1990; Goodinson & Singleton, 1989; Gotay, Korn, McCabe, Moore, & Cheson, 1992; Gunnars, Nygren, Glimelius, & Care, 2001; Holzner et al., 2001a; King et al., 1997; Larson, 1997; Leplege & Hunt, 1997; Mosconi et al., 2001; Nayfield et al., 1992; Osoba, 1994; Padilla, Ferrell, Grant, & Rhiner, 1990; Schipper, 1990a; Schraub, Mercier, & Arveux, 2000; Stewart, 1992; Ware, 1991). Clearly, the logic or validity link between definition and measurement of QOL is weak. That is, no one definition to date has established a list of essential characteristics or attributes that form the conceptual parameters for QOL definition.

Quality of Life Conceptualization and Measurement Issues

Mast (1995) described QOL as a primitive term with few directly observable and clearly identifying characteristics. There is continued discussion about whether defining and measurement of QOL is even possible, given the complexity of situational and demographic variables between patients and within patients over time (Albert, 1998; Frank et al., 1998; Leplege & Hunt, 1997). Clearly, at this point, QOL can only be communicated by variables or instances that *illustrate rather than define or specify the essential attributes of the concept.* For example, a health care provider who is concerned with the impact of illness treatment on physical functioning may focus on side effect characteristics as illustrative of the patients' QOL. Another health care provider with a desire to understand more about the impact of the illness on patients' overall happiness or satisfaction with life may focus on role performance or spirituality as illustrative of QOL. The number of potential illustrative indicators is large. It is not surprising that one set of exchanges among QOL researchers in the late 1980s was likened to the Tower of Babel (de Haes & van Knippenberg, 1989; Mor & Guadagnoli, 1988). Given the lack of clearly identified essential characteristics of QOL, the problem is to provide a meaningful way to differentiate related concepts from possible indicators that clearly identify the essential characteristics of QOL. QOL will cease to be a primitive term only when there is consensus about a set of clearly identifiable characteristics or attributes that will be consistently used as the basis for definition and measurement.

The number of articles on health-related quality of life of cancer patients has increased steadily. The proportion of randomized cancer trials incorporating QOL measures increased from 1.5 to 8.2% between 1980 and 1997 (Sanders et al., 1998). Although there is acceptance of a core set of broad domains that constitute health-related QOL (Gunnars et al., 2001), specific domains vary widely and measures are not always comparable (Holzner et al., 2001b). The QOL domains more or less agreed upon as broad domains in adult clinical trial QOL studies include: physical functioning, disease-related and treatment-related symptoms, and psychological and social functioning (Aaronson et al., 1991; Baker et al., 1994; Ferrans, 1990; Ferrell, 1990; King et al., 1997; Moinpour, 1994). Examples of other domains include satisfaction with care, feelings of well-being, and general life satisfaction (Aaronson & da Silva, 1987). Schipper (1990b) describes a QOL paradigm consisting of four components: physical and occupational function, psychological function, social interaction, and somatic sensation. Patrick and Erickson (1993) identify four core domains within which nine associated concepts are subsumed. The four core domains and nine component concepts form a health-related QOL framework. Opportunity, functional status, impairment, and death/duration of life are the relevant domains for identifying variables that are indicators of QOL. More recently, there is an increasing call for including spirituality in the basic list of domains for health-related quality of life (Brady et al., 1999; Mytko & Knight, 1999; Peterman et al., 2002).

In addition to variations in the domains that constitute QOL, there is still much debate about methods appropriate for defining the domains and variables that illustrate QOL (Gunnars et al., 2001; King et al., 1997; Koopmans, 2002). The level of consensus remains very general with the only solid source of agreement being the assumption that health-related QOL is a multidimensional construct (Faden & Leplege, 1992).

For the most part, the domains identified in QOL frameworks (Aaronson et al., 1991; Padilla et al., 1981; Patrick & Erickson, 1993; Patrick & Guttmacher, 1983) have little theoretical basis (King et al., 1997). Rather, sets of factors thought to indicate QOL are put together and items believed to represent the factors are developed or taken from existing scales designed to measure some other variable. Validity is sometimes assessed by exploratory factor analyses to deduce factors or to interpret agreement of the factors that emerge without a theoretical structure (Aaronson & da Silva, 1987; Bliss, Selby, Robertson, & Powles, 1992; Jenkins, Jono, Stanton, & Stroup-Benham, 1990). To illustrate, several studies comparing commonly used quality of life measures, scales, or subscales found the measures were not comparable across one or more domains (Cella, Hahn, & Dineen, 2002; Holzner et al., 2001b; Kemmler et al., 1999; Kuenstner et al., 2002). Frequently, there is no assessment made of the sensitivity of the factors to detect meaningful changes in a patient's QOL (Donovan et al., 1989; Gunnars et al., 2001; Testa & Simonson, 1996) and few studies address logistics such as timing of measurement (Hakamies-Blomqvist et al., 2001). Additionally, what patients find as meaningful factors that exemplify their QOL such as goals, dreams, and hopes is mostly left out of the multidimensional formulations developed by health care professionals (Corner, 1997; Costain et al., 1993; Padilla et al., 1990).

Acknowledgment that QOL is multidimensional is an insufficient basis to justify treatment choices and make judgments about the effects of therapeutic interventions, when a biomedical focused framework of QOL is primarily used (Corner, 1997; Costain et al., 1993; Molassiotis & Morris, 1998; Schipper, 1990). Such a focus results in a reliance on a functional living perspective with QOL domains selected on the basis of professional concerns about physical and psychological morbidity and the patient's capacity for active and independent function (Corner, 1997; Costain et al., 1993). By contrast, a patient-focused approach to QOL is based on the notion of the *meaning* of the cancer experience and its treatment. The patient perspective includes concerns about information, ideas about the nature of supportive and nonsupportive contacts, the nature of choice in decision making about treatment, and the changing perceptions of experience as the treatment continues or comes to an end. These perspectives go beyond merely the presence or absence of function. A meaning-based model can also be used as a basis for selecting treatment choices and for determining the effectiveness of therapeutic intervention (Levine & Ganz, 2002; Moinpour et al., 1989). A meaning-based model may also be a better perspective for guiding development of multidimensional frameworks for QOL (Costain et al., 1993; Somerfield, 2001).

For effective decision making, it is necessary to identify the most powerful predictors of QOL, beyond those measuring function (Bliss et al., 1992; Levine & Ganz, 2002). Bliss and colleagues (1992) concluded that further use of factor analysis will not help define QOL factors more precisely in cancer patients, because the findings are so similar to other measures that include psychological as well as physical distress domains. Thus, the problem with the existing general consensus about categories of variables represented in most health-related QOL frameworks is one of an increasing gap between sophisticated statistical analysis of data obtained from multidimensional questionnaires and the lack of conceptual sophistication reflected in the operational definition of variables thought to be illustrative of QOL (Costain et al., 1993). Faden and LePlege (1992) stated that the narrower conceptualization of QOL in terms of domains that illustrate health-related QOL does not resolve theoretical dilemmas about the nature or meaning of QOL. Thus, various measures and methods currently used to assess health-related QOL do not have congruent theoretical constructs or philosophic views.

Padilla and associates (1990) and Ferrell and colleagues (1992a, 1992b) offer inductive, patient-generated approaches to define the illustrative domains of QOL. The lists of categories and subcategories emerging from application of their essentially descriptive surveys converge on three very broad categories: physical, psychological, and interpersonal well-being. Ferrell and associates (Ferrell, 1992a, 1992b) add a spiritual well-being category based on their data. But, even Ferrell and colleagues (1992b) indicate that future inductive studies using more specific inductive approaches to collect data are necessary to obtain the depth, meaning, and experience of cancer treatment needed to understand QOL.

Padilla and colleagues' (1990) attention to subcategories under each of the broad domains emerging from their survey data provides some insight about which domains are most critical from the patient's point of view during the kind of life-changing events that cancer patients experience. These findings also support the idea that there is a middle road where a meaning-based model and a function-based model complement one another. For example, the data indicate that social role functioning composed of the themes of making others happy (satisfying others, giving of self, helping others) and fulfilling one's role (good parent, community member, churchgoer) are central to most patients' perception of what constitutes QOL in bad times as well as in good times. This finding fits well with several other researchers' conceptualizations, such as Ferrell and colleagues' (1992b) social well-being dimension that includes roles and relationships, affection/sexual function, leisure activities, and return to work aspects. It is also similar to Patrick and Erickson's (1993) health-related QOL concept of social function that fits within a broader domain of functional status. They defined roles in terms of social function (major activities), integration through participation in the community, contact (interaction with others) and intimacy, and sexual function. The data also fit with: (1) McBride's (1993) description of adult role outcomes as pivotal to the management of chronic illness conditions; (2) Braden's (1993) definition of self-help outcome in terms of involvement in the things one finds important in life, specifically social role activities; and (3) Leidy and Haase's (1999) conceptualization of Being Able and Being With as a means of preserving integrity or wholeness in chronic illness. Additionally, Faden and Leplege's (1992) observation that there is broad agreement on the general value of human experiences supports the importance of pursuing one's own life plans in any conceptualization of life quality.

Family relationships and social role performance as meaningful concepts for health-related QOL frameworks are supported by Costain and associates' (1993) comparison study of function-based and meaning-based perspectives on QOL. The focus of the meaning-based perspective of an illness experience includes personal relationships with close others. The measure contains nine items for family relationships and four for social life. By contrast, the measure used to index a function-based model (representing professional definitions of optimum functional status) contains one global item for family relationships. Results demonstrate a lack of fit between the two measures on family relationships and social life with the meaning-based measure providing more information about the context for family relationships including feelings of usefulness, expressing love and affection, sharing one's experience with a close other, and contact with children and parents. Additionally, the meaning-focused measure was more sensitive to detecting dissatisfaction in the domain, providing a better tool for problem identification and focusing of oncology support services. Another example of differences in function-based and meaning-based findings was demonstrated by Mackworth, Fobair, and Praelos (1992). They used a multidimensional QOL questionnaire that provides a more definitive assessment of health-related QOL than the assessment provided by the Karnofsky Performance Scale (KPS; Karnofsky & Burchenal, 1949). Specifically, the KPS was not sufficiently discriminatory to be sensitive to fine distinctions for two thirds of the subjects (Mackworth et al., 1992).

The issue of measure sensitivity or responsiveness to change is very important, given that a primary purpose for including QOL endpoints in clinical assessments of cancer treatment is to include the patient as well as the disease when assessing effectiveness of treatment (Costain et al., 1993; Moinpour et al., 1989; Ward et al., 1999).

Measures that are insensitive because they do not represent patients' views about their QOL during cancer experience fail in two regards: they will not inform clinicians about where and for whom intervention efforts need to be focused, and they will not be able to assess treatment effectiveness. A review of 17 scales commonly used as multidimensional QOL measures by Donovan and colleagues (1989) identified only three scales that could be linked to the cancer experience . The three scales that have enough items (Arvidson, Larsson, & Lonnerholm, 1999) and any type of domain subscores from which to detect changes in QOL are described by Izsak and Medalie (1971), Padilla and colleagues (1983), and Heinrich, Schag, and Ganz (1984).

Guidelines for Obtaining Clarity in Quality of Life Conceptualization and Measurement

A number of investigators offer criteria or guidelines that, if followed, will improve efforts to assess QOL for the purposes of justifying treatment choice and determining therapeutic intervention effectiveness. Several are discussed here and synthesized in Table 4-1.

Goodinson and Singleton (1989) list six criteria:

1. Data need to be based on patients' self-reports in order to reflect a patient perspective;
2. The conceptual orientation needs to give recognition to the fact that a patient's perspective cannot be abstracted from the individual in isolation from coping strategies, past experiences of illness, and other variables;
3. The weighing of dimension importance needs to reflect what is important to the patient;
4. The dimensions included need to have both a history of contribution to QOL and a definition base from which it is developed;
5. The design needs to ensure that the selected way of assessing QOL will be applicable across a range of times, e.g., in states of wellness, during illness diagnosis and treatment phases, and following treatment completion; and
6. Studies of QOL need to fit within an ongoing investigative framework that seeks to establish the influence of adaptation phenomenon and coping strategies on QOL.

Three of the four key policies adapted by the Cancer Control Research Committee of the Southwest Oncology group for guiding QOL definition demonstrate incorporation of many of the criteria offered by (Goodinson & Singleton, 1989):

1. Measure physical functioning, symptoms (Holland, 1991), and global QOL separately;

2. Include measures of social functioning and additional protocol-specific measures if resources permit; and

3. Use patient-based questionnaires with psychometric properties that have been documented in published studies.

An overview of the most commonly used quality of life questionnaires is provided by Gunnars and associates (2001). They include a discussion of the major characteristics, including number of items, scaling model, reliability and validity, differences in versions, and limited information on the specific subscales included in each instrument. These authors conclude there is little need for development of additional questionnaires. In addition to describing the questionnaires, this group also provides several conclusions:

1. Assessments are increasingly utilized and should primarily be done by self-reports.
2. A predicted hypothesis should determine the most appropriate questionnaires.
3. Despite difficulties in interpreting the relationship of objective endpoints in the light of subjective data, both perspectives are valuable.
4. QOL assessment continues to require methodological improvement. Timing, response shift, missing data, and difficulty comparing across protocols are all examples of the method problems that make the current state of knowledge tentative.
5. QOL assessments are resource demanding and should be used primarily in studies motivated by comparisons of treatments without major differences in objective endpoints.

A nursing state-of-the-knowledge conference on quality of life and the cancer experience resulted in guidelines related to both theory and measurement (King et al., 1997). Recommendations included:

1. The underlying mechanisms that explain how quality of life "works" should be considered.
2. Sources of items should be derived from patient-generated data.
3. Respondents should have the opportunity to weigh the importance as well as the occurrence of items in QOL instruments.
4. In addition to meeting established criteria for reliability and validity, instruments should be selected to fit the specific aims of the study.
5. Consideration should be given to the impact of culture and life experiences on basic perceptions of QOL.

As previously mentioned, general guidelines for achieving conceptual clarity in QOL assessment are outlined in Table 4-1. Three general steps are suggested: (a) specify the purpose, (b) identify the theoretical or conceptual framework, and (c) specify additional measurement criteria.

Table 4-1.   **Guidelines for Achieving Clarity in QOL Assessment**

---

1. Specify the purpose(s) for use of the QOL assessment

   a. Designate the population(s) of interest considering the following:

      - diagnostic groups
      - treatment option groups
      - groups experiencing specific phenomena such as specific symptoms
      - demographic characteristics such as gender, ethnicity, and age
      - consumer-focused populations such as HMO targeted populations

   b. Determine if the assessment is process- or endpoint-focused

      - Make decisions regarding issues of identifying and defining endpoints such as when the endpoint occurs and whose perspective of the endpoint will be measured.
      - Make decisions regarding issues of identifying and defining processes such as when data will be obtained and whose perspective(s) will be measured at each point.

   c. Identify design alternatives based on the state of knowledge development and the philosophical context of science

      - Options include: exploration, description, prediction, and evaluation
      - Contexts include: discovery or justification

2. Select a conceptual orientation or theoretical framework

   a. Variable (concept) specifications should be consistent with decision criteria about whether concept is "part of" or has a validity (logic) link to defining attributes of quality of life

      - decide on methods for clarification of variables (concept analysis, derivation, and synthesis; retrodiction process in middle range theory development; structural analysis of underlying measurement model to test alternative item sets)

   b. Relationship (statement) specification should be consistent with decision criteria about whether concepts are "illustrative of" QOL in terms of antecedents of ("cause of") or consequences of ("result of") QOL

      - decide on methods for clarification of relationships (statement analysis, derivation, and synthesis; alternative theory testing of multiple hypotheses using structural equation analysis or other methods)

3. Specify measurement criteria to include

   a. The current status of measurement of selected concepts
   b. The measurement burden
   c. Multiple stakeholders' perspective

      - critical multiplism
      - resources/access to multiple stakeholders

Specify the Purpose

Three general purposes for assessing QOL appear in the literature. Many authors (Bowling, 1991; Compas et al., 2001; de Haes & van Knippenberg, 1989; Faden & Leplege, 1992; Leplege & Hunt, 1997; Moinpour et al., 1989) indicate that the primary purpose for including QOL in clinical assessments of cancer treatment is to consider the patient as well as the disease when assessing treatment effectiveness or identifying treatment choices. Thus, the broad purposes are to provide a patient perspective of the cancer experience, identify treatment choices, and determine the effectiveness of therapeutic interventions. Examination of the goals for undertaking QOL assessment is essential as different goals can lead to different choices of measures as well as have implications for respondent and administrative burdens (Schag, Ganz, & Heinrich, 1991; Testa & Simonson, 1996; Somerfield, 2001).

A list of the most common reasons for undertaking QOL assessment was developed by Goodinson and Singleton (1989). These include: (1) "justify or refute different forms of medical treatment; (2) resolve disputes concerning different therapeutic approaches; (3) identify the sequelae of disease or treatment which may be resolved by other therapeutic interventions (e.g., nursing) and with regard to quality adjusted life year (QALY); and (4) provide a basis for allocating resources to those treatments judged to be most cost effective." The resource allocation reason for QOL assessment is an addition to the purposes stated earlier.

Goodinson and Singleton and others (Cascinu et al., 2001; Langenhoff, Krabbe, Wobbes, & Ruers, 2001) also suggested that QOL assessments serve as a basis for treatment selection between individuals, with preference given to those who have the potential for maximum benefit. The economic perspective inherent in QOL assessment as a basis for treatment selection clearly raises ethical issues that are a part of purpose identification (Goodwin, 2001; Sherbourne et al., 2001). However, there are moral issues surrounding any QOL assessment, regardless of purpose, which are not being addressed (Faden & Leplege, 1992; Leplege & Hunt, 1997). Thus, specifying the purpose for the QOL assessment is an important first step in working toward clarity, not only because of conceptual and measurement concerns but also because of significant ethical concerns. Specifying the purpose of QOL assessment is further enhanced when the population of interest, the focus as either process or endpoint, and the research design are clarified.

Population of Interest. One criterion to evaluate the adequacy of measures of QOL is that items are based on patient perspectives (Donovan et al., 1989). However, it is rare that the patient perspectives reflected in measures are population specific, even though QOL definitions and measures may change dramatically when the population is considered.

Quality of life populations are most often defined based on specific diagnoses and treatment groups (El-Serag, Olden, & Bjorkman, 2002; Trippoli et al., 2001). And, despite the lack of consensus in conceptualization or measurement, for some disease-specific groups, QOL assessment has influenced the nature of treatment. For example, Priestman (1987) concluded that studies of psychiatric morbidity associated with breast cancer patients have clearly influenced treatment decisions for surgeons toward lumpectomy and irradiation rather than disfiguring procedures.

Less frequently, QOL studies define population based on experiences with specific phenomena, often physical symptoms such as fatigue (Mast, 1998; Nail & Jones, 1995; Piper, 1991) and pain (Ferrell, Ferrell, Ahn, & Tran, 1994). Although nurses have studied and developed instruments for elusive but important concepts for patients with cancer, such as hope (Herth, 1989; Owen, 1989), courage (Haase, 1987), suffering (Gregory, 1994; Steeves & Kahn, 1987), spirituality (Kaczorowski, 1989), and self-transcendence (Coward, 1991), few studies have been conducted to study cancer patients by defining the population as those experiencing such phenomena. Yet, when such studies have been done, they yield important information on QOL, often identifying interventions that are specifically within nursing's domain. The importance of defining populations of interest in the study of QOL based on culture or ethnic group is well documented (Leininger, 1994; Marshall, 1990). When cultural group is defined as the population of interest, it is important that studies are culturally sensitive and appropriate. Quality of life itself is likely to be defined differently in different cultures (Iwamoto, 1994). Measures developed for one population may be very inappropriate in another. Erroneous conclusions can result from cultural bias about QOL, such as there are no differences attributable to culture, or that there are extreme differences which make cross-cultural studies futile (Bonomi et al., 1996; Cella, 1992).

Other demographic characteristics such as age and gender require special consideration. Developmental issues are especially important for children and adolescents when longitudinal studies are planned. For example, changes in functional status are difficult to track when the indicators of what a child can do change over the course of lengthy treatment periods (Bradlyn, Harris, & Spieth, 1995). Consumer-focused populations, such as those in Health Maintenance Organizations, are rapidly increasing. Even though dissatisfaction with the quality of care may be expressed in studies of QOL, important information may be obtained from which health care delivery systems can be revised. For example, QOL studies of cancer survivors imply long-term survivors may have a continued need for psycho-oncologic support (Holzner et al., 2001; Kiss et al., 2002; Kopp et al., 1998; Tomich & Helgeson, 2002).

People who are at later stages of cancer or in palliative care raise very different QOL questions than long-term survivors or those in early stages (Coates et al., 2000;

Frost et al., 2002; Tassinari et al., 2002). Although some understanding of quality of life in palliative care has been gained there are no well-established and validated QOL tools available to date (Tassinari et al., 2002).

Process or Outcome Focus. A second means of clarifying purpose of QOL assessment is to delineate whether QOL issues are process or outcome focused. While QOL factors are often labeled as "endpoints" or outcomes, they would be more appropriately labeled "treatment-related processes." Symptom distress and alterations in functional status—core domains in most cooperative group studies—occur most frequently during active treatment. While knowledge about the amount of symptom distress or the inability to carry out usual activities is important, patients may consider these conditions endurable with a perspective that the condition is temporary and accompanied by a hope of cure. Endpoint concerns might focus on such concepts as transcendence, role changes, and altered body image. Quality of life assessments that are meaning based, rather than function based, may yield very different information depending on whether variables are assessed as process or outcome. For example, patients' perspectives of their cancer experience and the meanings they derive from the experience, often change following the initial diagnosis and treatment phase. And, even after completion of treatments, the meaning of the experience may be evolving (Haase & Rostad, 1994).

One approach to addressing lack of sensitivity to the subtleties and complexities of human perception relative to quality of life is to incorporate the construct of response shift in QOL studies. Response shift is defined as the change in individuals' internal standards, values, and conceptualizations of QOL that accompany a change in health state (Schwartz & Sprangers, 2000). Lepore and Eton's (2000) test of two models of response shift effects on QOL in men treated for prostate cancer concluded response shifts may be an identifiable process of accommodation to disease-induced deterioration that preserves social and emotional well-being. Bernhard and colleagues (1999) reported similar conclusions in a study of patients with colon cancer who had radical resection with or without adjuvant chemotherapy. Further exploratory investigation of response shift in perception of health among newly diagnosed colon cancer patients indicated patients did substantively reframe their internal standards of health as well as their perceived QOL (Bernhard, Lowy, Maibach, & Hurny, 2001). Such studies offer a promising approach to researchers who seek to strengthen understanding of QOL as a standard outcome for oncology care.

In decisions about process and outcomes, two factors are key: timing and perspective (Huisman et al., 1987). In order to assess process, QOL factors must be assessed more than once and at times when the process is likely to vary. Relevant times depend on whose perspective is sought and for what purpose. As an example, from a physician's perspective, if the purpose for evaluation may be to determine which treatment produces the least symptom distress then the timing of measures is based on anticipated times of exacerbation following alternative treatments. A patient, on the other hand, may view QOL in terms of ability to resume desired activities. Relevant timing to assess symptom distress may be dictated based on, for example, whether an adolescent is able to go to a desired party on the weekend.

Clearly delineating processes by identifying phases of disease and treatment may increase the sensitivity of instruments as well as dictate variables of importance. Zittoun (1987) provided a good example of differences in patient perspectives of QOL based on the phases of acute leukemia disease and treatment. In the first phase, hospitalization and induction treatment, social context, hospital milieu, and personality and other individual psychological factors are considered. In the remission phase, when consolidation and maintenance treatments are conducted, Zittoun identified the struggle for cure and quality of survival as key issues. During this phase, side effects and returning to normal life are important. Failures of induction treatment or relapse present very different QOL issues, often marked by prolonged exacerbations of uncertainty. The end-of-life phase is also unique. Quality of life in the dying process requires a clear change of focus for the patient, his or her family, and the health care providers. In one study QOL was often affected in this phase by feelings of abandonment when physicians identified there was "nothing more to do" (Gregory, 1994). In fact, as physical condition deteriorates, spiritual issues commonly gain in importance as determinants of QOL, yet they are rarely studied (Gotay, 1985).

Specify a Conceptual or Theoretical Framework

The second step in achieving clarity in QOL assessment is to *explicitly* lay claim to and describe the conceptual/theoretical basis for the assessment. One way of dealing with very basic differences about the nature of QOL is to identify for one's self and others the assumptions that guide which dimensions are selected and the importance each is given.

Costain and associates (1993) assert that, by itself, a multidimensional approach to QOL assessment does not provide a conceptual basis for the QOL assessment. In their comparative study of two QOL models, even though measures selected to index each model were multidimensional and covered the same content (both assessed psychological, social, and physical function aspects of oncologic QOL) the resulting assessments produced markedly divergent information on some of the dimensions. Kemmler and colleagues (2002) also discuss the merits and drawbacks of multidimensional scaling as a tool for analyzing QOL data. If the conceptual/theoretical basis across all health-related QOL studies were explicit, it would be possible to compare findings in a way that would expand the understanding of QOL as a construct

(Costain et al., 1993). The result could be a change in the designation of QOL as a primitive construct to one that has definable attributes in its own right and that has the potential to provide a basis for development of a measure that could become the "gold standard" for indexing QOL in the future. King and colleagues (1997) provide a useful overview of beginning attempts to link concepts in explanatory models. Examples of emerging explanatory models include Mishel's uncertainty in illness theory (Mishel, 1990), discrepancy between expected and actual outcomes (Michalos, 1986), internalized standards (Breetvelt & Van Dam, 1991), distinctions between affective and cognitive components of QOL (de Haes & van Knippenberg, 1985), and meaning-making processes (Northouse & Northouse, 1987).

Variable Specification. As noted in the background section of this chapter, the only way to index QOL at this point is through identified dimensions that are illustrative of, rather than definers of, the construct. Stewart (1992) states that while it is safe to assume that persons who have fewer symptoms, more happiness, and better functioning in daily activities have a better QOL, it cannot be said that these concepts are components of QOL. For example, social well-being concepts appear to be predictors of QOL rather than a direct part of QOL. To date the conceptual muddiness across QOL studies has precluded identifying critical attributes of QOL. There are processes or methods available for clarifying the defining characteristics, in this case concepts, of an amorphous construct such as QOL.

A variety of methods for clarifying concepts are found in the nursing literature. While it is beyond the scope of this paper to describe each, we identify several in Table 4-1 (e.g., concept analysis, derivation, and synthesis). Inductive research approaches, such as *grounded theory* and *phenomenology*, have been used to study processes and experiences of cancer patients and concepts related to QOL. Examples include studying return-to-work experiences (Berry, 1993), experiences of completing treatment (Haase & Rostad, 1994; Weekes & Kagan, 1994), fatigue (Messias, Yeager, Dibble, & Dodd, 1997; Pearce & Richardson, 1994), and family communication in coping (Hilton, 1994). *Concept analysis*, in which critical attributes of the concept are identified and distinguished from antecedents and outcomes of the concept has been used to clarify concepts relevant to QOL (Haase et al., 1992). *Simultaneous concept analysis* provides a way of ferreting out subtle differences in concepts such as hope, self-transcendence, acceptance, and spiritual perspective (Haase et al., 1992). Deductive strategies also hold promise for clarifying concepts. *Structural analyses* of the underlying measurement model provides evidence about items that constitute specific domains in instrument development (Loehlin, 1992). Whatever method(s) is used, the goal is to distinguish the concept from all other concepts—related, contrary, antecedent, and outcome concepts.

Relationship Specification. Because most of the dimensions now specified to illustrate QOL represent variables that are related to, rather than definers of, QOL, description of patterns of relationships among the dimensions is particularly important for clarity. Again, the explicit identification of the underlying conceptual/theoretical perspective enables meaningful interpretation of the QOL assessment. An atheoretical approach to conceptualizing QOL as a multidimensional construct results in a laundry list of variables as can be seen in Table 4-2. Even though such a specification of variables is said to be atheoretical, there is an implied theoretical assumption underlying the specification that can be used as a framework for specifying relationships. An ontological perspective of humans as bio-psych-socio-spiritual-cultural beings forms the belief system for this particular type of multidimensional depiction of QOL. In this view, the whole of QOL is a compilation of the parts, a particularate–deterministic view that says every variable listed contributes to one's QOL. The relationship patterns that are implied in a laundry list of domains consist of multiple single-order associations with no means of indicating relationship patterns among the parts. Because each variable is considered necessary to predict the whole, there is no designation of which variables are *illustrative of* QOL versus designation of which variables are *related to* the illustrative variables.

There are many middle range theories that are consistent with the ontological belief that human experience is best represented by patterns that reflect reciprocal interaction of person and environment, an unfolding of life and context. Such theories seek to specify experience in terms of processes that move through and interact with a particular time/space frame. In this perspective, the selected dimensions of QOL are related in ways that represent a simultaneous stochastic process (Jones, Fayers, & Simons, 1987), whereby the choice of endpoint depends on what the particular theory identifies as the ultimate focus of concern. Thus, many psychosocial theories, such as Andersen, Kecolt-Glaser, and Glaser's (1994) model of cancer stress and psychosocial course specify psychosocial adjustment as the endpoint. In this

Table 4-2. **Atheoretical Dimensions of QOL**

Dimensions Related to Physical Problems	Dimensions Related to Psychological, Social, and Spiritual Factors	Wider Dimensions
Physical	Psychological	Individual
Toxicity	Interpersonal	Cultural
Body Image	Happiness	Political
Mobility	Spiritual	Philosophic
	Financial	Time

model QOL is a construct that is specified as affecting coping behaviors. However, one confounding problem that emerges from the relationship specifications posed is that the choice of measures for QOL as a construct include coping scales. The issue of confounding is a common problem in QOL studies because of the conceptual difficulties, but an explicit description of the models that underpin thinking about QOL assessment provide a way to identify sources of confounding and to rethink relationship specifications or measure choices.

Braden's Self-Help Model (Figure 4-1) provides an example of a model that specifies relationships among variables that influence QOL with the outcome, global QOL, defined as overall satisfaction with one's current circumstance. Thus, QOL conceptualized as a global variable, is the ultimate endpoint of a learned response to chronic illness within a specific time/space frame. Self-help and self-care are other interrelated outcome variables that contribute to overall life satisfaction. Self-help is

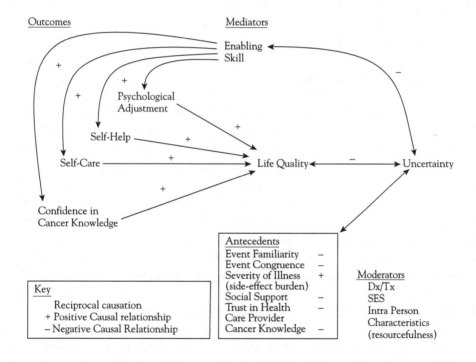

Figure 4-1.   **Combined self-help/uncertainty in illness model: essential variables and relationships of learned response to chronic illness experience and of uncertainty in illness.**

Dx = diagnosis; Tx = treatment; SES = socioeconomic status

defined in terms of social role function and self-care is defined in terms of adult role behaviors devoted to enhancing or maintaining health. The model variables that are often listed *within* a symptom/side effect dimension of a multidimensional QOL perspective measure the concept of severity of illness, which is the primary antecedent for initiation of learning in the cancer experience. Variables that are often listed in a physical functional status dimension of a multidimensional QOL perspective measure the concept of dependency, one of the adversities that can come with illness experience. Uncertainty is the other adversity that accompanies illness experience. Braden's theory identifies a positive relationship between symptom/side effects and uncertainty. Dependency levels increase in situations where the perceived severity of illness leads individuals to feel that they have to rely on others to carry out the functional activities of daily life. Thus, dependency (Eiser, Havermans, Craft, & Kernahan, 1995) operates as an adversity only in some, not all, illness experiences. For example, for most women, younger women in particular, the diagnosis and early treatment phase of breast cancer present greater adversity for uncertainty than for dependency. Dependency becomes a stronger aversive aspect of cancer experience with increased illness severity and/or more aggressive treatment protocols (e.g., late stage at time of diagnosis, recurrence, bone marrow transplant, and aggressive chemotherapy protocols). As previously noted patient demographic characteristics, such as age, can also moderate the relationship between severity of illness and dependency and the relationship between severity of illness and uncertainty.

In Braden's (1993) model symptom/side effects are not directly related to overall life satisfaction. Rather, the relationship of symptom/side effects with global life quality is mediated by uncertainty and dependency. That is, dependency and uncertainty have specified relationships with life quality that directly undermine one's satisfaction with life. The undermining effect of symptom/side effects relative to life quality is increased by the adversities that are operating in the particular situation. If the model contained only the four concepts—severity of illness, dependency, uncertainty, and life quality—and the relational statements linking severity of illness to dependency and to uncertainty and linking dependency and uncertainty to life quality, the model would be addressing only negative aspects of illness experience. Thus, the model incorporates personality/coping abilities as additional mediators. These potentially reduce the negative effect of uncertainty and dependency on life quality.

Enabling skills, the primary positive mediator in the Braden model, represent the opportunity dimension of a multidimensional health-related QOL framework as described by Patrick and Erickson (1993). Thus, across the process of learning to live with illness as depicted by the Self-Help Model (Figure 4-1) many of the dimensions commonly used in health-related QOL frameworks are addressed. The relationships among the dimensions are also specified. The problem of confounding is dealt with by clear definition and measure choice. For example, the measure for life quality is a global inventory of well-being scale. Additionally, the model incorporates feedback loops to depict the learning process over time and to allow assessment of variables illustrative of QOL over the cancer experience from diagnosis to long-term survival phases.

Specify Measurement Criteria

Desirable characteristics of QOL measures include: (1) developed from an appropriate conceptual or theoretical framework; (2) adequate evidence of validity and reliability; (3) responsive to changes; (4) based on client-generated data; and (5) are acceptable to clients, health providers, and researchers (Donovan et al., 1989). In applying these criteria to specific QOL instruments, Donovan and colleagues (1989) concluded that many QOL scales were clearly inadequate and that some met many of the criteria, but none met all. The situation is not different for concepts that are related to QOL. For example, in a review of the state of knowledge about fatigue, the authors concluded there is lack of theoretical models of fatigue (Winningham et al., 1994). It then follows that most fatigue measures lack a conceptual basis. The instruments do not clearly distinguish fatigue from depression or other mood situations. In order for instruments to be responsive to change, they must have reasonable total numbers of items and at least five items per domain (Donovan et al., 1989). These criteria often require a greater response burden, especially if several concepts related to QOL are of interest. To be acceptable to respondents and health care providers, QOL instrument(s) need to be completed in a reasonable amount of time, be easily administered and scored, readily understandable, and perceived as relevant and meaningful to the respondents (Donovan et al., 1989).

Summary

The conceptualization issues that continue to interfere with ability to adequately and appropriately assess the QOL of oncology clients are: (1) *conceptual inadequacy* relative to domains selected as illustrative of QOL and (2) *psychometric inadequacy* of measures with failure to use client-generated data to develop or to confirm scale items and to test reliability, validity, and sensitivity or responsiveness to change. Conceptual inadequacy can be attributed to failure to use a client perspective instead of a health care provider perspective about what is important for domain specification and the continued unquestioned selection of existing instruments that are not sensitive to the context. There is also failure to use theory to guide domain selection which decreases the ability to identify whether variables illustrating QOL are of equal weight relative to overall life satisfaction, cost, and quality of care outcomes. Atheoretical approaches fail in several ways: (1) one cannot assess if or how domains are related to one another; (2) there is no way to interpret the meaning of relationship patterns; and (3) there is no basis for specifying whether the dimensions are moderated or mediated by person-, disease-, and/or treatment-related factors relative to overall life satisfaction, cost, and quality of care outcomes. Psychometric inadequacy contributes to problems with credibility of findings, which then further undermine inclusion of QOL assessment in clinical trials.

Guidelines for achieving conceptual clarity include specification of the purpose of QOL assessment, specifically designating the population of interest and identifying whether the focus is on process or endpoint. Additionally, a conceptual or theoretical framework should be utilized. This requires identification of clearly defined concepts and the relationships among them. Finally, criteria for measurement should be specified. Instruments selected to measure concepts should have not only well-established psychometric properties, but should also include criteria regarding response burden.

REFERENCES

Aaronson, N. K., & da Silva, F. C. (1987). Prospects for the future: Quality of life evaluation in prostatic cancer protocols. *Progress in Clinical & Biological Research, 243B,* 501–512.

Aaronson, N. K., Meyerowitz, B. E., Bard, M., Bloom, J. R., Fawzy, F. I., Feldstein, M., Fink, D., Holland, J. C., Johnson, J. E., & Lowman, J. T. (1991). Quality of life research in oncology. Past achievements and future priorities. *Cancer, 67*(3 Suppl), 839–843.

Albert, S. M. (1998). Defining and measuring quality of life in medicine. [letter; comment.] *JAMA, 279*(6), 429, 431.

Andersen, B., Kiecolt-Glaser, J., & Glaser, R. A. (1994). A biobehavioral model of cancer stress and disease course. *American Psychologist, 49,* 389–404.

Arvidson, J., Larsson, B., & Lonnerholm, G. (1999). A long-term follow-up study of psychosocial functioning after autologous bone marrow transplantation in childhood. *Psycho-Oncology, 8*(2), 123–134.

Baker, F., Wingard, J. R., Curbow, B., Zabora, J., Jodrey, D., Fogarty, L., & Legro, M. (1994). Quality of life of bone marrow transplant long-term survivors. *Bone Marrow Transplantation, 13*(5), 589–596.

Ballatori, E. (2001). Unsolved problems in evaluating the quality of life of cancer patients. *Annals of Oncology, 12,* S11–S123.

Bernhard, J., Hurny, C., Maibach, R., Herrmann, R., & Laffer, U. (1999) Quality of life as subjective experience: Reframing of perception in patients with colon cancer undergoing radical resection with or without adjuvant chemotherapy. *Annals of Oncology, 10*(7), 775–782.

Bernhard, J., Lowy, A., Maibach, R., & Hurny, C. (2001). Response shift in the perception of health for utility evaluation: An explorative investigation. *European Journal of Cancer, 37*(14), 1729–1735.

Berry, D. (1993). Return to work experiences of people with cancer. *Oncology Nursing Forum, 20*, 905–911.

Bliss, J. M., Selby, P. J., Robertson, B., & Powles, T. J. (1992). A method for assessing the quality of life of cancer patients: Replication of the factor structure. *British Journal of Cancer, 65*(6), 961–966.

Bonomi, A.E., Cella, D. F., Hahn, E. A., Bjordal, K., Sperner-Unterweger, B., Bergman, B., Willems-Goot, J., Hanquet, P., & Zittoun, R. (1996). Multilingual translation of the functional assessment of cancer therapy (FACT) quality of life measurement system. *Quality of Life Research, 5*(3), 309–320.

Bowling, A. (1991). Health care research: Measuring health status. *Nursing Practice, 4*(4), 2–8.

Braden, C. J. (1993). Research program on learned response to chronic illness experience: Self-Help Model. *Holistic Nursing Practice, 8*(1), 38–44.

Bradlyn, A. S., Harris, C. V., & Spieth, L. E. (1995). Quality of life assessment in pediatric oncology: A retrospective review of phase III reports. *Social Science & Medicine, 41*(10), 1463–1465.

Brady, M. J., Peterman, A. H., Fitchett, G., Mo, M., & Cella, D. (1999). A case for including spirituality in quality of life measurement in oncology. *Psycho-Oncology, 8*(5), 417–428.

Breetvelt, I. S., & Van Dam, F. S. (1991). Underreporting by cancer patients: The case of response-shift. *Social Science & Medicine, 32*(9), 981–987.

Calman, K. C. (1987). *The Quality of Life of Cancer Patients*. New York: Raven Press.

Cascinu, S., Labianca, R., Daniele, B., Beretta, G., & Salvagni, S. (2001). Survival and quality of life in gastrointestinal tumors: Two different end points? *Annals of Oncology, 12*, S31–S36.

Cella, D. F. (1992). Quality of life: The concept. *Journal of Palliative Care, 8*(3), 8–13.

Cella, D. F., & Tulsky, D. S. (1990). Measuring quality of life today: Methodological aspects. *Oncology (Huntington), 4*(5), 29–38, 69.

Cella, D., Hahn, E. A., & Dineen, K. (2002) Meaningful change in cancer-specific quality of life scores: Differences between improvement and worsening. *Quality of Life Research, 11*(3), 207–221.

Coates, A. S., Hurny, C., Peterson, H. F., Bernhard, J., Castiglione-Gertsch, M., Gelber, R. D., & Goldhirsch, A. (2000). Quality-of-life scores predict outcome in metastatic but not early breast cancer. International Breast Cancer Study Group. *Journal of Clinical Oncology, 18*(22), 3768–3774.

Compas, B. E., Connor-Smith, J. K., Saltzman, H., Thomsen, A. H., & Wadsworth, M. E. (2001). Coping with stress during childhood and adolescence: Problems, progress, and potential in theory and research. *Psychological Bulletin, 127*(1), 87–127.

Corner, J. (1997). Beyond survival rates and side effects: Cancer nursing as therapy. The Robert Tiffany Lecture. 9th International Conference on Cancer Nursing, Brighton, UK, August 1996. *Cancer Nursing, 20*(1), 3–11.

Costain, K., Hewison, J., & Howes, M. (1993). Comparison of function-based model and a meaning-based model of quality of life in oncology: Multidimensionality examined. *Journal of Psychosocial Oncology, 11*(4), 17–37.

Coward, D. D. (1991). Self-transcendence and emotional well-being in women with advanced breast cancer. *Oncology Nursing Forum, 18*(5), 857–863.

Davis, G. C. (1989). *Development and testing of the pain management inventory.* Fort Worth: Harris College of Nursing, Texas Christian University.

de Haes, J. C., & van Knippenberg, F. C. (1989). Quality of life instruments for cancer patients: Babel's Tower revisited. *Journal of Clinical Epidemiology, 42*(12), 1239–1241.

de Haes, J. C., & van Knippenberg, F. C. (1985). The quality of life instruments for cancer patients: A review of the literature. *Social Science & Medicine, 20*(8), 809–817.

Donovan, K., Sanson-Fisher, R. W., & Redman, S. (1989). Measuring quality of life in cancer patients. *Journal of Clinical Oncology, 7*(7), 959–968.

Eiser, C., Havermans, T., Craft, A., & Kernahan, J. (1995). Development of a measure to assess the perceived illness experience after treatment for cancer. *Archives of Disease in Childhood, 72*(4), 302–307.

El-Serag, H. B., Olden, K., & Bjorkman, D. (2002). Health-related quality of life among persons with irritable bowel syndrome: A systematic review. *Alimentary Pharmacology & Therapeutics, 16*(6), 1171–1185.

Faden, R., & Leplege, A. (1992). Assessing quality of life. Moral implications for clinical practice. *Medical Care, 30*(5 Suppl), MS166–175.

Fallowfield, L. (1990). *The Quality of Life.* London, England: Souvenir Press Ltd (pp. 17–30).

Ferrans, C. C. (1990). Quality of life: Conceptual issues. *Seminars in Oncology Nursing, 6,* 248–254.

Ferrell, B. R. (1990). Development of a quality of life index for patients with cancer. *Oncology Nursing Forum, 17*(3)Supplement, 15–19.

Ferrell, B. R., Ferrell, B. A., Ahn, C., & Tran, K. (1994). Pain management for elderly patients with cancer at home. *Cancer, 74*(7 Suppl), 2139–2146

Ferrell, B., Grant, M., Schmidt, G. M., Rhiner, M., Whitehead, C., Fonbuena, P., & Forman, S. J. (1992a). The meaning of quality of life for bone marrow transplant survivors. Part 1.The impact of bone marrow transplant on quality of life. *Cancer Nursing, 15*(3), 153–160.

Ferrell, B., Grant, M., Schmidt, G. M., Rhiner, M., Whitehead, C., Fonbuena, P., & Forman, S. J. (1992b). The meaning of quality of life for bone marrow transplant survivors. Part 2. Improving quality of life for bone marrow transplant survivors. *Cancer Nursing, 15*(4), 247–253.

Frank, L., Kleinman, L., Leidy, N. K., Legro, M., Shikiar, R., & Revicki, D. (1998). Defining and measuring quality of life in medicine. [letter; comment.] *JAMA, 279*(6), 429–430; discussion 431.

Frost, M. H., Bonomi, A. E., Ferrans, C. E., Wong, G. Y., Hays, R. D., & Clinical Significance Consensus Meeting (2002). Patient, clinician, and population perspectives on determining the clinical significance of quality-of-life scores. *Mayo Clinic Proceedings, 77*(5), 488–494.

Ganz, P. A., Schag, C. A., & Cheng, H. L. (1990). Assessing the quality of life—a study in newly-diagnosed breast cancer patients. *Journal of Clinical Epidemiology, 43*(1), 75–86.

Goodinson, S. M., & Singleton, J. (1989). Quality of life: A critical review of current concepts, measures and their clinical implications. *International Journal of Nursing Studies, 26*(4), 327–341.

Goodwin, P.J. (2001). Economics, quality of life and breast cancer outcomes—is balance possible? *Breast 10*, 190–198.

Gotay, C. C. (1985). Why me? Attributions and adjustment by cancer patients and their mates at two stages in the disease process. *Social Science & Medicine, 20*(8), 825–831.

Gotay, C. C., Korn, E. L., McCabe, M. S., Moore, T. D., & Cheson, B. D. (1992). Quality-of-life assessment in cancer treatment protocols: Research issues in protocol development. *Journal of the National Cancer Institute, 84*(8), 575–579.

Gregory, D. (1994). *Narratives of suffering in the cancer experience*. Tucson: University of Arizona College of Nursing.

Gunnars, B., Nygren, P., Glimelius, B., & SBU Group Swedish Council of Technology in Assessment in Health Care (2001). Assessment of quality of life during chemotherapy. *Acta Oncologica, 40*(2–3), 175–184.

Haase, J. (1987). The components of courage in chronically ill adolescents. *Advances in Nursing Science, 9*(2), 64–80.

Haase, J. E., Britt, T., Coward, D. D., Leidy, N. K., & Penn, P. E. (1992). Simultaneous concept analysis of spiritual perspective, hope, acceptance and self-transcendence. *Image—The Journal of Nursing Scholarship, 24*(2), 141–147.

Haase, J., Leidy, N., Coward, D., Penn, P., & Britt, T. (1993). Simultaneous Concept Analysis: A Strategy for Developing Multiple Interrelated Concepts. In

E. Rodgers & K. Knafl (Eds.), *Concept Development in Nursing: Foundations, Techniques and Applications*. Orlando, FL: W. B. Saunders.

Haase, J. E., & Rostad, M. (1994). Experiences of completing cancer therapy: children's perspectives. *Oncology Nursing Forum, 21*(9), 1483–1492; 1493–1494.

Hakamies-Blomqvist, L., Luoma, M. L., Sjostrom, J., Pluzanska, A., Sjodin, M., Mouridsen, H., Ostenstad, B., Mjaaland, I., Ottosson, S., Bergh, J., Malmstrom, P. O., & Blomqvist, C. (2001). Timing of quality of life (QoL) assessments as a source of error in oncological trials. *Journal of Advanced Nursing, 35*(5), 709–716.

Heinrich, R. L., Schag, C. C., & Ganz, P. A. (1984). Living with cancer: The Cancer Inventory of Problem Situations. *Journal of Clinical Psychology, 40*(4), 972–980.

Herth, K. (1989). The relationship between level of hope and level of coping response and other variables in patients with cancer. *Oncol. Nurs. Forum, 16*, 67–72.

Hilton, B. A. (1994). Family communication patterns in coping with early breast cancer. *Western Journal of Nursing Research, 16*(4), 366–388; 388–391.

Holland, J. C. (1991). Progress and challenges in psychosocial and behavioral research in cancer in the twentieth century. *Cancer, 67*(3 Suppl), 767–773.

Holzner, B., Kemmler, G., Kopp, M., Dachs, E., Kaserbacher, R., Spechtenhauser, B., Vogel, W., & Sperner-Unterweger, B. (2001a). Preoperative expectations and postoperative quality of life in liver transplant survivors. *Archives of Physical Medicine & Rehabilitation, 82*(1), 73–79.

Holzner, B., Kemmler, G., Kopop, M., Moschen, R., Schweigkofler, H., Dunser, M., Margreiter, R., Fleischhacker, W. W., & Sperner-Unterweger, B. (2001b). Quality of life in breast cancer patients—Not enough attention for long-term survivors? *Psychosomatics, 42*(2), 117–123.

Huisman, S., van Dam, F., Aaronson, N. K., & Hanewald, G. (1987). (1987). On measuring complaints of cancer patients: Some remarks on the time span of the question. In N. K. Aaronson & J. Beckman (Eds.), *Quality of Life of Cancer Patients* (pp. 101–109). New York: Raven Press.

Iwamoto, R. (1994). Cultural influences on quality of life. *Quality of Life: A Nursing Challenge, 3*, 68–73.

Izsak, F. C., & Medalie, J. H. (1971). Comprehensive follow-up of carcinoma patients. *Journal of Chronic Diseases, 24*(2), 179–191.

Jenkins, C. D., Jono, R. T., Stanton, B. A., & Stroup-Benham, C. A. (1990). The measurement of health-related quality of life: Major dimensions identified by factor analysis. *Social Science & Medicine, 31*(8), 925–931.

Jones, D. R., Fayers, P. M , & Simons, J. (1987). Measuring and analyzing quality of life in cancer clinical trials. In N. K. Aaronson & J. Beckman (Eds.), *Quality of Life of Cancer Patients* (pp. 41–61). New York: Raven Press.

Kaczorowski, J. M. (1989). Spiritual well-being and anxiety in adults diagnosed with cancer. *Hospice Journal—Physical, Psychosocial, & Pastoral Care of the Dying, 5*(3–4), 105–116.

Karnofsky, D. A., & Burchenal, J. H. (1949). The clinical evaluation of chemotherapeutic agents in cancer. In I. C. M. McCleod (Ed.), *Evaluation of Chemotherapeutic Agents*. New York: Columbia University Press.

Kemmler, G., Holzner, B., Kopp, M., Dunser, M., Margreiter, R., Greil, R., & Sperner-Unterweger, B. (1999). Comparison of two quality-of-life instruments for cancer patients: The functional assessment of cancer therapy–general and the European Organization for Research and Treatment of Cancer Quality of Life Questionnaire–C30. *Journal of Clinical Oncology, 17*(9), 2832–2940.

Kemmler, G., Holzner, B., Kopp, M., Dunser, M., Greil, R., Hahn, E., & Sperner-Unterweger, B. (2002). Multidimensional scaling as a tool for analysing quality of life data. *Quality of Life Research 11*(3), 223–233.

King, C. R., Haberman, M., Berry, D. L., Bush, N., Butler, L., Dow, K. H., Ferrell, B., Grant, M., Gue, D., Hinds, P., Kreuer, J., Padilla, G., & Underwood, S. (1997). Quality of life and the cancer experience: The state-of-the-knowledge. *Oncology Nursing Forum, 24*(1), 27–41.

Kiss, T. L., Abdolell, M., Jamal, N., Minden, M. D., Lopton, J., & Messner, H. A. (2002). Long-term medical outcomes and quality-of-life assessment of patients with chronic myeloid leukemia followed at least 10 years after allogeneic bone marrow transplantations. *Journal of Clinical Oncology, 20*(9), 2334–2343.

Koopmans, P. P. (2002). Clinical endpoints in trials of drugs for cancer: Time for a rethink? *British Medical Journal, 324,* 1389–1391.

Kopp, M., Schwigkofler, H., Holzner, B., Nachbaur, D., Niederwieser, D., Fleischhacker, W. W., Sperner-Unterweger, B. (1998). Time after bone marrow transplantation as an important variable for quality of life results of a cross-sectional investigation using two different instruments for quality-of-life assessment. *Annals of Hematology, 77*(1–2), 27–32.

Kuenstner, S., Langelotz, C., Budach, V., Possinger, K., Krause, B., & Sezer, O. (2002). The comparability of quality of life scores: A multitrait multimethod analysis of the EORTC QLQ-C30, SF-36 and FLIC questionnaires. *European Journal of Cancer, 38,* 339–348.

Langenhoff, B. S., Krabbe, P. F. M., Wobbes, T., & Ruers, T. J. M. (2001). Quality of life as an outcome measure in surgical oncology. *British Journal of Surgery, 88*(5), 643–652.

Larson, J. S. (1997). The MOS 36-item short form health survey. A conceptual analysis. *Evaluation & the Health Professions, 20*(1), 14–27.

Leidy, N. K., & Haase, J. E. (1999). Functional status from the patient's perspective: The challenge of preserving personal integrity. *Research in Nursing & Health*, *22*(1), 67–77.

Leininger, M. (1994). Quality of life from a transcultural nursing perspective. *Nursing Science Quarterly*, *7*(1), 22–28.

Leplege, A., & Hunt, S. (1997). The problem of quality of life in medicine. *JAMA*, *278*(1), 47–50.

Lepore, S. J., & Eton, D. T. (2000). Response shifts in prostate cancer patients: An evaluation of suppressor and buffer models. In C. Schwartz & M. A. Sprangers (Eds.), *Adaptation to Changing Health Response Shift in Quality-of-Life Research*. American Psychological Association, Washington, D.C., 37–51.

Levine, M. N., & Ganz, P. A. (2002). Beyond the development of quality-of-life instruments: Where do we go from here? *Journal of Clinical Oncology*, *20*(9), 2215–2216.

Loehlin, J. C. (1992). *Latent variable models: An introduction to factor, path, and structural analysis*. Hillsdale, NJ: Lawrence Erlbaum Associates, Inc.

Mackworth, N., Fobair, P., & Praelos, M. D. (1992). Quality of life self-reports from 200 brain tumor patients: Comparisons with Karnofsky performance scores. *Journal of Neuro-Oncology*, *14*(3), 243–253.

Marshall, P. A. (1990). Cultural influences on perceived quality of life. *Seminars in Oncology Nursing*, *6*(4), 278–284.

Mast, M. E. (1995). Definition and measurement of quality of life in oncology nursing research: Review and theoretical implications. *Oncology Nursing Forum*, *22*(6), 957–964.

Mast, M. E., (1998). Correlates of fatigue in survivors of breast cancer. *Cancer Nursing 21*(2), 136–142.

McBride, A. B. (1993). Managing chronicity: The heart of nursing care. Key Aspects of Caring for the Chronically Ill. In S. Funk, E. Tornquist, M. Champagne, & R. Wiese (Eds.), *Hospital and Home*. New York: Springer.

Messias, D. K., Yeager, K. A., Dibble, S. L., & Dodd, M. J. (1997). Patients' perspectives of fatigue while undergoing chemotherapy. *Oncology Nursing Forum*, *24*(1), 43–48.

Michalos, A. C. (1986). Job satisfaction, marital satisfaction and quality of life: A review and a preview. In F. M. Andrews (Ed.), *Research in Quality of life* (pp. 57–83). Ann Arbor, MI: Institute for Social Research, University of Michigan.

Mishel, M. H. (1990). Reconceptualization of the uncertainty in illness theory. *Image—The Journal of Nursing Scholarship*, *22*(4), 256–262.

Moinpour, C. M. (1994). Measuring quality of life: An emerging science. Seminars in Oncology, *21*(5 Suppl 10), 48–60; 60–43.

Moinpour, C. M., Feigl, P., Metch, B., Hayden, K. A., Meyskens, F. L., & Crowley, J. (1989). Quality of life end points in cancer clinical trials: Review and recommendations. *Journal of the National Cancer Institute, 81*(7), 485–495.

Molassiotis, A., & Morris, P. J. (1998). The meaning of quality of life and the effects of unrelated donor bone marrow transplants for chronic myeloid leukemia in adult long-term survivors. *Cancer Nursing, 21*(3), 205–211.

Mor, V., & Guadagnoli, E. (1988). Quality of life measurement: A psychometric Tower of Babel. *Journal of Clinical Epidemiology, 41*, 1055–1058.

Mosconi, P., Colozza, M., Laurentiis, M. D., DePlacido, S., & Maltoni, M. (2001). Survival, quality of life and breast cancer. *Annals of Oncology, 12*, S15–S19.

Mytko, J. J., & Knight, S. J. (1999). Body, mind and spirit: Towards the integration of religiosity and spirituality in cancer quality of life research. *Psycho-Oncology, 8*(5), 439–450.

Nail, L., & Jones, L. (1995). Fatigue as a side effect of cancer treatment: Impact on quality of life. *Quality of Life: A Nursing Challenge, 4*, 8–13.

Nayfield, S. G., Ganz, P. A., Moinpour, C. M., Cella, D. F., & Hailey, B. J. (1992). Report from a National Cancer Institute (USA) workshop on quality of life assessment in cancer clinical trials. *Quality of Life Research, 1*(3), 203–210.

Northouse, P. G., & Northouse, L. (1987). Communication and cancer: Issues confronting patients, health professionals and family members. *Journal of Psychosocial Oncology, 5*(3), 17–46.

Osoba, D. (1994). Lessons learned from measuring health-related quality of life in oncology. *Journal of Clinical Oncology, 12*(3), 608–616.

Owen, D. (1989). Nurses' perspectives on the meaning of hope in patients with cancer: A qualitative study. *Oncology Nursing Forum, 16*, 75–79.

Padilla, G. V., Ferrell, B., Grant, M. M., & Rhiner, M. (1990). Defining the content domain of quality of life for cancer patients with pain. *Cancer Nursing, 13*(2), 108–115.

Padilla, G., Presant, C. A., Grant, M., Baker, C., & Metter, G. (1981). Assessment of quality of life in cancer patients. *Proceedings American Association of Cancer Research., 22*, 397.

Padilla, G. V., Presant, C., Grant, M. M., Metter, G., Lipsett, J., & Heide, F. (1983). Quality of life index for patients with cancer. *Research in Nursing & Health, 6*(3), 117–126.

Patrick, D. L., & Erickson, P. (1993). *Health Status and Health Policy.* New York, Oxford University Press.

Patrick, D. L., & Guttmacher, S. (1983). Socio-political issues in the uses of health indicators. In A. J. Culyer (Ed.), *Health Indicators.* Oxford, England: Martin Robertson and Company (pp. 165–173).

Pearce, S., & Richardson, A. (1994). Fatigue and cancer: A phenomenological study. *Journal of Clinical Nursing, 3*(6), 381–382.

Peterman, A. H., Fitchett, G., Brady, M. J., Hernandez, L., Cella, D. (2002). Measuring spiritual well-being in people with cancer: The functional assessment of chronic illness therapy-spiritual well-being scale (FACIT-Sp). *Annals of Behavioral Medicine, 24*(1), 49–58.

Piper, B. (1991). Alterations in energy: The sensation of fatigue. In R. S. Baird & R. M. G. McCorkle (Eds.), *Cancer nursing: A comprehensive texbook.* Philadelphia: W. B. Saunders.

Priestman, T. (1987). Evaluation of quality of life in women with breat cancer. In N. K. Aaronson & J. Beckman (Eds.), *Quality of Life of Cancer Patients,* (pp. 193–199). New York: Raven Press.

Sanders, C., Egger, M., Donovan, J., Tallon, D., & Frankel, S. (1998). Reporting on quality of life in randomised controlled trials: Bibliographic study. *BMJ, 317*(7167), 1191–1194.

Schag, C. A., Ganz, P., & Heinrich, R. L. (1991). Cancer Rehabilitation Evaluation System—short form (CARES-SF). A cancer specific rehabilitation and quality of life instrument. *Cancer, 68*(6), 1406–1413.

Schipper, H. (1990). Definition and conceptual issues. In I. B. Spilker (Ed.), *Quality of life assessments in clinical trials* (pp. 11–24). New York: Raven Press.

Schipper, H. (1990). Quality of life: Principles of the clinical paradigm. *Journal of Psychosocial Oncology, 8*(2/3), 171–185.

Schraub, S., Mercier, M., Arveux, P. (2000). Quality of life assessment in cancerology. *Presse Medicale, 29*(6), 310–318.

Schwartz, C. E., & Sprangers, M. A. G. (2000). Introduction. In C. E. Schwartz & M. A. G. Sprangers (Eds), *Adaptation to Changing Health Response Shift in Quality-of-Life Research,* Washington, D.C.: American Psychological Association, xiii–xvi.

Sherbourne, C. D., Unutzer, J., Schoenbaum, M., Duan, N., Lenert, L. A., Sturm, R., Wells, K. B. (2001). Can utility-weighted health-related quality-of-life estimates capture health effects of quality improvement for depression? Medical Care, 39(11), 1246–1259.

Somerfield, M. (2001). Hazards of quality-of-life data for clinical decision making. *Journal of Clinical Oncology, 19*(2), 594–595.

Steeves, R. H., & Kahn, D. L. (1987). Experience of meaning in suffering. *Image—The Journal of Nursing Scholarship, 19*(3), 114–116.

Stewart, A. (1992). Conceptual and methodological issues in defining quality of life: State of the art. *Progress in Cardiovascular Nursing* (Vol. 7, pp. 3–10).

Tassinari, D., Panzini, I., Ravaioli, A., Maltoni, M., & Sartori, S. (2002). Quality of life at the end of life: How is the solution far away? *Journal of Clinical Oncology,* *20*(6), 1704–1705.

Testa, M. A., & Simonson, D. C. (1996). Assesment of quality-of-life outcomes. *New England Journal of Medicine, 334*(13), 835–840.

Tomich, P. L. & Helgeson, V. S. (2002). Five years later: A cross-sectional comparison of breast cancer survivors with healthy women. *Psycho-Oncology, 11*(2), 154–169.

Trippoli, S., Vaiani, M., Linari, S., Longo, G., Morfini, M., Messori, A., (2001). Multivariate analysis of factors influencing quality of life and utility in patients with hemophilia. *Haematologica, 86*(7), 722–728.

Ward, W. L., Hahn, E. A., Mo, F., Hernandez, L., Tulsky, D. S., & Cella, D. (1999). Reliability and validity of the Functional Assessment of Cancer Therapy-Colorectal (FACT-C) quality of life instrument. *Quality of Life Research,* 8(3), 181–195.

Ware, J. E. (1991). Measuring functioning, well-being and other generic health concepts. In I. D. Osoba (Ed.), *Effect of cancer on quality of life* (pp. 7–23). Boca Raton, FL: CRC.

Weekes, D. P., & Kagan, S. H. (1994). Adolescents completing cancer therapy: Meaning, perception, and coping. *Oncology Nursing Forum, 21*(4), 663–670.

Winningham, M. L., Nail, L. M., Burke, M. B., Brophy, L., Cimprich, B., Jones, L. S., Pickard-Holley, S., Rhodes, V., St. Pierre, B., & Beck, S. (1994). Fatigue and the cancer experience: The state of the knowledge. *Oncology Nursing Forum, 21*(1), 23–36.

Zittoun, R. (1987). *Quality of life in adults with acute leukemia.* In N. K. Aaronson & J. B. (Eds.), New York: Raven Press (pp. 183–192).

Spiritual *Quality of Life*

ELIZABETH JOHNSTON TAYLOR

Mrs. Lee is a 58-year-old woman who is receiving chemotherapy for ovarian cancer. When asked about the quality of her life, she reports that she is adversely affected by nausea, sluggishness, worry, and sadness. She wistfully describes how her cancer and its treatments have limited her social interactions. She doesn't have the energy to romp with her grandkids or to have sex with her husband. Her once weekly lunch dates with friends are on hold, she is unable to cook or clean now, and she is very disappointed that a planned vacation cruise with her husband had to be cancelled. Mrs. Lee then confides: "What's really getting to me, is the part that people can't see—the questions I have inside. Like, what's the purpose for this happening to me? Why would God allow this to happen to me? And some days, all I do is lie in bed, and as you stare at the ceiling, you wonder a lot of things. But I do keep praying, and I sometimes do get a feeling that God is out there watching out for me."

Mrs. Lee's descriptive statements and questions illustrate how spirituality is connected with the quality of the life of a person living with cancer. Her questions also demonstrate how a person's religious background can provide him or her with helpful coping strategies, such as prayer, as well as the assumptions that prompt asking distressing questions like "Why would God allow this to happen to me?" Mrs. Lee also demonstrates how overtly spiritual concerns are often difficult for individuals to voice because personal spirituality is an intimate topic.

The spiritual aspect of quality of life is increasingly being recognized as an important domain of health-related quality of life (HRQOL). Until this past decade, the core dimensions of HRQOL included physical, emotional, social, and functional well-being (Brady, Peterman, Fitchett, Mo, & Cella, 1999). Now that researchers report qualitative data that indicate spirituality is considered by clients to be essential to their overall quality of life, a spiritual domain is being included in conceptualizations of HRQOL and HRQOL instruments.

Included in this chapter are a discussion about the spiritual domain of HRQOL and its importance to those who receive cancer care. Also included are a description of the elements of spiritual quality of life (SpQOL), a review of the available research about SpQOL in individuals receiving cancer care and a description of the clinical implications that are derived from this research. A discussion of how SpQOL can be empirically investigated concludes this chapter.

Conceptualizing Spiritual Quality of Life

Spirituality Defined

Because the term "spiritual" is an abstraction that often causes confusion, it is important that it be defined before any discussion of spiritual quality of life. *Spirituality* refers to that part of being human that seeks meaningfulness through intra-, inter-, and trans-personal connection (Reed, 1992). Or, as Dossey and Guzzetta (2000) define it, spirituality is that "unifying force of a person . . . [that involves] interconnectedness with self, others, nature, and God/Life" (p. 7).

Elements of Spiritual Quality of Life

As with physical, social, and other domains of HRQOL, spiritual quality of life is comprised of several elements. Table 5-1 presents the elements of SpQOL identified by three research teams who interviewed cancer patients to develop or refine their models of HRQOL. Cohen and colleagues' (1996) identification of existential well-being as an important determinant of HRQOL elucidates how issues of existence and meaning can occur regardless of client religiosity. Ferrans' (2000) model does not distinguish clearly between what is spiritual and what is psychological, indicating that the overlap or interrelatedness of the spiritual and psychosocial domains is great. Ferrell and Grant's (Ferrans, 2000; Ferrell, Dow, Leigh, Ly, & Gulasekaram, 1995) model confirms a reciprocal relationship between spiritual well-being and HRQOL, and equates spiritual well-being with SpQOL. In addition, the review of elements of spirituality found in definitions in nursing literature by Martsolf and Mickley (1998) provides similar conclusions to the research summarized in Table 5-1. These authors identify five frequently reported elements: meaning (i.e., having purpose, making sense of life), value (i.e., having cherished beliefs and standards), transcendence (i.e., appreciating a dimension that is beyond self), connecting (i.e., relating), and becoming (which involves reflection, allowing life to unfold, and knowing who one is).

Table 5-1.   **Elements of Spiritual Quality of Life**

Researcher/Terminology for Domain	Elements
Cohen, Mount, Tomas, & Mount (1996)/ Existential Well-being	• Concerns regarding death (existential obliteration) • Freedom (the absence of external structure) • Isolation (the unbridgeable gap separating self from all else) • Questions of meaning (the dilemma of recognizing the possibility of a cosmos without meaning)
Ferrans (2000)/ Psychological/Spiritual Domain	• Satisfaction with life • Happiness in general • Satisfaction with self • Achievement of personal goals • Peace of mind • Personal appearance • Faith in God
Ferrell & Grant (e.g., Ferrell, Grant, Funk, Otis-Green, & Garcia, 1998; in Ferrans, 2000)/ Spiritual Well-being	• Hopefulness • Suffering • Meaning of illness • Religiosity • Transcendence • Feelings of uncertainty

Related Concepts

Because these models suggest various elements comprise SpQOL, it is useful to review these elements. *Religiosity*, often used interchangeably with spirituality, is a narrower concept that is more easily observed directly. Religions are systems of beliefs and practices that reflect spiritualities; they can also function as a bridge for developing spiritual awareness. Whether or not a person's religion is of an organized form, religion offers a participant a specific worldview and answers to questions about ultimate meaning. Religion responds to, and provides mechanisms for, attending to spiritual yearnings (Taylor, 2002a).

Hope has been described in nursing literature as an emotion, an experience, or a need (Kylma, Vehvilainen, & Julkunen, 1997). A concept analysis of hope in adults yielded this definition: "a process of anticipation that involves the interaction of thinking, acting, feeling and relating, and is directed toward a future fulfillment that is personally meaningful" (Stephenson, 1991). Study findings suggest that levels of hope remain rather constant between diagnosis and recurrence of cancer (Ballard, Green, McCaa, & Logsdon, 1997) and throughout the dying process (Herth, 1990).

In nursing literature, *transcendence* is often used interchangeably with *self-transcendence*, which Coward (1990) defined as: "the capacity to reach out beyond oneself, to extend oneself beyond personal concerns and to take on broader life perspectives, activities, and purposes" (162). Transcendence is also thought to involve a person's recognition that there is something other or greater than the self and a seeking and valuing of that greater other, whether it is an ultimate Being, Force, or Value. In western society, transcendence often involves recognition of a Greater Other typically called God, or "faith in God" as it is labeled in Ferrans' model. Coward (1990) observed that experiences of self-transcendence foster a sense of meaning among persons with cancer. *Meaning* is often used simultaneously with purpose. Frankl (1984) proposed that the "will to meaning" is the most basic concern and motivating force for humans. Several scholars have differentiated between ultimate, cosmic meaning and the need to make sense of life on a more personal level—the meaning *of* life versus the meaning *in* life. The need for meaning among persons with cancer at any stage has been well documented (Taylor, 2000). The search for meaning often manifests itself in the asking of questions about causality (e.g., "What caused my cancer?"), selective incidence (e.g., "Why did *I* get it?"), responsibility, and significance (e.g., "How will I let this cancer make me a better person?").

Empirical Research about Spiritual Quality of Life

Indicators of Spiritual Quality of Life

Because of the subjective nature of HRQOL (Brady et al., 1999), and because spirituality is a particularly ethereal phenomenon, it is helpful to understand what phenomenon may reveal SpQOL among persons with cancer. In addition to research investigating cancer patients' perceptions of what quality of life encompasses, research about what comprises spiritual needs for cancer patients, will be reviewed.

Ferrell's research teams (Ersek, Ferrell, Dow, & Melancon, 1997; Ferrell, Grant, Funk, Otis-Green, & Garcia, 1998) have studied what cancer patients think quality of life means. Content analysis of 130 ovarian cancer patients' written responses to a questionnaire revealed the following themes that explicitly show the interrelatedness of spirituality and HRQOL:

- To have happiness and enjoyment, to live life to its fullest, to appreciate the small things (the most frequently cited theme with 46 of the respondents indicating this);

- To engage in relationships, to love and be loved; to be close to God, to be spiritual, to have meaning in life, to have hope;

- To be able to make a contribution, to feel worthwhile, to participate, to feel useful;

- To prioritize what's important in life, to maintain balance; and

- To let go of control (Ersek et al., 1997).

These informants were also able to identify how having cancer positively influenced their quality of life. For example, having cancer helped nearly half of them to change their attitude about life, live for the present, reprioritize, and appreciate life more fully. Women living with breast cancer have been observed to have similar responses to inquiries about their SpQOL (Ferrell et al., 1998b). These women described how their illness made them recognize inner spiritual qualities and spiritual coping strategies that assisted them during the challenges of illness.

Research findings about what constitute spiritual needs of cancer patients also offer information about what may contribute to their SpQOL. For example, Peteet (1985) identified "religious issues" observed among cancer patients during psychiatric consultations. These issues (found in 32 of 50 consecutively seen hospitalized patients) included: loss of religious support; pressure from others to adopt a religious position other than their own; bizarre expressions of religious belief; conflict between religious views and view of oneself as ill; and preoccupation with the ultimate meaning of illness and life.

Data from in-depth interviews with 28 cancer patients and family caregivers, suggest seven categories of spiritual needs that would determine SpQOL (Taylor, unpublished data). These "needs" involved:

- Relating to God (the language of these informants). Examples of such needs include needing to know God's will, remembering how God has guided, getting right with God, believing God has or will heal, and resigning to God being in control of the illness.

- Having hope, gratitude, and being positive. Examples of such needs include needing to have hope for healing, keep a positive outlook, and count blessings.

- Giving and receiving love from other persons. Examples of such needs include needing to make the world a better place, help others, and get right with others.

- Reviewing beliefs. Examples of such needs include wondering if your beliefs about God are correct, and asking "why?" questions.

- Creating meaning, finding purpose. Examples of such needs include needing to get past asking "why me?", become aware of positive things that have come with illness, reevaluate life, and sense that there is a reason for being alive now.

- Having religious needs met. Examples of such needs include needing to pray or receive a religious ritual from a religious leader, or have quiet time or space to reflect or meditate.

- Preparing for death. Examples of such needs include needing to make sure personal business is in order, and balance thoughts about dying with hoping for health.

These research findings provide a rich description of many of the spiritual needs that persons living with cancer experience. These needs reflect spiritual experiences that can be distressful or euphoric. These negative and positive spiritual needs can occur simultaneously. Individuals can, for example, concurrently be engaged in a spiritually distressing wrestle with God about what is the purpose of their suffering, while experiencing forgiveness with others or sensing God's providence. These needs, in concert, are what determine an individual's state of spiritual health or well-being, hence SpQOL.

Degree of Spiritual Quality of Life

The levels and patterns of SpQOL among persons with cancer are now being documented. Because several instruments for quantitatively measuring HRQOL among persons with cancer include items assessing SpQOL, it is now possible to identify a person's level or degree of SpQOL and to compare SpQOL with other domains of HRQOL. These data are helpful for clinicians who seek to understand who may need additional spiritual support or when an individual may be at risk for spiritual distress.

Several studies have found that persons with cancer rank SpQOL second, after the physical domain, as the most important domain of HRQOL. In a study of women with all stages of ovarian cancer, Ersek and colleagues (1997) found that spiritual well-being ranked second, after physical well-being, and higher than psychological and social well-being. The average score for this subscale, in fact, was higher than the overall HRQOL score. This subscale mean score is all the more remarkable because responses to one of its items (about uncertainty) were much lower than the other spiritual well-being subscale items, therefore lowering the subscale score. Saleh and Brockopp (2001) reported that bone marrow transplant survivors (n = 41) also ranked SpQOL second to physical well-being using Ferrell and Grant's scale. Whereas spiritual and religious activities, sense of purpose, hope, and peace highly influenced their HRQOL, these cancer survivors were likewise troubled by a sense of uncertainty.

Similarly, 188 long-term female cancer survivors reported moderately high levels of SpQOL, making the "spiritual/philosophical view of life" subscale the second highest mean score (Wyatt & Friedman, 1996). Evidence from testing the McGill Quality of Life Questionnaire (Cohen, Mount, Tomas, & Mount, 1996) also showed the existential well-being subscale mean to rank second (after a two-item subscale measuring support in ways that could be linked with spiritual perspective), and higher than the tool's overall mean. McMillan and Weitzner (2000) also found the "social/spiritual well-being" subscale to rank highest while testing a HRQOL tool among hospice patients with cancer.

While there is growing evidence that SpQOL may consistently rank first or second among the various domains of HRQOL, there is scant documentation about how SpQOL may change during the cancer trajectory. Ferrell and colleagues (1995) reported that SpQOL in 687 cancer survivors was significantly higher for survivors who had lived at least five years since their initial diagnosis than their more recently diagnosed counterparts. Two studies suggest SpQOL may remain fairly constant. Ersek and colleagues (1997) noted no significant differences in SpQOL between patients with ovarian cancer and patients without evidence of cancer. Similarly, McMillan and Weitzner (1998) observed only a minimal difference in the social/spiritual well-being scores of hospice patients with cancer and scores of healthy adults.

Factors Related to Spiritual Quality of Life

Certain demographic factors have been found to be associated with SpQOL. Three studies reported that younger cancer patients (those less than 40 years old) have lower SpQOL (Gioiella, Berkman, & Robinson, 1998; Wyatt and Friedman, 1996) or "spiritual health" (Highfield, 1992). Ferrell and colleagues (1995) document higher SpQOL in female cancer survivors than in male survivors (who comprised only 19% of their sample). There is weak support suggesting a positive relationship between SpQOL and being married and/or living with children (Ferrell et al., 1995; Gioiella, Berkman, & Robinson, 1998). Although similar findings are reported in a limited number of other research studies exploring spirituality in the context of health, there are other studies that have not demonstrated these relationships. Thus, these findings musts be interpreted cautiously.

A growing body of evidence can be interpreted as indicating that SpQOL is an integrative and unifying force within humans. SpQOL is strongly and positively related to overall HRQOL. Ferrell and colleagues (1998a; Ersek, Ferrell, Dow, & Melancon, 1997), for example, documented correlations of 0.39 and 0.45 between SpQOL and overall HRQOL. Other investigations exploring the direct relationship between spiritual well-being and HRQOL are presented in Table 5-2, as are selected

Table 5-2.   **Factors Related to Spiritual Quality of Life**

Author	Concept Studied/ Empirical Indicator	Sample	Findings with Significant Correlations
Kaczorowski (1989)	Spiritual well-being/ Paloutzian and Ellison Spiritual Well-Being Scale (SWBS)	114 with cancer diagnosis	• SWB correlated with state-trait anxiety (−0.44)
Yates, Chalmer, St. James, Follansbee, & McKegney (1981)	Religious belief/10-item Religious Belief Index (RBI) Religiosity/ 4 items developed by investigators to assess activity and connection	71 with advanced cancer	• RBI and religiosity correlated (0.25–0.41) with satisfaction with life • RBI and religiosity negatively correlated (−0.22 to −0.37) with pain level • Attendance at religious services correlated with happiness and positive affect (0.34 and 0.32)
Cohen, Mount, Tomas, & Mount (1996)	Existential well-being/ McGill Quality of Life Existential Well-being subscale (EWB)	254 cancer patients and survivors	• EWB correlated with physical symptoms (0.37), psychological symptoms (0.45), feeling supported (0.54), overall QOL (0.48)
Fehring, Miller, & Shaw (1997)	Spiritual well-being, religiosity/ SWBS and Gorsuch & McPherson Intrinsic–Extrinsic Religiosity Scale	100 elderly cancer patients	• Positive correlations found among SWB, intrinsic religiosity, hope, and positive mood states • Negative correlations observed among intrinsic religiosity, depression, and other negative mood states • E.g., correlation between hope and SWB (r = 0.75) and intrinsic religiosity (r = 0.58) • E.g., correlation between depression and SWB (r = −0.52) and intrinsic religiosity (r = −0.44)

Table 5-2.   (continued)

Author	Concept Studied/ Empirical Indicator	Sample	Findings with Significant Correlations
Ferrell, Grant, Funk, Otis-Green, & Garcia (1998)	Spiritual well-being/ Spiritual well-being subscale of Ferrell & Grant Quality of Life–Breast Cancer Version	298 breast cancer survivors	• SWB correlated with depression (0.35*) and psychological well-being (0.29) *Presumably a negative correlation. There are no negative correlations in the large table where these finds were reported. Depression was also positively correlated, surprisingly, with overall QOL and other variables.
Riley, Perna, Tate et al. (1998)	Spiritual well-being/ SWBS	216 rehabilitation hospital patients which included 71 with cancer	• "Nonspiritual" subjects (vs. religious and existential clusters of subjects) reported lower HRQOL and life satisfaction
Brady, Peterman, Fitchett, Mo, & Cella (1999)	Spiritual well-being/ Functional Assessment of Chronic Illness Therapy-Spiritual Well-Being (FACIT-Sp)	1,610 patients with current or past diagnosis of cancer or HIV	• FACIT-Sp correlated with overall QOL as measured by Functional Assessment of Cancer Therapy–General ($r = 0.58$) and item stating "I am content with the quality of my life right now" ($r = 0.48$) • Regression analysis indicated SWB remained a significant contributor to QOL even after controlling for physical, emotional, and social well-being were controlled

Table 5-2.   (continued)

Author	Concept Studied/ Empirical Indicator	Sample	Findings with Significant Correlations
Cotton, Levine, Fitzpatrick, Dold, & Targ (1999)	Spiritual well-being/ FACIT-Sp	142 currently with invasive breast cancer	• SWB correlated with fighting spirit (0.46), helplessness/ hopelessness (–0.55), fatalism (0.62), and anxiety (–0.49) • Regression analysis showed small, but significant impact of SWB on QOL (after demographic variables and psychological adjustment were entered)
Fernsler, Klemm, & Miller (1999)	Spiritual well-being/ Paloutzian & Ellison's Spiritual Well-Being Scale (SWBS; which includes Religious and Existential subscales)	121 persons with colorectal cancer	• No correlations between Religious well-being and Demands of Illness (DOI) • Negative correlations (–0.28 to –0.36) between Existential well-being and DOI (including physical symptoms, personal meaning, family functioning, social relations, monitoring symptoms and treatment issues subscales)
Thomson (2000)	Spiritual well-being/ FACT-Spiritual Well-being subscale	16 hospice patients assessed 4 times over 6-month period	• FACT-Sp scores averaged higher than overall QOL and ranked second to social well-being

studies that demonstrate the relationship between spirituality and religiosity, and other domains of HRQOL.

In addition to the above studies that focus on HRQOL in persons with cancer, there are numerous other studies reporting positive relationships between spirituality and HRQOL in healthy individuals and in those with other chronic illnesses (e.g., Poloma & Gallup, 1991; Ayele, Mulligan, Gheorghiu, & Reyes-Ortiz, 1999; Miller, 1985). These studies provide ample support for the importance of considering SpQOL in HRQOL discussions.

This review of research exploring SpQOL among persons with cancer suggests several important points. First, human spirituality can manifest in numerous ways. The elements that contribute to SpQOL (or spiritual well-being or health) among cancer patients can include helpful cognitive perspectives and coping strategies, as well as distressing questions and inner conflicts. Also, what comprises a spiritual phenomenon is often confused with a psychosocial phenomenon. HRQOL instruments that have been factor analyzed are often composed of items that could be argued as reflective of either the spiritual or psychosocial domain.

Second, there is some evidence that SpQOL may remain fairly high throughout the cancer and survivorship experiences. The research indicating that SpQOL ranks first or second among the various domains comprising HRQOL suggests that cancer care recipients perceive their spiritual well-being as quite important to their overall well-being. It is also intriguing that when physical symptoms become less of a concern, spiritual aspects of having lived with cancer can remain. When survivors are told their cancer is cured, they still may wonder why God allows cancer to happen. Or they may be savoring the spiritual blessings of having a serious illness such as the increased inner strength, the improved relationships, and the new or invigorated sense of mission and purpose for life.

Third, the little available evidence describing the patterns of SpQOL among cancer patients suggests that it either remains constant or it adapts quickly to life transitions such as cancer. Whether these findings reflect the response shift phenomenon observed in other HRQOL research (Breetvelt & Van Dam, 1991) or the indomitable nature of the human spirit—or both—is an intriguing topic for further study. Regardless, it is impressive that SpQOL remains high despite declines in physical functioning (see especially, Brady et al., 1999).

Fourth, several studies investigating SpQOL or spiritual well-being of cancer patients suggest that it is a significant factor that contributes to overall HRQOL. Spiritual well-being, measured in its varied forms, appears to be indirectly associated with depression, anxiety, negative moods, pain level, and demands of illness. Conversely, a healthy spiritual state appears to be associated with a fighting spirit, hope, life satisfaction, happiness, and other positive moods.

While most study findings present strong, unified support for SpQOL contributing significantly to HRQOL, there is still room for further investigation. Some discrepant findings across studies illuminate the need for improved design and methods for specifically understanding SpQOL in relation to other HRQOL phenomena. For instance, is SpQOL associated with physical pain or well-being? Ferrell and colleagues (1998b) observed no relationship, while Yates and colleagues (1981) observed significant low-moderate correlations between aspects of religiosity and pain ($r = -0.22$ to -0.33).

Future oncology nursing research should also address what factors contribute to SpQOL. There is evidence that intrinsic religiosity (religiosity that is motivated by internal yearnings, in contrast to socially driven extrinsic religiosity) is associated with spiritual well-being among cancer patients (Fehring, Miller, & Shaw, 1997; Mickley, Soeken, & Belcher, 1992). But what other characteristics that may be supported by nurses may contribute to spiritual well-being?

Clinical Implications

In part, because of the swelling chorus of research findings demonstrating that SpQOL is a significant contributor to HRQOL, nursing literature is replete with affirmations for nurses to support spiritual well-being in their patients and, to provide spiritual care. The Joint Commission for the Accreditation of Health Care Organizations (JCAHO) now mandates spiritual assessments be completed for all patients, and that spiritual support be available to those who request it (JCAHO, 2000). Because of the nature of the work of nursing—the intimacy and availability required of a nurse to provide nursing care—the nurse can be an ideal professional for providing spiritual care. This section will discuss not only some specific strategies nurses can employ to support SpQOL, but client perspectives on what promotes SqQOL.

Client Perspectives

Before discussing what nurses can do to support SpQOL, it is imperative that nurses understand the client perspective. Ferrell and colleagues' (1998) study of breast cancer survivors directly documents what spiritual care some perceive will improve HRQOL. When asked what aspects of care were most helpful in improving their HRQOL, respondents first indicated supportive, cheerful, positive, caring hospital staff (154 of 243 patients), then identified support from family and friends (n = 45) and spiritual support (n = 30) as the next most important aspects of care. Yet when asked what resources they did not get that are most necessary to improving HRQOL, only 5 of 72 respondents indicated spiritual support. Greisinger and colleagues (1997), however, learned from 74 terminally ill cancer patients that existential and spiritual aspects of illness are rarely the focus of care, and that patients wish they were.

Certain studies indicate that some patients do want spiritual support from a nurse; however, many patients may *not* expect or want their nurses to address their spiritual needs. From a survey of 161 women with ovarian cancer, Fitch, Gray, and Franssen (2001) observed that 57% wanted to talk about the challenges of living with cancer. Of these women, only 13% identified nurses as the persons with whom they would talk of these concerns. An apparent reticence of clients to share their spiritual concerns, in particular with nurses, has been documented by other studies with oncology patients. When Reed (1991) asked 100 cancer patients "In what ways could hospital nurses help you in your spiritual needs?" only 14% marked "talk with you about your beliefs and concerns." In two studies with small samples, cancer patients ranked nurses fourth (after family, friends, and clergy) as spiritual resource persons (Highfield, 1992; Sodestrom & Martinson, 1987). Although clients rarely identify nurses as primary spiritual resource persons, clients do recognize them as potential spiritual caregivers.

Several survey studies have documented the complementary and alternative medicine (CAM) approaches that Americans use. "Spiritual healing," faith, and prayer are often identified as some of more frequently utilized CAM approaches (e.g., Eisenberg et al., 1993). Studies of CAM use among persons with cancer indicate that such approaches may be especially prevalent. VandeCreek, Rogers, and Lester (1999) learned from 112 outpatients with breast cancer that 85% used prayer and 48% used spiritual healing of some type. Similarly, Sparber and colleagues (2000) found "spirituality" to be the most-used CAM in a sample of 100 cancer patients.

Parallel findings are found in studies exploring coping strategies used by cancer patients (see Pargament, 1997 for a review.) When investigating spiritual coping strategies, in particular, there is evidence that spiritual beliefs and practices are fundamental, cherished, and influential mechanisms for coping with cancer (e.g., Cohen, Headley, & Sherwood, 2000; Halstead & Fernsler, 1994; Sodestrom & Martinson, 1987; Taylor & Outlaw, 2002).

Nursing Approaches to Promoting SpQOL

Although the recipients of cancer care may not expect spiritual support from nurses, they generally do seek it privately and they do desire it. Individuals who are not overtly aware of personal spirituality or receptive to spiritual care will still want care that "boosts their spirits," gives them a "fighting spirit," or inner peace, meaningfulness, and hope." So how can nurses assist their patients to maintain or develop spiritual well-being?

The nursing literature that describes approaches to nurturing the spirit is filled with a variety of "interventions" to include in spiritual care. Examples of these approaches or mechanisms for nurturing the spirit are:

- Presencing
- Being empathic and respectful
- Story listening or storytelling
- Encouraging self-expression through art (e.g., drawing, singing, dancing, flower arranging) or journal writing
- Facilitating recreation through play and sabbatarian rest periods
- Prayer, meditation, and guided spiritual imagery
- Providing spiritually edifying reading material or music or visual focal points
- Humor
- Facilitating religious practices
- Encouraging dream analysis
- Introducing nature
- Healing rituals
- Respecting spiritual beliefs.

For in-depth descriptions of these approaches to spiritual care, readers are encouraged to consult excellent recent nursing texts on spiritual care (see Burkhardt & Nagai-Jacobson, 2002; Taylor, 2002a).

Because a comprehensive discussion of how to promote spiritual well-being or SpQOL is beyond the scope of this chapter, a brief review of a few specific approaches that are perhaps most pertinent to persons living with cancer are offered. Research findings suggest that assisting cancer patients to transcend their suffering and find meaning, supporting their spiritual beliefs and practices, and "simply" being caring, may be especially helpful (e.g., Feher & Maly, 1999; Ferrell et al., 1998b; Miller, 1985; Post-White et al., 1996).

Transcending Suffering: Finding Meaning

Persons experiencing cancer often ask spiritually painful questions in an attempt to find meaning. These questions can include questions of causality (e.g., "Why do bad things happen?"), selective incidence (e.g., "Why me—instead of someone else?"), responsibility (e.g., "Did I do something to allow this to happen to me?"), and significance (e.g., "How can I become a better person because of this?") (Taylor, 2002a). Although some persons with cancer get "stuck" in the process of searching for meaning, many are able to transcend this suffering and ascribe some positive meaning (Taylor, 2000).

The positive meanings that persons ascribe to their cancer experience parallel those of persons who have suffered other serious losses (Violanti, Paton, & Dunning, 2000). That is, positive meanings that can be ascribed to cancer include:

- Perceived changes in self (e.g., development of news skills, confidence, inner strength)
- Changed sense of relatedness to others (e.g., more receptivity, sensitivity, and compassion for others, deeper relationships)
- Change in philosophy of life (e.g., more spiritual awareness, increased faith or religiousness, greater appreciation and perspective for life).

It is this transformation of the tragedy of cancer that allows some cancer patients to remark, "Cancer was the best thing that happened to me" or "Cancer made me a better person!"

Although nurses cannot make a patient find meaning, they can encourage or facilitate activities that promote a sense of meaningfulness. These activities that can help a person sense that his or her life is meaningful include altruistic deeds of service to others or the world, dedication to a cause, creative experiences of any type, and pleasurable activities. For example, bored, bedridden patients can find some meaning when they write a poem, taste gourmet food, pray for others, donate time or money for a campaign, or call to encourage another cancer survivor.

A nurse can also facilitate meaning-making by allowing patients to discuss their search for meaning. Nurses who ask thoughtful questions and listen attentively to responses may help clients to gain self-awareness. A nurse might ask, for example, "What are some of the good things that have come out of your cancer experience?" or "What sorts of lessons about life have you learned from this experience?" Sensitive responses to patients asking questions about meaning must not be superficial or avoidant. Questions of meaning are ultimately unanswerable. By being compassionately present to those who seek meaning, the nurse can support patients while they attempt to "be patient towards all that is unsolved . . . and . . . to love the questions themselves. . . . [to] live the questions. . . . [and] then gradually, without noticing it, live along some distant day into the answer" (p. 149, Rilke, in Wismer, 1995).

Supporting Spiritual Beliefs and Practices

There are numerous ways a nurse can support spiritual beliefs and practices for religious and nonreligious patients. First, however, the nurse must assess how spiritual beliefs and practices influence the illness experience and how they need to be supported (Taylor, 2002a). A spiritual assessment can include looking at the patient's environment (e.g., Are there religious items present in the room or being worn?) or reflecting on the patient's verbal conversation. Nurses can gain information about spiritual beliefs and practices during social chats with patients when beliefs and practices are often mentioned in passing. More formal assessment questions, which may or may not use religious language, can also be used. For example, "What helps you to cope during difficult times like this?" and "What can we nurses do to lift your spirits?" are nonthreatening questions. Such questioning also conveys to the patient that the nurse is sensitive and interested in supporting his or her spiritual well-being. This act will, in itself, convey care and help to create a spirit-healing environment.

Supporting spiritual beliefs does not require that a nurse alter or devalue personal spiritual beliefs. Neither does it mean that a nurse unethically impose his or her beliefs (Taylor, 2002a). Rather, the nurse can allow the patient to explore spiritual beliefs, remember how these beliefs are helpful, and determine what beliefs may need revision. The nurse accomplishes this by remaining present, actively listening, and when appropriate, asking questions that allow the patient to probe within further. When a patient recognizes discordant beliefs, it is likely that the services of a trained chaplain will be beneficial. Indeed, nurses often support spiritual beliefs by involving chaplains, clergy, or other spiritual care experts in the care of their patients.

Supporting spiritual practices may involve assisting a patient with prayer or devotional practices, educating them about how to attend religious services when neutropenic, safeguarding religious clothing, talismans, or other personal objects. A nurse need not be an expert in comparative religions. Rather, the nurse allows the patient to give instructions for how to help and follows them respectfully. While some religious practices may not be right for a nurse to support, many are rituals that a nurse who shares similar beliefs can participate in or support. Questions that can guide a nurse in determining when to support a religious practice include: Is this spiritual practice harmful to my patient? Is there an underlying commonality in the spiritual beliefs of my patient and my own beliefs that would allow me to participate in this religious ritual? Would it be therapeutic or damaging to this nurse–patient relationship if I participated in this ritual? Usually, the ritual is not harmful. And usually a nurse and patient have some fundamental commonality in their beliefs that would allow a nurse to authentically participate in a ritual. Furthermore, patients who invite their nurse to participate in a ritual are usually deeply grateful when the nurse does participate (Taylor, 2001; Taylor, 2002a).

Being Caring

Although being caring may appear to be a simpleton's suggestion for enhancing SpQOL, it is not easy given current health care system stressors and given the psycho-spiritually challenging work of oncology nursing. Findings from a qualitative study of cancer patients' and family caregivers' (n = 28) perspectives on how a nurse can provide spiritual care support this approach (Taylor, 2002b). When asked how a nurse could help them with their spiritual needs, these informants almost invariably first replied with statements like "just be nice," "it's the little things," "show care and concern," or "a smile does a lot."

These informants also described how they wanted to have a degree of connectedness with their nurse. Symmetry (e.g., "I want her to not be my nurse, but be my friend"), physical presence (e.g., "just stay for a few minutes"), and authenticity (e.g., "Be genuine . . . if you're talking and connecting [with the nurse], it's a spiritual thing") were all important desired aspects of the nurse–patient relationship (Taylor, 2002b). These statements underscore what chaplains and spiritual care nurse experts have often espoused: spiritual care is ultimately about *being*, not *doing*.

Considering the spiritual need for connectedness with others who sincerely care, cancer nurses will promote patient SpQOL when they:

- Develop and use empathic listening skills
- Use full or transcendent presencing (when the nurse is present to the client not only physically, but emotionally and spiritually)
- Use appropriate nonprocedural, caring touch while maintaining an attitude of genuine care
- Explore personal barriers that may prevent personal warmth and concern
- Take measures to prevent work burnout
- Purposely nurture personal spiritual health.

Nurses are a very significant factor in determining the degree to which a patient's environment is a healing one. Showing authentic care and compassion is elemental to creating a healing environment.

Empirically Investigating Spiritual Quality of Life

Studying any concept presents challenges. Studying SpQOL is no exception. Whether investigating SpQOL qualitatively or quantitatively, the researcher must address certain challenges to enhance the credibility of study findings. A few of these challenges are described and several instruments for quantifying SpQOL are presented.

Qualitative Research

Issues that pertain especially to qualitative research exploring SpQOL are confusion about terminology, cultural bias, and social desirability. Not only do professionals confuse religiosity with spirituality, but laypersons do so as well. While asking about spiritual well-being, for example, informants may limit their responses to include only descriptions of personal religiosity. Even for informants who can distinguish spirituality from religiosity, it is often difficult for them to identify what comprises the spiritual domain. Concepts such as meaning in life and transcendence are complex to think about, let alone put into language.

The interviewer is essentially the instrument for collecting data during a qualitative study. The researcher[s] who designs the study and analyzes the data, likewise, personally influences the research process. Those who conduct qualitative research about SpQOL are especially prone to coloring their findings with their cultural backgrounds. A white, educated, Christian researcher will inevitably design, use language, and interpret data through these culturally colored lenses. Trustworthiness of findings will depend on the researcher's openness, flexibility, and ability to recognize and control personal biases. Getting informants' feedback on preliminary analyses of data may be especially helpful when the researcher and informant represent significantly different cultural or religious backgrounds.

Although social desirability plagues much social research, it may be a special threat to research about SpQOL. For many, recognizing spiritual distress or concerns is very disconcerting personally and/or socially embarrassing. A sensitive, respectful interviewer's prolonged engagement may allow an informant to verbalize such private spiritual pain.

Quantitative Research

During the 1990s, several instruments were developed to measure quality of life with subscales that recognized the spiritual domain. These subscales are summarized in Table 5-3. While McMillan and Weitzner's (2000) and Ferrans and Powers' (1992) subscales combine the spiritual domain with other psychosocial quality of life concerns, the Cella/Fitchett (Brady, Peterman, Fitchett et al., 1996), McGill (Cohen, Mount, Tomas et al., 1996), World Health Organization (Brady et al., 1996), and Ferrell and colleagues' (Ferrell, Grant, Funk et al., 1998) quality of life instruments all include a subscale dedicated to spiritual well-being.

During the past two decades, dozens of quantitative measures for assessing spirituality or aspects of spirituality and religiosity have been developed by social scientists and health care professionals. These instruments measure concepts as diverse as purpose in life, hope, mysticism, daily spiritual experience, prayer experience, religious beliefs and practices, spiritual or religious coping, and forgiveness. Some of these tools may measure a concept similar to SpQOL, spiritual well-being (Brady et al., 1999).

As Table 5-2 illustrates, the gold standard thus far in social research, for measuring spiritual well-being has been the 20-item Spiritual Well-Being scale developed by Paloutzian and Ellison (Ellison, 1983). This scale has been used in over 300 studies.

Table 5-3.   Subscales Measuring Spiritual Quality of Life

Authors/Instrument/ Subscale Title	Basic Descriptors	Examples of Content for Items
Fitchett et al. (1996) and Cella (1997) (in Cotton et al., 1999)/ Functional Assessment of Chronic Illness Therapy (FACIT)/FACIT– Spirituality	• 12 items • 2 subscales: meaning/peace and faith • internal consistency Cronbach alpha = 0.87	• Having a reason for living • Finding purpose or meaing in life • Finding strength or comfort in faith • Effect of illness on faith
Cohen, Mount, Tomas, & Mount (1996)/ McGill Quality of Life Questionnaire (MQOL)/ MQOL Existential Well-being	• 6 items with 10-point response options • Cronbach alpha = 0.87	• Existence meaningful • Achieve goals • Life worthwhile • Control over life • Like self • Every day a gift
Ferrell & Grant (e.g., in Ferrell et al., 1998)/ Quality of Life-Spiritual Well-being	• 7 items with 10-point response options • Cronbach alpha = 0.71	• Feelings of hopefulness • Sense of purpose • Positive changes because of illness • Spiritual life changed • Importance of church or temple • Importance of meditation or praying • Uncertainty about the future
McMillan (in McMillan and Weitzner, 2000)/ Hospice Quality of Life Index/HQLI social/spiritual domain	• 8 items, some of which may be tangential to spirituality • 0–10-point response options • Cronbach alpha between 0.82 and 0.86	• Meaning in life • Spiritual support from health care team • Support from family and friends • Emotional support • Relationship with God (however defined)

Table 5-3. **(continued)**

Authors/Instrument/ Subscale Title	Basic Descriptors	Examples of Content for Items
Ferrans & Powers (1992)/ Quality of Life Index (QLI)/ Psychological/Spiritual domain	• Factor analysis confirmed four domains, including 7 items reflecting emotional and spiritual concerns • 6-point response scales • original testing done with dialysis patients • Cronbach alpha for this subscale = 0.90	• Satisfaction with life • Happiness in general • Satisfaction with self • Achievement of personal goals • Peace of mind • Personal faith in God • Personal appearance

The scale consists of two subscales: the "vertical" dimension (i.e., how one relates to God) is measured by religious well-being (RWB); and the "horizontal" dimension of spirituality (or how well one relates to self, community, and environment) is measured by the existential well-being subscale (EWB). The RWB items all use the term "God," which can be problematic for the less than 10% of Americans who avow they do not believe in a "God" (Poloma & Gallup, 1991). Each subscale contains 10 items with 6-point Likert response options. Satisfactory psychometric properties have been observed when the tool was used with cancer patients. Permission to use the SWB can be addressed to Life Advance, Inc., 81 Front St., Nyack, NY 10960.

Summary

This literature review provides overdue recognition for a domain of HRQOL that is extremely important to persons with cancer. Spirituality, an interior and integrative aspect of human life, contributes fundamentally to overall HRQOL. Oncology nurses, therefore, must provide spiritual care in clinical arenas that cultivates SpQOL. Also, oncology nurse researchers must investigate further what promotes SpQOL and how nurses can effectively nurture spiritual well-being.

REFERENCES

Ayele, H., Mulligan, T., Gheorghiu, S., & Reyes-Ortiz, C. (1999). Religious activity improves life satisfaction for some physicians and older patients. *Journal of the American Geriatrics Society, 47*, 453–455.

Ballard, A., Green, T., McCaa, A., & Logsdon, M. C. (1997). A comparison of the level of hope in patients with newly diagnosed and recurrent cancer. *Oncology Nursing Forum, 24,* 899–904.

Brady, M. J., Peterman, A. H., Fitchett, G., Mo, M., & Cella, D. (1999). A case for including spirituality in quality of life measurement in oncology. *Psycho-Oncology, 8,* 417–428.

Breetvelt, I. S., & Van Dam, F. S. A. M. (1991). Underreporting by cancer patients: The case of response-shift. *Social Science and Medicine, 32*(9), 981–987.

Burkhardt, M. A., & Nagai-Jacobson, M. G. (2002). *Spirituality: Living our connectedness.* Albany, NY: Delmar.

Cohen, M. Z., Headley, J., & Sherwood, G. (2000). Spirituality and bone marrow transplantation: When faith is stronger than fear. *International Journal for Human Caring, 4*(2), 40–46.

Cohen, S. R., Mount, B. M., Tomas, J. J. N., & Mount, L. F. (1996). Existential well-being is an important determinant of quality of life. *Cancer, 77,* 576–586.

Cotton, S. P, Levine, E. G., Fitzpatrick, C. M., Dold, K. H., & Targ, E. (1999). Exploring the relationships among spiritual well-being, quality of life, and psychosocial adjustment in women with breast cancer. *Psycho-Oncology, 8,* 429–438.

Coward, D. D. (1990). The lived experience of self-transcendence in women with advanced breast cancer. *Nursing Science Quarterly, 3*(4), 162–169.

Dossey, B. M., & Guzzetta, C. E. (2000). Holistic nursing practice (Chapter 1). In B. M. Dossey, L. Keegan, and C. E. Guzzetta (Eds.), *Holistic nursing: A handbook for practice* (3rd ed.). pp. 5–26. Rockville, MD: Aspen.

Eisenberg, D. M., Kessler, R. C., Foster, C., Norlock, F. E., Calkins, D. R., & Delbanco, T. L. (1993). Unconventional medicine in the United States: Prevalence, costs, and patterns of use. *New England Journal of Medicine, 328,* 246–252.

Ellison, C. W. (1983). Spiritual well-being: Conceptualization and measurement. *Journal of Psychology and Theology, 11,* 330–340.

Ersek, M., Ferrell, B. R., Dow, K. H., & Melancon, C. H. (1997). Quality of life in women with ovarian cancer. *Western Journal of Nursing Research, 19*(3), 334–350.

Fehring, R. J., Miller, J. F., & Shaw, C. (1997). Spiritual well-being, religiosity, hope, depression, and other mood states in elderly people coping with cancer. *Oncology Nursing Forum, 24,* 663–671.

Feher, S., & Maly, R. C. (1999). Coping with breast cancer in later life: The role of religious faith. *Psychooncology, 8,* 408–416.

Fernsler, J. I., Klemm, P., & Miller, M. A. (1999). Spiritual well-being and demands of illness in people with colorectal cancer. *Cancer Nursing, 22,* 134–140.

Ferrans, C. E. (2000). Quality of life as an outcome of cancer care (Chapter 12). In C. H. Yarbro, M. H. Frogge, M. Goodman, & S. L. Groenwald (Eds.), *Cancer Nursing: Principles and practice* (5th ed.). Sudbury, MA: Jones and Bartlett.

Ferrans, C. E., & Powers, M. (1992). Psychometric assessment of the Quality of Life Index. *Research in Nursing and Health, 15*(1), 29–38.

Ferrell, B. R., Dow, K. H., Leigh, S., Ly, J., & Gulasekaram, P. (1995). Quality of life in long-term cancer survivors. *Oncology Nursing Forum, 22*, 915–922.

Ferrell, B. R., Grant, M. M., Funk, B., Otis-Green, S., & Garcia, N. (1998a). Quality of life in breast cancer survivors: Implications for developing support services. *Oncology Nursing Forum, 25*, 887–895.

Ferrell, B. R., Grant, M., Funk, B., Otis-Green, S., & Garcia, N. (1998b). Quality of life in breast cancer: Part II: Psychological and spiritual well-being. *Cancer Nursing, 21*(1), 1–9.

Fitch, M. I., Gray, R. E., & Franssen, E. (2001). Perspectives on living with ovarian cancer: Older women's views. *Oncology Nursing Forum, 28*, 1433–1442.

Frankl, V. (1984). *Man's search for meaning.* New York: Washington Square Press.

Gioiella, M. E., Berkman, B., & Robinson, M. (1998). Spirituality and quality of life in gynecologic oncology patients. *Cancer Practice, 6*, 333–338.

Griesinger, A. J., Lorimor, R. J., Aday, L. A., Winn, R. J., & Baile, W. F. (1997). Terminally ill cancer patients: Their most important concerns. *Cancer Practice, 5*, 147–154.

Halstead, M. T., & Fernsler, J. I. (1994). Coping strategies of long-term cancer survivors. *Cancer Nursing, 17*, 94–100.

Herth, K. (1990). Fostering hope in terminally-ill people. *Journal of Advanced Nursing, 15*, 1250–1259.

Highfield, M. F. (1992). Spiritual health of oncology patients: Nurse and patient perspectives. *Cancer Nursing, 15*(1), 1–8.

Joint Commission on Accreditation for Health Care Organizations. (2000). *Hospital accreditation standards.* Oakbrook, IL: Author.

Kaczorowski, J. M. (1989). Spiritual well-being and anxiety in adults diagnosed with cancer. *Hospice Journal, 5*(3/4), 105–116.

Kylma, J., Vehvilainen, J. K., & Julkunen, K. (1997). Hope in nursing research: A meta-analysis of the ontological and epistemological foundations of research on hope. *Journal of Advanced Nursing, 25*, 364–371.

Martsolf, D. S., & Mickley, J. R. (1998). The concept of spirituality in nursing theories: Differing world-views and extent of focus. *Journal of Advanced Nursing, 27*, 294–303.

McMillan, S. C., & Weitzner, M. (2000). How problematic are various aspects of quality of life in patients with cancer at the end of life? *Oncology Nursing Forum, 27*, 817–823.

McMillan, S. C., & Weitzner, M. (1998). Quality of life in cancer patients: Use of a revised hospice index. *Cancer Practice, 6,* 282–288.

Mickley, J. R., Soeken, K., & Belcher, A. (1992). Spiritual well-being, religiousness, and hope among women with breast cancer. *Image, 24,* 267–272.

Miller, J. F. (1985). Assessment of loneliness and spiritual well-being in chronically ill and healthy adults. *Journal of Professional Nursing, 1*(2), 79–85.

Pargament, K. I. (1997). *The psychology of religion and coping.* New York: Guilford.

Peteet, J. R. (1985). Religious issues presented by cancer patients seen in psychiatric consultation. *Journal of Psychosocial Oncology, 3*(1) 53–66.

Poloma, M. M., & Gallup, G.H., Jr. (1991). *Varieties of prayer: A survey report.* Philadelphia, PA: Trinity Press International.

Post-White, J., Ceronsky, C., Kreitzer, M. J., Nickelson, K., Drew, D., Mackey, K. W., Koopmeiners, L., & Gutknecht, S. (1996). Hope, spirituality, sense of coherence and quality of life in patients with cancer. *Oncology Nursing Forum, 23,* 1571–1579.

Reed, P. G. (1992). An emerging paradigm for the investigation of spirituality in nursing. *Research in Nursing and Health, 15,* 349–357.

Reed, P. G. (1991). Preferences for spiritually related nursing interventions among terminally ill and nonterminally ill hospitalized adults and well adults. *Applied Nursing Research, 4,* 122–128.

Riley, B. B., Perna, R., Tate, D., Forchheimer, M., Anderson, C., & Luera, G. (1998). Types of spiritual well-being among persons with chronic illness: Their relation to various forms of quality of life. *Archives of Physical Medicine and Rehabilitation, 79,* 258–264.

Saleh, U. S., & Brockopp, D. Y. (2001). Quality of life one year following bone marrow transplantation: Psychometric evaluation of the Quality of Life Bone Marrow Transplant Survivors Tool. *Oncology Nursing Forum, 28,* 1457–1464.

Sodestrom, K. E., & Martinson, I. M. (1987). Patients' spiritual coping strategies: A study of nurse and patient perspectives. *Oncology Nursing Forum, 14*(2), 41–45.

Sparber, A, Bauer, L, Curt, G., Eisenberg, D, Levin, T., Parks, S., Steinberg, S. M., &Wootton, J. (2000). Use of complementary medicine by adult patients participating in cancer clinical trials. *Oncology Nursing Forum, 27,* 623–632.

Stephenson, C. (1991). The concept of hope revisited for nursing. *Journal of Advances in Nursing, 16,* 1456–1461.

Taylor, E. J. (2002a). *Spiritual care: Nursing theory, research, and practice.* Upper Saddle River, NJ: Prentice Hall.

Taylor, E. J. (2002b). Nurses caring for the spirit: Cancer patient and family caregiver expectations. Podium presentation at the Oncology Nursing Society congress, April 18, 2002, Washington, DC.

Taylor, E. J. (unpublished). Spiritual needs of cancer patients and family caregivers. Research project funded by Oncology Nursing Society/Glaxo-Wellcome Small Research Grant.

Taylor, E. J. (2001). Spirituality, Culture, and Cancer Care. *Seminars in Oncology Nursing, 17*(3), 197–205.

Taylor, E. J. (2000). Transformation of tragedy among women surviving breast cancer. *Oncology Nursing Forum, 27,* 781–788.

Taylor, E. J., & Outlaw, F. H. (2002). Use of Prayer Among Persons with Cancer. *Holistic Nursing Practice, 16*(3), 46–60.

Thomson, J. E. (2000). The place of spiritual well-being in hospice patient's overall quality of life. *Hospice Journal, 15*(2), 13–27.

VandeCreek, L., Rogers, E., & Lester, J. (1999). Use of alternative therapies among breast cancer outpatients compared with the general population. *Alternative Therapies in Health and Medicine, 5*(1), 71–76.

Violanti, J. M., Paton, D., & Dunning, C. (Eds.). (2000). *Posttraumatic stress intervention.* Springfield, IL: C. C. Thomas.

Wismer, P. (1995). For women in pain: A feminist theology of suffering. In A. O. Graff (Ed.), *In the Embrace of God: Feminist approaches to theological anthropology.* Maryknoll, NY: Orbis Books.

Wyatt, G., & Friedman, L. L. (1996). Long-term female cancer survivors: Quality of life issues and clinical implications. *Cancer Nursing, 19,* 1–7.

Yates, J. W., Chalmer, B. J., St. James, P., Follansbee, M., & McKegney, F. P. (1981). Religion in patients with advanced cancer. *Medical and Pediatric Oncology, 9,* 121–128.

6

Quality of Life and Culture

GERALDINE V. PADILLA

Increasing cultural/ethnic diversity of people within the borders of all countries, the growing communication network around the globe, and the age-old problem of racial discrimination underscore the relevance of cross-cultural comparisons to better understand disparities in health status and quality of life (QOL). The weight of scientific evidence underscores the unequal burden of disease endured by ethnic minorities and by socioeconomically poorer countries and peoples. An exemplar is the case for HIV/AIDS. Karon and colleagues (2001) examined U.S. surveillance data on AIDS cases, particularly, after 1996 with the introduction of antiretroviral (HAART) treatment. Among other findings, they reported ". . . increasing proportions of HIV infections and disease in communities of color, especially African Americans; and unequal reductions in morbidity and mortality by race/ethnicity, gender, and socioeconomic status . . ." (p. 1060). Disparities in health outcome include health-related quality of life which is worse for ethnic minorities. The case of African American men with prostate cancer is a representative example. This population presents with worse clinical characteristics and poorer health-related quality of life (HRQOL) even after controlling for age, education, and income (Lubeck et al., 2001). Black men with prostate cancer who have recently completed treatment also experience poorer prostate-specific and general HRQOL (Eton et al., 2001). Disparities in health and QOL extend to other ethnic groups. For example, Gee (2002) reported that individual (perceived) and institutional (segregation and redlining) racial discrimination against Chinese Americans is associated with poorer health status and worse quality of life as measured by the MOS SF-36 and the Symptom Checklist 90. The investigator controlled for acculturation, sex, age, social support, income, health insurance, employment status, education, neighborhood poverty, and housing value.

   Cross-national studies are important because of the interest in multinational drug trials, multinational health care programs, international allocation of scarce resources, and the interest of scientists in crosscultural comparisons (Fox-Rushby & Parker, 1994).

Definitions of Quality of Life and Culture

The influence of culture on one's quality of life has often been overlooked, and when these concepts are used in relation to each other, they have eluded precise definition. Since culture, as described in this chapter, is a major determinant of quality of life it is important to clarify the meaning of culture in the context of quality of life.

Culture

Erroneously assumed to be interchangeable with race and ethnicity, the use of the term culture is further clouded by the restrictive application of the "other" label. That is, groups other than Western and European Americans are assumed to have cultures that interfere with access and use of western biomedicine. The lack of recognition of the influence of the values of the dominant American and northern European cultures on the concept of "quality of life" as currently measured has hindered its application abroad as well as in the United States among the multicultural and minority populations.

Culture is fundamental to human life. It serves two functions: it prescribes the ways of life for a group of people to ensure their survival and well-being, and it provides the beliefs and values that give life meaning and purpose (Kagawa-Singer & Blackhall, 2001; Kagawa-Singer & Chung, 1994; Orlandi, 1992; Spector, 1991). Every culture is designed to fulfil three universal needs: (1) safety and security, (2) a sense of integrity and meaning or purpose in life, and (3) a sense of belonging as an integral member of ones social network (Kagawa-Singer & Chung, 1994). Each culture, however, has a set of beliefs, values, and practices that are unique to each group's identity, and are usually not isomorphic with other cultural groups. Often many similarities exist between cultural groups, along with gradations of differences. For example, the influence and variations in Buddhism on the life ways across South, Southeast, and far East Asia or the variations in Christianity and its effects on cultures in the West and East.

Culture is not the same as ethnicity or race. Race is an antiquated, scientifically flawed concept that was assumed to identify genetically different groups of people (Hirschman, Alba, & Farley, 2000; Kagawa-Singer, 2001; Montagu, 1962, 1997). More differences exist genetically within groups than between. However, genetic variations do exist between groups, with particular genetic polymorphisms that occur more frequently in particular population groups, such as PD deficiency or Tay-Sachs disease. Race, understood as assumptions about group differences of character, behavior, and physiology, based on phenotypic characteristics, does affect QOL in the form of racism. Racism is the exertion of power and discriminatory action by particular groups against others based on these phenotypic differences. Health outcomes and differential care have been demonstrated to result from such beliefs and actions (Institute of Medicine, 2002).

Ethnicity is the relationship of multicultural groups within a particular power structure. Multicultural societies result in ethnic identification by members of groups for solidarity and assurance of their life ways and meaning in life when the three universal needs are threatened. Cultural and ethnic mores also specify the strategies that promote or maintain health and prevent disease or illness, and play an important role in times of crisis by helping members to understand and manage events that appear to be uncontrollable and unpredictable (Kagawa-Singer, 1995). Race also affects how individuals are able to access and utilize health care. As such, the quality of one's life is fundamentally influenced by ones cultural, ethnic, and racialized identity (Kagawa-Singer, 2001) and is a determinant of health-related QOL.

Culture defines "good" behavior, assures people a valued place in their social network, provides them with a purpose in life, and promotes their well-being (Kagawa-Singer & Chung, 1994). Cultural mores also specify the strategies that promote or maintain health and prevent disease or illness, and play an important role in times of crisis by helping members to understand and manage events that appear to be uncontrollable and unpredictable (Kagawa-Singer, 1995). Thus, culture is an important determinant of QOL since it defines the purpose of and prescriptions for living a meaningful life in sickness and in health.

Quality of Life and Health-related Quality of Life

Definitions of QOL abound in the literature but seldom mention culture. This omission is understandable, since culture/ethnicity are generally viewed as factors that shape the meaning of QOL, but are not attributes or dimensions of the construct. The Division of Mental Health of the World Health Organization (WHO) offers one of the few definitions that explicitly identifies culture as an important determinant of quality of life. The WHO defines QOL very broadly as people's ". . . perception of their position in life in the context of the culture and value systems in which they live and in relation to their goals, expectations, standards and concerns" (1993, p. 1). A broad definition seems preferable since QOL can mean different things to people of different cultural/ethnic backgrounds. A broad definition of QOL admits a diversity of meanings of well-being that can accommodate those cultures for which there is no direct translation of the concept of QOL. For example, the Japanese language has no direct equivalent for the English phrase, "quality of life" (Yoshida, 1985). Yet, the notion of QOL resonates with the Japanese who use the English phrase to express the feeling that life is worth living. In discussing health and illness in the context of QOL, Higuchi (1985, p. 89) emphasizes the importance of ". . . the patient's harmony with the world, with others, with himself, and with death" (p. 89). No English language measure of QOL captures the notion of harmony. Instead, the constructs of acceptance, adaptation, and adjustment are used in relation to disease and QOL.

Other explanations of HRQOL acknowledge the influence of culture by defining QOL in terms of personal perceptions of what it is about one's life that makes it worthwhile. For instance, Patrick and Erickson (1993) defined HRQOL as ". . . the value assigned to duration of life as modified by the impairments, functional states, perceptions and social opportunities influenced by disease, injury, treatment or policy" (p. 22). Perceptions and social opportunities occur in a cultural context. After reviewing the theoretical, clinical, and research literature concerning HRQOL, Shumaker and Naughton (1995) proposed the following definition: "Health-related quality of life refers to people's subjective evaluations of the influences of their current health status, health care, and health promoting activities on their ability to achieve and maintain a level of overall functioning that allows them to pursue valued life goals and that is reflected in their general well-being. The domains of functioning that are critical to HRQOL, include: social, physical and cognitive functioning; mobility and self-care; and emotional well-being" (p. 7). Culture is implied in the phrases, ". . . subjective evaluations of the influences of their current health status . . . that allows them to pursue valued life goals. . . ."

In August 1992, an international Advisory Board of experts (i.e., behavioral scientists and health care providers) met in North Carolina with the support of the Burroughs Wellcome Company and the Bowman Gray School of Medicine to discuss client-based measures of individual function, well-being, and satisfaction within the context of cross-cultural, clinical research. The Advisory Board, composed primarily of representatives of white Euro-American cultures from Canada, the United States, and western Europe, recognized that culture influences variations in perceptions of health and sickness, interpretations of symptoms, the meaning of quality of life, and expectations of care (Berzon & Shumaker, 1995). The Advisory Board turned its attention to the definition, measurement, and use of HRQOL in cross-national clinical trials. Considering cultural diversity in the conceptualization of HRQOL, four fundamental dimensions were identified: physical, mental/psychological, social, and global perceptions of function and well-being. Additional possible attributes were described as pain, energy/vitality, sleep, appetite, and symptoms associated with the disease or treatment (Berzon & Shumaker, 1995).

Two investigators who were not part of the international Advisory Board of experts, Parker and Fox-Rushby (1995), believe that it is inappropriate to assume that dimensions of health are identical or comparable across cultures. They question ". . . whether it is appropriate to assume that there is a cultural universality in the definition of HRQOL, and whether the research methods used to date have been capable of unearthing universal dimensions of HRQOL" (p. 154). For example, participants at the 1984 WHO conference on QOL held in Tokyo (Yoshida, 1985) spent a great deal of time attempting to reach consensus on a QOL definition and struggling with an appropriate translation of quality of life into Japanese since an equivalent concept did not exist in that language. In a study of Japanese-American and Anglo-American cancer clients, Kagawa-Singer (1988) found that instruments standardized in the Anglo-American culture did not measure the cultural differences between the groups in the conceptualization and meaning of QOL. However, ethnographic interviews showed that clients from both cultures viewed a life of quality as one that enabled them to maintain their sense of self-integrity and continue to fulfill their role responsibilities; yet, these views of life quality were interpreted according to their own cultural background. For example, Japanese Americans viewed side effects of treatment as expected outcomes to be endured; while Anglo Americans perceived side effects as problems to be eliminated/overcome (Kagawa-Singer, 1993).

An aspect of QOL gaining in support and which may be useful cross-culturally is the dimension of existential/spiritual well-being (Brady et al., 1999; Kaczorowski, 1989; Reed, 1987; Tuck, McCain, & Elswick, 2001). This dimension refers to the meaning that disease and treatment impart to one's life, feelings of hope/despair, personal beliefs about the value of life, religiosity, and inner strength (Ferrell et al., 1992). This dimension may capture cultural elements of quality of life better than other recognized attributes of HRQOL. The conditions that give meaning to life, that provide a reason for living are not just personal, but cultural (Kashiwagi, 1985; Taylor, 2001). Culturally based values about the relationship between life and death and health and illness are at the heart of QOL assessments. Finding meaning in one's state of ill health, may be perceived cross-culturally as essential to maintaining quality of life, yet the conditions that bestow meaning may be very different or even contradictory across cultures. Thus, Kagawa-Singer proposed a transcultural framework of QOL that is heuristic in its focus on fulfillment of role responsibilities. Within Kagawa-Singer's (1988) heuristic framework, the broad domains of quality of life address the need for safety and security (i.e., food, shelter, clothing, physical comfort), a sense of integrity and meaning or purpose in one's life (i.e., perceiving oneself to be a contributing member of one's group), and a sense of belonging (i.e., connection to others).

Issues in the Definition of HRQOL

Shumaker and Naughton (1995) identified some issues surrounding the construct, HRQOL. One issue concerns the distinction between QOL and HRQOL. Quality of life is a subjective, multidimensional experience that involves a summary evaluation of the positive and negative attributes that characterize one's life (Padilla, Grant, Ferrell, & Presant, 1996). It is a dynamic construct affected by one's ability to adapt to discrepancies between expected and experienced well-being (Padilla, Grant, Ferrell, & Presant, 1996), as well as one's ability to maintain an overall level of functioning that allows the individual to pursue valued life goals (Shumaker & Naughton, 1995). Quality of life is also reflected in general well-being (Shumaker & Naughton, 1995). HRQOL means that the summary evaluation of attributes that characterize one's life is made at a point in time when health, illness, and treatment conditions are relevant (Padilla, Grant, Ferrell, & Presant, 1996). The relevant characteristics of a healthy person's QOL may not include physical, emotional, or biomedically defined health, but rather social relationships, financial success, and a satisfying job. On the other hand, a person whose health is threatened by acute or chronic illness will likely attribute certain dimensions of life quality to the influence of health problems, health status, health care, and health-promoting activities.

The definition of health in the context of quality of life should not be limited to the biomedical model of physiologic integrity or to the WHO model (1946) of absence of disease and complete physical, mental, and emotional well-being. Instead, health should be viewed in the context of self-integrity along the dimensions of physical status and social function (Kagawa-Singer, 1993). Thus, persons with cancer can maintain a sense of self-integrity and perceive themselves as healthy along the social functioning dimension even as they acknowledge the effects of the disease and treatment on their physical status (Kagawa-Singer, 1993).

A second issue concerns the distinction between determinants (predictors) and dimensions (attributes) of HRQOL (Shumaker & Naughton, 1995; Stewart, 1992; Strickland, 1992). The lack of a distinction between determinants and dimensions of HRQOL in definitions of the construct leads to conceptual and operational confusion. For example, pain is identified as a symptom of cancer or side effect of treatment that has an impact on QOL. At the same time, evaluations of pain distress, intensity, and frequency are used as a basis for QOL scores. Generally, pain should not be treated as both the cause and effect. The distinction between predictors and attributes is important to future understanding of interventions that can maintain or improve HRQOL in persons with acute or chronic illness. What attributes of HRQOL are most salient to ill people? How do these characteristics differ between people of different cultural orientations? What aspects of culture are most likely to affect

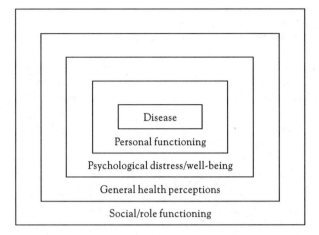

Figure 6-1.   **Ware model of the progressive relationship between disease and quality of life domains.**

Source: Ware, J. E., Jr. (1984). Methodology in behavioral and psychological cancer research. Conceptualizing disease impact and treatment outcomes. *Cancer, 53 (10 Suppl),* 2316–2326.

elements of HRQOL? These questions are associated with the third issue discussed next regarding models and measures.

The distinction between conceptual models and measures of HRQOL is the third concern expressed in the literature (Shumaker & Naughton, 1995). At issue is the kind of relationship that exists between determinants and dimensions of HRQOL. How specific are these relationships? Are current HRQOL instruments able to measure these relationships? For example, do the instruments include the specific dimensions of QOL (e.g., perceived physical/psychological support from family/friends) that can be affected by the predictors (e.g., network of actual social resources)? Keeping in mind that investigators are constantly revising their models of HRQOL as they learn more about the construct, the models described here are illustrations of different ways of viewing the relationships between determinants and dimensions of HRQOL.

The model proposed by Ware in 1984 (Figure 6-1) suggests that disease has its most immediate impact on personal functioning, then psychological distress/well-being, followed by general health perceptions and social/role functioning. Should HRQOL dimensions that reflect these factors be weighted accordingly? In contrast, the model proposed by Ferrell and colleagues in 1991 (Figure 6-2) conceptualizes pain from cancer and its treatment as having an independent impact on the HRQOL dimensions of physical well-being and symptoms, psychological, social, and spiritual well-being. In 1985, Padilla and Grant included a number of process, mediating

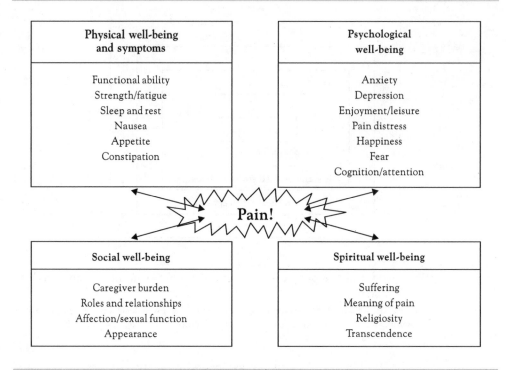

Figure 6-2.　**Ferrell, Grant, Padilla, Vemuri, & Rhiner model of relationship between pain and dimensions of quality of life.**
Source: Ferrell, B. R., Grant, M., Padilla, G., Vemuri, S., Rhiner, M. (1991). The experience of pain and perceptions of quality of life: Validation of a conceptual model. *Hospice Journal, 7*(3), 9–24. Fig. 2. p. 21.

cognitive, extraneous, and HRQOL outcome variables in their model (Figure 6-3). The relationships between process or mediating or extraneous variables to HRQOL outcomes are specific. For example, extraneous variables concerning diagnosis (e.g., stage of cancer) are predicted to have their most immediate impact on physical well-being and the diagnosis/treatment response. On the other hand, implementing the nursing process (e.g., colostomy care) has a direct impact on body image concerns surrounding the colostomy as well as on physical well-being. Padilla and colleagues' model includes examples of the kinds of measures required and predicts the specific relationships between determinants and dimensions of HRQOL. The 1996 Spilker model (Figure 6-4) illustrates how medical treatments can result in adverse reactions (safety measures), benefits (efficacy measures), and costs (other measures). These in turn are filtered through the client's belief and value structure before affecting QOL domains.

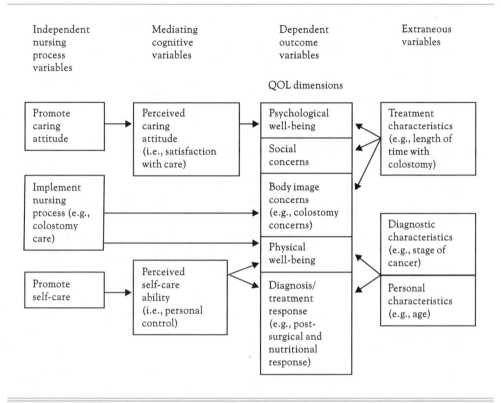

Figure 6-3. **Padilla and Grant model of nursing process and quality of life outcomes.**

Source: Padilla, G. V., & Grant, M. M. (1985). Quality of life as a cancer nursing outcome variable. *Advances in Nursing Science*, 8(1), 45–60, Fig. 1. p. 53.

In 1999, Sprangers and Schwartz proposed a theoretical model of response shift and HRQOL (Figure 6-5). Response shift concerns an alteration in the meaning of one's assessment of a construct because of a change in ones: (a) internal standards of measurement concerning the construct (i.e., scale recalibration); (b) values relative to the construct (i.e., the relative worth of aspects of one's life in relation to the construct); or (c) definition of the construct (i.e., reconceptualization of the construct)(see also Schwartz & Sprangers, 1999). The theoretical model of response shift and QOL includes five components. A catalyst such as a diagnosis of cancer activates behavioral, cognitive, or affective mechanisms. These mechanisms may include goal reordering or reframing of expectations or other accommodation processes that are used to adjust to the catalyst. Successful accommodation mechanisms result in a response shift, or a change in ones internal standards, values, or conceptualizations.

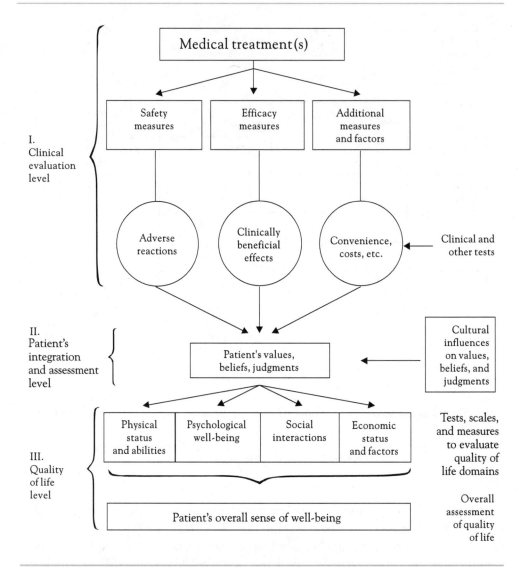

Figure 6-4.   **Spilker model of clinical evaluation, integration/assessment, and quality of life.**

Source: Spilker, B. (1996). Introduction. In Spilker, B. (Ed.), *Quality of Life and Pharmacoeconomics in Clinical Trials* (pp. 1–10). New York: Lippincott-Raven. Fig. 2, p. 6.

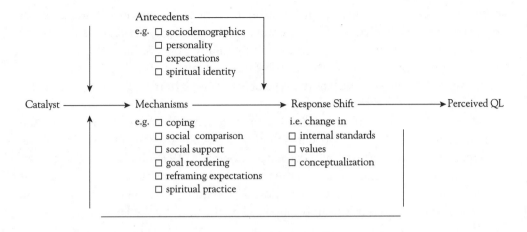

Figure 6-5. **Sprangers and Schwartz theoretical model of response shift and quality of life (QOL).**

Source: Sprangers, M. A. G., & Schwartz, C. E. (1999). Integrating response shift into health-related quality of life research: A theoretical model. *Social Science and Medicine, 48,* 1507–1515, Fig. 1. Reprinted with permission from Elsevier Science.

Response shift permits the individual to maintain or improve HRQOL despite the catalytic negative change in health status. The relationships between the catalyst and accommodation mechanisms and response shift can be affected by antecedent factors such as sociodemographics (e.g., age), personality (e.g., optimism), expectations, and spiritual identity.

The Spilker model is the only one of the five examples that explicitly accommodates cultural determinants of HRQOL outcomes. However, the other four models do not exclude cultural considerations. The Ware model (Figure 6-1) assumes that there exists a specific progression of immediacy and intensity of the impact of disease. In fact, the progression of disease impact may be different across cultures. In some cultures the impact of disease may be greater on social/role functioning than on general health perceptions. Ferrell & colleagues' (1991) model (Figure 6-2) suggests that the disease experience is separate from other human responses in cause-and-effect order. Other cultures may conceptualize disease as an integral part of the whole human response to life events. Thus, the disease experience may be perceived as less central to life's quality. The issues raised concerning the Ware (Figure 6-1) and Ferrell and colleagues (Figure 6-2) models can also be applied to the Padilla and Grant (Figure 6-3) model. In addition, the Padilla and Grant framework reduces QOL responses to specific antecedents that may or may not be relevant across cultures. The Sprangers and Schwartz model (Figure 6-5) conceptualizes the disease experience as the trigger that starts an accommodation process resulting in a response shift. Culture is an important determinant of the impact of the catalyst. Culture also shapes expectations concerning the catalyst, as well as the type of accommodation mechanisms to be used, and the nature of the response shift.

As investigators continue to develop their frameworks of HRQL, including the authors of the models described here, there is a more consistent recognition of the influence of culture. For example, Patrick and Bergner (1990) included culture as an environmental factor that influences the chain of effects from disease and impairment to opportunity for health. Federal policy that requires the inclusion of women, minorities, and children in research supported by the U.S. Public Health Service and U.S. Military (*http://www.washingtonfax.com/p1/frarchive.html*) has played a very important role in the growing attention to cultural/ethnic factors in all research conducted in the United States.

A broad, flexible definition of QOL can accommodate diverse cultural orientations toward well-being, life, death, health, and illness. However, in translating broad, conceptual definitions into predictive models of HRQOL, it is important to consider the cause-and-effect fit between determinants and dimensions of HRQOL within and across cultural groups. For example, one might predict a similar effect of disease on physical function in Hispanics and Anglos. However, it might be important to add belief in fate to predict the effect of disease severity on perceived distress in Hispanics as compared to Anglos, and degree of threat to one's sense of control for Anglos compared to Hispanics.

Comparability of Quality of Life Across Cultures

Relevance and Usefulness of Cross-cultural Comparisons

Examining a concept such as HRQOL across cultures helps the scientist and clinician to better understand the construct and its utility for particular groups. The cultural context of cancer risk factors, prevention/intervention strategies, and treatment-related outcomes affects HRQOL responses. For example, cigarettes may be more relevant to economic and social well-being in some cultures as compared to others (Jenkins et al., 1997). An ostensibly objective measure such as physical function can be perceived differently by different cultures (Folmar, 1995). For example, a measure such as the Activities of Daily Living (ADL) Scale is culturally biased and needs to be recast to fit the way in which functional ability is interpreted by different cultural/ethnic groups (Beall & Eckert, 1986). The Kagawa-Singer (1993) study of ADL in Japanese and Anglo American male and female cancer clients is particularly revealing. She found that Anglo men and Japanese women experienced more ADL disruption due to cancer than Japanese men and Anglo women. The ADL scores could be interpreted in light of interview data relevant to cultural expectations of the Anglo males and Japanese females. While chemotherapy, surgery, or radiation therapy to treat cancer can be standardized across countries, the meaning of cancer and its treatment in terms of life's quality differs across cultures.

Cross-culturally appropriate and valid measures of HRQOL are necessary before cross-national/cross-cultural studies can proceed, as noted by Parker and Fox-Rushby (1995) who caution that generic instruments of HRQOL are essentially culture-bound instruments. Measures tended to be biased in the direction of the culture in which they were developed and tested. The process of translation, back-translation, and review may not be sufficient to ensure a cross-culturally sensitive measure if the assumptions that led to the development of the instrument in the original version are not challenged. Parker and Fox-Rushby believed that it is inappropriate to assume that dimensions of health are identical or comparable across cultures. They cautioned that most generic instruments of HRQOL were developed in the United States or western Europe where health, well-being, individuality, and autonomy are linked. However, this may not be the case in non-western cultures. Numerous studies in end-of-life care demonstrate that values about life or about sustaining life are not universal (Blackhall et al., 1999; Kagawa-Singer & Blackhall, 2001). Thus, development of cross-culturally valid instruments is essential.

Conceptual and Operational Equivalence of HRQOL

As discussed, HRQOL is not an equivalent concept across cultures nor are the individual dimensions equivalent. Cross-cultural studies of HRQOL can only be undertaken when researchers achieve equivalence of instruments to measure HRQOL (Hui & Triandis, 1985; Meadows, 1994). *Conceptual* (functional) equivalence means that the content of a measure should carry the same connotation across the different cultural groups being measured. *Operational* equivalence means that the measure should have content, semantic, technical, scalar/metric, and criterion equivalence across cultural groups.

- *Content equivalence*—the same information is covered and is equally representative for the different cultural groups.
- *Semantic equivalence*—the different language versions of the instrument should agree.

- *Technical equivalence*—the procedure for administration, scaling, scoring, length, time to completion, etc. should be the same across groups.

- *Scalar or metric equivalence*—the measure is able to rank order persons from different language or cultural groups in equivalent ways.

- *Criterion equivalence*—the standard against which the measure is compared should be the same across groups.

Translations of English questionnaires into other languages have attempted to achieve, at the very least, operational equivalence. However, this level of equivalence is inadequate for cross-cultural comparisons. Cross-cultural conceptual equivalence is essential. A useful strategy for arriving at operational equivalence was demonstrated by Hendricson and colleagues (1989) who translated the Arthritis Impact Measurement Scale for use in a South Texas population. For each item, the Spanish translation was printed alongside the English version. This format made it easy to see and compare content, semantic, technical, and criterion equivalence. It also made it easier for bicultural and bilingual focus groups to evaluate conceptual equivalence. The domains of the instrument applied to both Spanish- and English-speaking groups. The three basic strategies used to achieve conceptual and operational equivalence across cultures include sequential, parallel, and simultaneous development approaches (Bullinger, Anderson, Cella, & Aaronson, 1995). These are described in Table 6-1. Minimal requirements for cross-cultural translations and validation of HRQOL measures involve translation, psychometric, sample size, procedural, and testing criteria (Table 6-2).

Issues in Cross-Cultural Research in Quality of Life

Role of Acculturation

Acculturation means learning the beliefs, values, and standards of behavior of another cultural group to function comfortably in that group, typically the dominant culture, and, in the case of immigrants—the host culture. Assimilation means taking on the beliefs, values, and practices of the host culture and giving up those of one's own native culture. Most individuals tend to acculturate to varying degrees without assimilating to the host culture. Acculturation can modify the significance of any of the variables listed in Table 6-3 that contribute to disparities in disease incidence and mortality between ethnic groups. A common conceptualization of acculturation is comprised of domains such as one's preferred language, self-identity, friendship choices that determine social boundaries, standards of acceptable behavior, genera-

Table 6-1. **Strategies for Developing Cross-Cultural HRQOL* Measures**

Sequential	Translate an HRQOL instrument developed in one language into another language.
Parallel	Use an international (cross-cultural) team to conceptualize HRQOL and construct new items and/or select items from existing scales that reflect within the same item pool the HRQOL in different nations (cultures).
Simultaneous	Use an interactive approach to construct a new HRQOL instrument that subsumes the specific contents and assessment strategies of each participating nation (culture). The HRQOL instrument will include cross-culturally universal dimensions of the construct as well as culture-specific components.

Source: Based on Bullinger et al., 1995. Used with permission from Lippincott-Raven Publishers.

*HRQOL = Health-Related Quality of Life

Table 6-2. **Minimal Requirements for Cross-Cultural Translation and Validation of HRQOL* Measures**

Translation	Forward and backward translation in each language under study.
Psychometrics	Test of reliability, validity, and sensitivity in each country (culture) using appropriate comparison groups (e.g., healthy versus ill persons).
Sample size	A minimum of 100 persons per cultural group.
Procedure	A clear description of the number of translators (more than one), forward-backward translation process, evaluation process including critique by translators, focus group discussions, and response scaling for evaluation.
Design	A well-designed, common study protocol for use in different countries (cultures) such as in a multinational clinical trial.
Analysis	Innovative statistical procedures to evaluate international (cross-cultural) comparability.

Source: Based on Bullinger et al., 1995. Used with permission from Lippincott-Raven Publishers.

*HRQOL = Health-Related Quality of Life

Table 6-3. **Variables That Contribute to the Differences between Ethnic Populations in Disease Incidence and Mortality**

Physiological and Biochemical Differences
  Genetic differences
    Consanguinity
    Mutation rates
    Genetic predispositions or protective factors
  Environmental factors
    Exposure to toxic elements
    Dietary influences
  Exposure to infectious agents

Socioeconomic Factors
  Poverty
    Differential access to diagnostic facilities/medical treatments
    Work exposure to toxic elements
    Available, affordable healthy food in adequate quantities
    Educational base
      Knowledge about current treatment and adherence
      Value of early detection
    Discrimination
  Insurance (underinsured and uninsured)
  Costs of family and home care (direct and indirect)
    Shifts from hospital to home for semiacute and long-term care

Structural Aspects of the Health Care System
  Documentation
    Errors of measurement
    Completeness of morbidity and mortality data
    Lack of completeness and detail in coding categories
    Lack of representativeness in the ethnic samples
  Availability issues
    Lack of facilities within reasonable distances
    Lack of facilities that address cultural needs
  Accessibility (see Socioeconomic Factors)
  Practitioner/patient interactions
    Time restrictions in clinical encounters
    Clinic settings in which different doctors seen at each visit
    Focus only on chief complaint to detriment of other problems
    Institutional racism
    Insensitivity to needs/diseases of diverse ethnic groups

Cultural Factors for Patients and Practitioners
  Misconceptions concerning culture
  Acculturation and assimilation variation
  Acceptability of recommendation
  Differential use of available facilities

Table 6-3. **continued**

Culturally competent practitioners
Attitudes, beliefs, behaviors about illness/specific diseases
    Early detection
    Consequences of late diagnosis
    Treatment plans
    Role of health care practitioner
    Social stigma
Lifestyle differences in personal customs or habits
    Reproductive, nursing habits
    Sexual practices
    Smoking, alcohol, drug use, diet
Response to racism

Source: Based on Kagawa-Singer, 1995, p. 110. Copyright 1995 W. B. Saunders.

tion since family immigration to the host country, country of origin, and attitudes (willingness to behave in certain ways) (Suinn, Rickard-Figueroa, Lew, & Vigil, 1987). Acculturation is also defined by the length of residence, age at arrival in the host country, and by media influence (Marin et al., 1987). However, these last are less important indicators of HRQOL. To these lists Alarcon and colleagues (1999) expanded on language proficiency including usage and preferences, and added type of neighborhood. Hishinuma and colleagues (2000) measured Hawaiian acculturation as knowledge and practices about the Hawaiian way of life, valuation and maintenance of Hawaiian beliefs and non-Hawaiian beliefs, Hawaiian blood quantum, and specific cultural traditions using seven subscales (lifestyles, customs, activities, folklore, causes-locations, causes-access, and language proficiency).

It is important to note that people can acculturate without assimilating into the host culture. The ability to gain sufficient knowledge about a culture to transact easily within that culture does not necessarily mean that one gives up his/her original culture. In fact, an individual can belong to several cultural groups. An understanding of the influence of culture on HRQOL needs to consider ethnic affiliation as well as level of acculturation and assimilation into another, usually the host, culture (Berry and Kim, 1988; Oetting and Beauvais, 1990–91).

Knowledge of acculturation and assimilation provides insight into health-seeking attitudes of ethnic groups, reasons for success or failure of prevention and treatment regimens, ways to best reach diverse ethnic groups with health-related messages, and strategies for opening access to health care for ethnic groups (Padilla & Perez, 1995). Consequently, acculturation influences HRQOL, and may itself be a risk factor for illness (Kagawa-Singer, 1995). All cross-cultural studies need to include a measure of acculturation.

Reliability of Group Identification Labels

To more accurately assess the influence of culture on concepts of QOL, cross-cultural studies need to attend to the validity and reliability of cultural/ethnic or racial coding schemes. Coding schemes tend to identify broad categories of people by a mixture of racial, geographic, and ethnic labels. Typical coding categories in the United States are: White, Black (or African American), Asian, Pacific Islander, Hispanic (or Latino), and Native American. Like any classification scheme, there are errors in the manner in which these racial/ethnic codes are applied (Hahn, 1992). For example, a Latino may be classified as African American. Notably, these broad racial/ethnic categories are not culturally valid. For example, when it comes to reliance on the health care system, a recent West African immigrant to the United States is culturally very different from a middle class African American professional in Los Angeles whose heritage in the United States goes back to the African slaves over 400 years ago. Two first generation Asian Americans, one from the Philippines and one from Korea, are likewise different in beliefs and values about quality of life. Any coding scheme needs to be checked against self-identified cultural labels in determining the validity of the code.

Epidemiology and Prevalence of Disease in Relation to Cultural/Ethnic Diversity

Cultural/ethnic or racial groups exhibit differences in disease prevalence, incidence, mortality, and morbidity. It is, therefore, logical to examine cross-cultural differences in the epidemiology and prevalence of a physical or mental illness prior to assessing its impact on HRQOL. The four categories of variables that influence the distribution of cancer prevalence, incidence, mortality, and morbidity across different cultural/ethnic or racial groups discussed by Kagawa-Singer (1995) generalize to other diseases. These include physiologic and biochemical, socioeconomic, health care system structure, and cultural factors. Specific sources of ethnic diversity within each of these factors are listed in Table 6-3. These major sources of variability are seldom independent of one another, but instead exercise an interactive effect on disease incidence and mortality in culturally/ethnically diverse populations (Kagawa-Singer, 1995). Consequently, they are also expected to exert an interactive influence on HRQOL. However, due to errors in racial/ethnic classification, investigators need to be cautious when using national databases in determining differences between ethnic

Table 6-4.   **Limitations of National Databases for Ethnic Research**

- Racial misclassification
- Undercounting due to sampling
- Insufficient sample size of particular ethnic groups for statistical analyses
- Geographic uniqueness which precludes generalizations
- Lack of uniformity in the operationalization of key variables

Source: Based on Kagawa-Singer, 1995, p. 110. Copyright 1995 W. B. Saunders.

groups in mortality, morbidity, socioeconomic indicators, and other variables (Hahn, 1992). The five major limitations described by Kagawa-Singer (1995) in relation to cancer also apply to other diseases (Table 6-4).

Summary

Culture prescribes the ways of life for a group of people to ensure their survival and well-being, and provides the beliefs and values that give life meaning and purpose (Kagawa-Singer & Blackhall, 2001; Kagawa-Singer & Chung, 1994; Orlandi, 1992; Spector, 1991). Culture also provides consistency and predictability in everyday social interactions and inevitable stressful life events, such as cancer (Kagawa-Singer, 1996). HRQOL is a subjective, multidimensional experience that involves a summary evaluation of positive and negative attributes, such as health and illness conditions, that characterize one's life (Padilla, Grant, Ferrell, & Presant, 1996). Quality of life is culturally constructed as individuals seek to fulfill the three universal needs for: (1) safety and security; (2) a sense of integrity and meaning or purpose in life; and (3) a sense of belonging as an integral member of ones social network (Kagawa-Singer, 1994). Evaluations of these life attributes are influenced by personal goals, expectations, standards, and concerns that occur in a specific cultural context (World Health Organization, 1993). The individual is engaged in a dynamic evaluation process (Padilla, Grant, Ferrell, & Presant, 1996).

In examining QOL in the context of culture it is important to consider the different cultural definitions of HRQOL; the cultural fit of determinants and dimensions of HRQOL (Shumaker and Naughton, 1995; Stewart, 1992; Strickland, 1992); the conceptual and operational equivalence of HRQOL measures across cultures (Bullinger, Anderson, Cella, & Aaronson, 1995); the role of acculturation and assimilation in HRQOL outcomes (Kagawa-Singer, 1995); the reliability of cultural/ethnic/racial labels (Hahn, 1992); and the epidemiology and prevalence of disease, specifically cancer, in different cultural/ethnic groups (Kagawa-Singer, 1995).

Due to the pervasiveness of cultural/ethnic diversity within countries, the extent of global communication, and the impact of racial discrimination around the world, cross-cultural comparisons to better understand disparities in health status and QOL are essential. Selection of treatment regimens, design of public policies, and programs for cancer care are based on evidence of efficacy and effectiveness, including the comparative impact of treatments on quality of life. Therefore, the weight of scientific evidence that underscores the unequal burden of disease endured by ethnic minorities and by socioeconomically poorer countries and peoples mandates that the cross-cultural validity of measures of QOL be demonstrated.

References

Alarcon, G. S., Rodriguez, J. L., Benavides, G. Jr., Brooks, K., Kurusz, H., & Reveille, J. D. (1999). Systemic lupus erythematosus in three ethnic groups. V. Acculturation, health-related attitudes and behaviors, and disease activity in Hispanic patients from the LUMINA cohort. LUMINA Study Group. Lupus in Minority Populations, Nature versus Nurture. *Arthritis Care Res, 12*(4), 267–76.

Beall, C. M., & Eckert, J. K. (1986). Measuring functional status cross culturally. In Fry, C. L., & Keith, K. (Eds.), *New Methods for Old Age Research* (pp. 21–55). South Hadley, MA: Bergin and Garvey.

Berry, J. W., & Kim, U. (1988). Acculturation and mental health. In Dasen, P. R., Berry, J.W., & Satorius, N. (Eds.), *Health and Cross-Cultural Psychology: Toward Applications, 10* (pp. 207–236). Newbury Park: Sage Publications.

Berzon, R. A., & Shumaker, S. A. (1995). Preface. In Shumaker, S. A., & Berzon, R. A. (Eds.), *The International Assessment of Health-related Quality of Life: Theory, Translation, Measurement and Analysis* (pp. v–vi). Oxford: Rapid Communication.

Blackhall, L. J., Frank, G., Murphy, S. T., Michel, V., Palmer, J. M., & Azen, S. P. (1999). Ethnicity and attitudes towards life sustaining technology. *Social Science and Medicine, 48*(12), 1779–89.

Brady, M. J., Peterman, A. H., Fitchett, G., Mo, M., & Cella, D. (1999). A case for including spirituality in quality of life measurement in oncology. *Psychooncology, 8*(5), 417–28.

Bullinger, M., Anderson, R., Cella, D., & Aaronson, N. (1995). Developing and evaluating cross-cultural instruments from minimum requirements to optimal models. In Shumaker, S. A., & Berzon, R. A. (Eds.), *The International Assessment of Health-related Quality of Life: Theory, Translation, Measurement and Analysis* (pp. 83–91). Oxford: Rapid Communication.

Eton, D. T., Lepore, S. J., & Helgeson, V. S. (2001). Early quality of life in patients with localized prostate carcinoma: an examination of treatment-related demographic and psychosocial factors. *Cancer, 92*(6), 1451–1459.

Ferrell, B., Grant, M., Padilla, G., Vemuri, S., & Rhiner, M. (1991). The experience of pain and perceptions of quality of life: Validation of a conceptual model. *Hospice Journal, 7*(3), 9–24.

Ferrell, B., Grant, M., Schmidt, G. M., Whitehead, C., Fonbuena, P., & Forman, S. J. (1992). The meaning of quality of life for bone marrow transplant survivors. Part 1. The impact of bone marrow transplant on quality of life. *Cancer Nursing, 15*(3), 153–160.

Fox-Rushby, J. A., & Parker, M. (1994). Accounting for culture in the measurement of health-related quality of life. *Quality of Life Research, 3*, 41–45.

Folmar, S. (1995). Culture and health-related quality of life. In Shumaker, S. A., & Berzon, R. A. (Eds.), *The International Assessment of Health-related Quality of Life: Theory, Translation, Measurement and Analysis* (pp. 157–158). Oxford: Rapid Communication.

Gee, G. C. (2002). A multilevel analysis of the relationship between institutional and individual racial discrimination and health status. *Am J Public Health, 92*(4), 615–23.

Hahn, R. A. (1992). The state of federal health statistics on racial and ethnic groups. *Journal of the American Medical Association, 267*(2), 268–271.

Hendricson, W. D., Russell, I. J., Prihoda, T. J., Jacobson, J. M., Rogan, A., Bishop, G. D., & Castillo, R. (1989). Development and initial validation of a dual-language English-Spanish format for the Arthritis Impact Measurement Scales. *Arthritis and Rheumatology, 32*, 1153–1159.

Higuchi, K. (1985). Quality of life in cancer patients and their psychological care. In Takeda, F., Hinohara, S., Iio, M. et al. (Eds.), *Quality of Life in Cancer Patients: A Current Topic in Cancer Treatment and Care* (pp. 87–92). Proceedings of the Workshop on Quality of Life in Cancer Patients-Tokyo 1984.

Hirschman, C., Alba, R., & Farley, R. (2000). The meaning and measurement of race in the U.S. census: glimpses into the future. *Demography, 37*(3), 381–93.

Hishinuma, E. S., Andrade, N. N., Johnson, R. C., McArdle, J. J., Miyamoto, R. H., Nahulu, L. B., Makini, G. K. Jr., Yuen, N. Y., Nishimura, S. T., McDermott, J. F. Jr., Waldron, J. A., Luke, K. N., & Yates, A. (2000). Psychometric properties of the Hawaiian Culture Scale—Adolescent Version. *Psychol Assess, 12*(2), 140–57.

Hui, C., & Triandis, H. C. (1985). Measurement in cross-cultural psychology: A review and comparison of strategies. *Cross Cultural Psychology, 16*, 131–150.

Institute of Medicine. (1999). The Unequal Burden of Cancer: An assessment of NIH Research and Programs for Ethnic Minorities and the Medically Underserved. M. Alfred Haynes and Brian D. Smedley (Eds.). Committee on Cancer Research among Minorities and the Medically Underserved. Washington DC: National Academy Press.

Institute of Medicine. (2002). Unequal Treatment: Confronting Racial and Ethnic Disparities in Health Care. Smedley BD, Stith AY, & Nelson AR. Eds. Committee on Understanding and Eliminating Racial and Ethnic Disparities in Health Care, Board on Health Sciences Policy. Washington, DC: National Academy Press.

Jenkins, C. N., Dai, P. X., Ngoc, D. H., Kinh, H. V., Hoang, T. T., Bales, S., Stewart, S., & McPhee, S. J. (1997). Tobacco use in Vietnam. Prevalence, predictors and the role of the transnational tobacco corporations. *Journal of the American Medical Association, 277*(21), 1726–1731.

Kaczorowski, J. M. (1989). Spiritual well-being and anxiety in adults diagnosed with cancer. *The Hospice Journal, 5*, 105–116.

Kagawa-Singer, M. (1988). Bamboo and Oak: A comparative study of adaptation to cancer by Japanese-American and Anglo-American cancer patients. Los Angeles: University of California at Los Angeles, Dissertation.

Kagawa-Singer, M. (1993). Redefining health: Living with Cancer. *Social Science and Medicine, 37*, 295–304.

Kagawa-Singer, M. (1995). Socioeconomic and cultural influences on cancer care of women. *Seminars in Oncology Nursing, 11*(2), 109–119.

Kagawa-Singer, M. (1996). Cultural systems related to cancer. In McCorkle, R., Grant, M., Frank-Stromborg, M., & Baird, S. B. (Eds.), *Cancer Nursing: A Comprehensive Textbook*, 2nd ed. (pp. 38–52). Philadelphia: W.B. Saunders Company.

Kagawa-Singer, M. (2001). From genes to social science: impact of the simplistic interpretation of race, ethnicity, and culture on cancer outcome. *Cancer, 1*(1 Suppl), 226–32.

Kagawa-Singer, M., & Blackhall, L. J. (2001). Negotiating cross-cultural issues at the end of life: "You got to go where he lives." JAMA, 286(23), 2993–3001.

Kagawa-Singer, M., & Chung, R. (1994). A paradigm for culturally based care for minority populations. *Journal of Community Psychology, 22*(2), 192–208.

Kagawa-Singer, M., & Chung, R. C.-Y. (1994). A paradigm for culturally based care. *Community Psychology, 22*, 192–208.

Karon, J. M., Fleming, P. L., Steketee, R. W., & De Cock, K. M. (2001). HIV in the United States at the turn of the century: an epidemic in transition. *Am J Public Health, 91*(7), 1060–1068.

Kashiwagi, T. (1985). A report from Yodogawa Christian Hospital. In Takeda, F., Hinohara, S., Iio, M., et al. (Eds.), *Quality of Life in Cancer Patients: A Current Topic in Cancer Treatment and Care. Proceedings of the Workshop on Quality of Life in Cancer Patients-Tokyo 1984* (pp. 114–118). Tokyo: Office Organizing Committee Workshop on Quality of Life in Cancer Patients-Tokyo.

Lubeck, D. P., Kim, H., Grossfeld, G., Ray, P., Penson, D. F., Flanders, S. C., & Carroll, P. R. (2001). Health related quality of life differences between black and white men with prostate cancer: data from the cancer of the prostate strategic urologic endeavor. *Journal of Urology, 166*(6), 2291–2292.

Marin, G., Sabogal, F., Van Oss-Marin, B., Otero-Sabogal, R., & Perez-Stable, E. J. (1987). Development of a short acculturation scale for Hispanics. *Hispanic Journal of Behavioral Sciences, 9*, 183–199.

Meadows, K. (1994). Criteria for translations of health measurement instruments. *Quality of Life Research, 3*, 67.

Montagu, A. (1962). The concept of race. *American Anthropologist, 64*, 919–928.

Montagu, A. (1997). *Man's Most Dangerous Myth: The Fallacy of Race.* Newbury Park: Sage Press.

Oetting, E. R., & Beauvais, F. (1990–1991). Orthogonal and cultural identification theory: The cultural identification of minority adolescents. Special Issue: Use and misuse of alcohol and drugs. Ethnicity Issues. *International Journal of the Addictions, 25*(5A–6A), 655–685.

Orlandi, M. A. (1992). The challenge of evaluating community-based prevention programs: A cross-cultural perspective. In Orlandi, M. A., Weston, R., & Epstein, L. G. (Eds.), *Cultural Competence for Evaluators: A Guide for Alcohol and Other Drug Abuse Prevention Practitioners Working with Ethnic/Racial Communities. OSAP Cultural Competence Series I* (pp. 1–22). Office of Substance Abuse Prevention, USDHHS Publication No (ADM) 92–1884.

Padilla, G. V., & Grant, M. M. (1985). Quality of life as a cancer nursing outcome variable. *Advances in Nursing Science, 8*(1), 45–60.

Padilla, G. V., Grant, M. M., Ferrell, B. R., & Presant, C. A. (1996). Quality of Life—Cancer. In Spilker, B. (Ed.), *Quality of Life and Pharmacoeconomics in Clinical Trials* (pp. 301–308). New York: Lippincott-Raven.

Padilla, G. V., & Perez, E. (1995). Minorities and arthritis. *Arthritis Care and Research, 8*(4), 251–256.

Parker, M., & Fox-Rushby, J. A. (1995). International comparisons in health-related quality of life: Acquiescence in academia. In Shumaker, S. A., & Berzon, R. A. (Eds.), *The International Assessment of Health-related Quality of Life: Theory, Translation, Measurement and Analysis* (pp. 153–154). Oxford: Rapid Communication.

Patrick, D. L., & Bergner, M. (1990). Measurement of health status in the 1990s. *Annual Review of Public Health, 11*, 165–183.

Patrick, D. L., & Erickson, P. (1993). Health status and health decisions. In Patrick, D. L., & Erickson, P. (Eds.), *Health Status and Health Policy: Quality of Life in Health Care Evaluation and Resource Allocation* (pp. 3–26). New York: Oxford University Press.

Reed, P. (1987). Spirituality and well-being in terminally ill hospitalized adults. *Research in Nursing and Health, 10*, 335–344.

Schwartz, C. E., & Sprangers, M. A. G. (1999). Methodological approaches for assessing response shift in longitudinal quality of life research. *Social Science and Medicine, 48*, 1531–1548.

Shumaker, S. A., & Naughton, M. J. (1995). The international assessment of health-related quality of life: A theoretical perspective. In Shumaker, S. A., & Berzon, R. A. (Eds.), *The International Assessment of Health-related Quality of Life: Theory, Translation, Measurement and Analysis* (pp. 3–10). Oxford: Rapid Communication.

Spilker, B. (1996). *Quality of Life and Pharmacoeconomics in Clinical Trials.* New York: Lippincott-Raven, pp. 1–10.

Spector, R. E. (1991). *Cultural Diversity in Health and Illness*, 3rd ed. San Mateo, CA: Appleton & Lange.

Sprangers, M. A. G., & Schwartz, C. E. (1999). Integrating response shift into health-related quality of life research: a theoretical model. *Social Science and Medicine, 48*, 1507–1515.

Stewart, A. L. (1992). Conceptual and methodologic issues in defining quality of life: State of the art. *Progress in Cardiovascular Nursing, 7*(1), 3–11.

Strickland, O. L. (1992). Measures and instruments. In *Patient Outcomes Research: Examining the Effectiveness of Nursing Practice, Proceedings of the State of the Science Conference*, sponsored by the National Center for Nursing Research, September, 1991, NIH Publication No. 93–3411.

Suinn, R. M., Rickard-Figueroa, K., Lew, S., & Vigil, P. (1987). The Suinn-Lew Asian self-identity acculturation scale: An initial report. *Educational and Psychological Measurement, 47*, 401–407.

Taylor, E. J. (2001). Spirituality, culture, and cancer care. *Seminars in Oncology Nursing, 17*(3), 197–205.

Tuck, I., McCain, N. L., & Elswick, R. K., Jr. (2001). Spirituality and psychosocial factors in persons living with HIV. *Journal of Advances in Nursing, 33*(6), 776–83.

Ware, J. E., Jr. (1984). Methodology in behavioral and psychological cancer research. Conceptualizing disease impact and treatment outcomes. *Cancer, 53 (10 Suppl)*, 2316–2326.

World Health Organization. (1993). WHOQOL Study Protocol: The development of the World Health Organization Quality of Life assessment instrument. Geneva, Switzerland: Division of Mental Health, World Health Organization, publication No. MNH/PSF/93.9

World Health Organization. (1946). *Preamble of the Constitution of the WHO*. Geneva, Switzerland: World Health Organization.

Yoshida, O. (1985). Medical decision-making in palliative care. In Organizing Committee of the Workshop Quality of Life in Cancer Patients-Tokyo 1984: Takeda, F., Hinohara, S., Iio, M., et al. (Eds.), *Quality of Life in Cancer Patients: A Current Topic in Cancer Treatment and Care. Proceedings of the Workshop on Quality of Life in Cancer Patients-Tokyo 1984* (pp. 93–97). Tokyo: Office Organizing Committee Workshop on Quality of Life in Cancer Patients-Tokyo.

Quality of Life
in Children and Adolescents with Cancer

PAMELA S. HINDS • JOAN E. HAASE

Nurses have rapidly and enthusiastically accepted the importance of quality of life (QOL) for children and adolescents experiencing cancer. In addition, we are making progress in learning how QOL information should be gathered from children, adolescents, and their families and used to improve their cancer experience. Our enthusiasm and eagerness are well intended and convey the caring nature of our discipline, but could lead to frustrating clinical or research experiences. These frustrations stem from the advancing but as-yet-unfinished conceptual and empirical work on QOL.

The lack of sufficiently accurate and sensitive ways to determine QOL in children and adolescents from point of diagnosis to cure and survival or to end of life is an opportunity to advance the work in this area. For example, critical evaluation of the extensive QOL work completed with adult oncology patients is helping us to devise improved avenues for extending that work to children and adolescents, while hopefully avoiding some of the pitfalls. In this chapter we: (1) describe the current conceptual and empirical work on QOL in children and adolescents diagnosed with cancer; (2) discuss the significance of QOL to nursing care, education, administration, and research; and (3) make recommendations for future conceptual, research, and clinical work with QOL in children and adolescents.

The Concept of Quality of Life in Pediatric Oncology: Can It Be Precisely Defined?

How accurately a concept is measured and evaluated is directly related to the clarity with which it is first defined (Knafl & Deatrick, 1993). Existing work addressing the definition of QOL does not yet adequately distinguish this concept in children and adolescents from related concepts (e.g., coping and adaptation), from the quality of life of parents and other family members, or from one defined point in treatment to another. This unfinished conceptual work could slow or impede efforts to measure and document QOL in children and adolescents. The research leading to these distinctions between QOL and related concepts may yield exciting and useful new knowledge. Work to clarify the conceptual overlap is moving forward through carefully planned programs of research by nurses and scientists working in collaboration with clinicians.

The conceptual challenges with QOL in pediatric oncology patients include the need to: (1) discover the meaning, importance, and characteristics of QOL for children and adolescents; (2) use descriptive terms and clear language when defining and referring to QOL for these developmentally diverse age groups; and (3) determine whether, for the purposes of complete description, this definition should reflect contextual differences such as diagnosis, prognosis, or point on the continuum of care for childhood cancer.

The urgency to discover the meaning and importance of QOL for children and adolescents makes obvious the need to ask them directly about their cancer experience and its effects on their feelings, thoughts, choices and decisions, and other health-related outcomes. Reports in the literature generally agree that the child's or youth's view of his or her QOL should be solicited (Eiser et al., 1999; Bradlyn et al., 1995; Raphael, 1996), and creative efforts to directly obtain child and youth perspectives are being explored with some success (Haase, Heiney, Ruccione, & Stutzer, 1999; Hockenberry-Eaton & Hinds, 2000). In addition, when family members or health care providers are asked for QOL information, there is increasing effort to compare their perspectives for congruence with the child or adolescent's perspective (Levi & Drotar, 1999; Parsons, Barlow, Levy, Supran, & Kaplan, 1999; Phipps, Dunavant, Jayawardene, & Srivastiva, 1999). An example of such work is a comparison of two measures of QOL completed by children and compared with parent reports of their child's and their own QOL (Vance, Morse, Jenny, & Eiser, 2001). This study, which found good correspondence between the two child report measures and poor to moderate correspondence between the parent and child ratings, also provided a way to sort out parent characteristics that influence child QOL. Conducting more such comparison studies will help shed light on questions of how QOL experiences for patients are distinct from, or highly influenced by, those of the family. An additional need is to determine how the developmental levels of both the child and family contribute to their unique and shared perceptions of QOL. Completing the conceptual work on the construct of quality of life in pediatric oncology patients will necessarily involve soliciting comparisons of the perceptions of developmentally and culturally diverse patients and families. That knowledge will ultimately provide a basis for nursing care of pediatric oncology patients and their families and will enable nurses to decide whether the patient or the family is the most effective target for intervention.

Defining or describing QOL for children and adolescents with cancer requires clear language. This requirement is especially important because of the present difficulty in distinguishing QOL from related, but different, concepts. Other terms currently used interchangeably with QOL for children and adolescents include well-being (Bradlyn, Harris, Warner, Ritchey, & Zaboy, 1993; Czyzewski et al., 1994; Haase, Heiney, Ruccione, & Stutzer, 1999) and global health status (Feeny et al., 1993; Barr et al., 1993). Some works neglect to conceptually define QOL and other apparently equivalent terms (Cadman, Goldsmith, & Torrance, 1986; Bradlyn et al., 1993; Czyzewski et al., 1994; see Table 7-1). This failure may arise because: (1) the construct is considered to have a widely known and universally accepted meaning, thereby making efforts to define it redundant and unnecessary; (2) the necessary but time-consuming work for its conceptual definition is incomplete; or (3) the term is thought to be too nebulous to define.

Despite inherent difficulties with conceptual clarity and completeness, the definitions in the literature do have important similarities, including attributes of multidimensionality, subjectivity, dynamism, inclusivity, and comparison of past and current circumstances with desired future outcome. Dimensions specified by different authors vary (Table 7-1) but generally include physical health (including symptoms and health conditions), psychological/spiritual health (such as satisfaction with self and orientation to the future), social relationships (including friendships and activities), and family relationships (such as the coping abilities of parents and siblings). Differences in the specificity of each of the dimensions indicate the need to continue to refine these broad domains to capture the components most important to the child/adolescent and parent. There is increasing recognition that the specific QOL dimensions valued by individuals are unique and dependent on past experiences, current circumstances, and future hopes and expectations (Eiser & Morse, 2001).

Conceptualizing about QOL dimensions is a cognitive tool that helps us organize our thoughts and knowledge about QOL in children and adolescents; it also serves a practical function for nursing care interventions. For example, QOL may be reported by the parent and/or family member as quite high in the dimension of physical health, but low in psychological/spiritual health. Such a report would direct the nurse's assessment and intervention skills to the dimension of the lower score.

Dimensions found in the current literature are distinguishable, but not discrete, from each other. Even when there is distinction, a change in one dimension may affect another. This influence of change also has implications for nursing care, because an intervention directed at one dimension could also influence other dimensions of QOL.

Table 7-1. **Definition and Dimensions of Quality of Life in Children and Adolescents**

Definition	Dimensions	Source
None Offered	Sensory and communication ability, happiness, self-care ability, freedom from moderate to severe chronic pain or discomfort, learning and school ability, physical ability	Cadman, Goldsmith, Torrance, Boyle, & Furlong, 1986
Children's and adolescent's subjective and changeable sense of well-being which reflects how closely their desires and hopes match what is actually happening, and their orientation toward the future, both their own and that of others.	Hopefulness, self-esteem/self-efficacy, symptom distress, adverse physical effects of treatment	Hinds, 1990, p. 285
The impact of illness and predicament of a biological disorder	Incidence, prevalence, physiological dysfunction, or mortality rate	Rosenbaum, Cadman, & Kerpalani, 1990, p. 207
A term describing the total existence of an individual or group, including the more positive aspects of health	External conditions, internal conditions, personal psychological conditions	Lindstrom & Kohler, 1991, p. 121
None offered	Mobility, physical activity, social activity	Bradlyn, Harris, Warner, Ritchey, & Zaboy, 1993, p. 250
"Quality of life is a multidimensional construct, incorporating both objective and subjective data, including (but not limited to) the social, physical, and emotional functioning of the child and, when indicated, his/her family. QOL measurement must be sensitive to changes that occur throughout development."	Social functioning, physical functioning, emotional functioning	Pediatric Oncology Group, 1993

Table 7-1. **continued**

Definition	Dimensions	Source
None offered	Physical symptoms and functionality in the areas of mobility, physical activity, and social activity	Czyzewski, Mariotto, Bartholomew, LeCompte, & Sockrider, 1994, p. 966
Personal opinions reflecting satisfaction with current circumstances, participation in activities and relations, and the opportunity to have control over one's life and to make choices	Satisfaction, well-being, social belonging, empowerment/control	Keith & Schalock, 1994, p. 84
The way in which individuals view their own health and the degree to which they are satisfied with it	None specified	Vivier, Bernier, & Starfield, 1994, p. 532
Impact of disease and treatment on self-perceptions of functioning	Core: physical, psychological, social Symptom: pain, nausea	Seid, Varni, Rode, & Katz, 1999, p. 72
Discrepancy between what the child can and would like to be able to do	Social, physical, actual self, ideal self	Eiser, Cotter, Oades, Seamark, & Smith, 1999, p. 87
Preference-based valuation of overall disability reported by each subject and reported in a single summary utility score	Global	Barr, Chalmers, DePauw, Furlong, Weitzman, & Feeny, 2000, p. 3281

The available literature also helps to identify differences or disagreements in the conceptual work with QOL in pediatric patients. Differences in conceptual definitions include the extent to which objective aspects are included, the positive or negative slant reflected, the sense of time (past, present, or future) conveyed, and the extent to which context such as setting or culture influence quality of life (Table 7-1). Definitions or descriptions generated by nurses tend not to include the objective aspects (e.g., socioeconomic status, neighborhood, or type of dwelling) that other disciplines include. Nursing's efforts to focus only on those aspects of QOL directly influenced by nursing care may account for this difference.

There remain many challenges in QOL research for children, adolescents, and their families. Both creative and systematic efforts to determine how pediatric oncology patients describe or define their QOL are needed. Triangulation of methods (qualitative and quantitative), sources (i.e., self-, parent-, health care provider-reports), and research/clinicians are needed to continue our progress in understanding the quality of life of children and adolescents experiencing cancer.

Significance of Quality of Life in Children and Adolescents Who Have Cancer

Some researchers view QOL for children and adolescents with cancer as an endpoint indicator, a measure that could determine whether one area of a clinical trial is more demanding on a patient than another. In contrast, nursing sees QOL as a process and outcome variable that is influenced directly and indirectly by nursing care (Hinds, 1990; Grant, Padilla, & Creimel, 1996). Consequently, QOL has implications for nursing care, education, administration, and research. The full significance of quality of life for children and adolescents is unknown in part because of the unfinished conceptual work. Increasingly, there is an emphasis on viewing quality of life more holistically, acknowledging a link between physical and psychosocial domains (Eiser & Morse, 2001). Nursing's interest in the relevance of the concept is remarkably high, and nurses' clinical interest results from the sincere desire for valid knowledge and understanding of the care-related experiences of a child or youth (Hinds & Varricchio, 1996; King, Hinds, Dow, Schum, & Lee, 2002). Nurses want to use this knowledge to provide more sensitive care that is tailored to each child or adolescent, and they believe that QOL information can assist them in providing the most appropriate intervention.

Incorporating QOL issues into all levels of formal nursing education is also an interest in nursing. Because of the nature of our discipline's work (giving sensitive, competent, individualized care that helps a care recipient to achieve the most positive health outcomes possible), most nursing curricula already contain certain philosophic and practice based assumptions similar to, consistent with, or at least parallel to, those of QOL. A more formal, focused emphasis on QOL also encourages nurses to view their care and research with care recipients as needing to reflect: (1) the interrelated aspects of the various dimensions of a child's or youth's being; (2) actual or at least possible change (situational or developmental) in any of the identified dimensions of the child's or youth's quality of life; (3) the opinion or perception of the child or youth; (4) the influencing context within which the child or youth lives and experiences health-related situations; and (5) the role of nursing care in facilitating QOL for children and adolescents as a way of promoting their health.

The administrative interest in QOL is twofold. First, nurse administrators are aware that nurses experience job-related meaning and satisfaction when they feel they have contributed to the QOL of their patients (Jones, 1990; Wakefield, Curry, Price, Mueller, & McCloskey, 1988). The importance to nurses of making a positive difference to pediatric patients and their families is often reflected in the findings from nursing role and function studies (Hinds, Quargnenti, Hickey, & Mangum, 1994; Olson et al., 1998). Second, nurse administrators want to justify the importance of QOL work by nurses, the outcomes of which may be difficult to define and quantify. How may quality of life work by nurses be figured into a patient acuity system? What is the cost of that kind of care or the lack of it?

Research interests are derived from the clinical, educational, and administrative questions and concerns in nursing. The significance here is nursing's determination to carefully and completely determine (conceptually and empirically) the nature and characteristics of QOL for children and adolescents who are experiencing or have experienced cancer. Building on that work, nursing's related intention is to develop and test interventions designed to promote QOL in these children and youths, with systematic focus on the processes by which QOL is affected and the outcomes of those interventions.

Conceptual Models of Quality of Life in Children and Adolescents with Cancer

Several conceptual models and frameworks that may contribute to our understanding of QOL for children and adolescents are presented here. Function- and meaning-based models represent differing conceptual approaches to QOL. Function-based models primarily emphasize functions (such as ability to attend school and keep up with friends) as indicators of QOL, whereas meaning-based models rely on subjective reports of meaning (such as finding meaning in life or strengthening friendships as a result of having cancer). The Life-Span Development Framework provides a basis for understanding the dynamic nature of QOL within a context of universal and unique developmental experiences. In addition, four substantive models specific to QOL in pediatric oncology patients are described. These models offer descriptive detail about the process and outcomes of the components comprising QOL.

Function- and Meaning-Based Models

Function-based models predominate in QOL research in adult oncology (Costain, Hewison, & Howes, 1993). Function-based models are most often used to examine outcomes of treatments from a biomedical perspective of objectivity and reductionism. They emphasize goal setting to manage clinical concerns, toxicity of treatments, and role-related tasks or functions. In adult oncology, acceptance of the function-based models seems to be occurring without critical evaluation of the underlying assumptions of function as the basis for QOL and without a clear definition of QOL and its dimensions. In particular, function-based models have not been examined for their congruence with nursing's philosophic perspectives of holism or the expressed needs of children and adolescents.

Meaning-based models focus on the experience of the illness from the perspective of the child/adolescent or parent and incorporate a more holistic view. Meaning-based models view QOL as enabling patients to choose and realize their own goals through the exploration of meanings derived from the personal experiences of illness and its treatment. Meaning can also be derived from patients' understanding of their situation, autonomy, beliefs, choices, and relationships with others.

Because research on QOL in children and adolescents is lagging behind that in adults, the pressing need to measure QOL in children and adolescents with cancer may lead to a premature acceptance of a function-based model in nursing. Several recent publications on pediatric oncology QOL assert the importance of function-based models forming the minimum data set for QOL assessment (Eiser, 1997; Bradlyn & Pollock, 1996). For example, the guidelines for QOL research put forth by the Pediatric Oncology Group (POG) are derived in part from the definition of health offered by the World Health Organization (1947). The POG guidelines define QOL as "a multi-dimensional construct . . . that includes, but is not limited to, social, physical, and emotional functioning of the child and, when indicated, his or her family" (Pediatric Oncology Group, 1993). This definition appears to be holistic, but it emphasizes functioning, whether physical, psychological, or social. This emphasis is more behavioral than holistic in nature, in that how well a child or adolescent functions does not necessarily reveal the meaning, value, importance, or satisfaction that he/she derives from those functions. Two examples may help distinguish these important differences between function- and meaning-based models. The loss of hair for one adolescent may have an important negative impact on her QOL and, indeed, may negatively influence social functioning. For another adolescent, the meaning of hair loss may be minor and have very little influence on her evaluation of quality of life. For a third, the loss of hair could conceivably have a positive impact on quality of life, if friends communicated their strong connectedness by shaving off their own hair. When social function is assessed in terms of the child's or adolescent's ability to carry out typical social activities, often the assessment does not consider whether the activities are meaningful to him or her. Thus, when a child or adolescent is asked if he or she is able to continue with school activities, a "no" answer may be interpreted as an indicator of decreased QOL. Missing from this response is the meaning that staying at home has for the pediatric oncology patient, or the meaning that parents find in staying at home with an ill child. Although such isolation is assumed to be un- pleasant and burdensome, qualitative data from one study indicated that some chil- dren and families use the isolation as an opportunity to be together and strengthen family ties, and to focus on the strength of friendships that endure in spite of the iso- lation (Haase & Rostad, 1994). In that same study, one adolescent who was unable to attend school reported feeling cheated of an important time in high school, but an- other adolescent described positive outcomes from her home schooling. Both patients had a decrease in social functioning, but their experiences of the decrease differed be- cause of the meaning attached to the change. Meaning is not likely to be assessed in a function-based model, and potentially misleading conclusions could be drawn about the QOL of pediatric oncology patients.

When meaning-based models are used with QOL research, functioning is con- sidered within the greater context of the meaning of the cancer experience. The per- ceptions of the child and the family about the meaning of the altered functioning are the essential research data. Did the child and family consider the altered functioning to be a loss or an opportunity? Is the particular social activity that is being used as an indicator of QOL important to the child and family? These are the kinds of questions reflected in research that are guided by meaning-based models and would likely con- tribute substantially to efforts to develop conceptual completeness of QOL in pedi- atric oncology patients. In addition, interventions to enhance QOL would look very different if the emphasis was on helping a child make meaning from the experience, rather than improving function. For example, many of the expressive therapies, such as journaling, music therapy, or art, are focused on helping participants to form mean- ing, and improvement in function often follows. Further, emphasis on either function or meaning in isolation sets up an artificial dichotomy, and such a dichotomy is not reflective of child/adolescent experiences.

The Life-Span Development Framework

An additional conceptual approach that may be valuable in QOL work with children and adolescents with cancer is the Life-Span Developmental Framework. This frame- work "seeks to determine the historical and contemporary influences on development as well as the quantitative and qualitative aspects of (child) and adolescent responses to illness" (Weekes, 1991, p. 42). The important principles of life-span development are that, (1) development is change that has an underlying temporal and logical order that results in systematic and progressive alterations in organization; (2) developmental changes arise from a combination of influences (e.g., biological, psychological, social, historical, or evolutionary); (3) the person and environment or context are embedded in, and interact to influence, each other; and (4) developmental factors are normative age-graded (e.g., children typically begin walking between 12 and 16 months), normative history- or experienced-graded (e.g., school-age children in the United States whose first exposure to terrorism was the September 11, 2001, attacks on New York City and Washington, DC), and nonnormative universal occurrences (e.g., illness; Baltes, 1979; Lerner, 1986). The life-span perspective recognizes the nonnormative aspects of developmental change that can be caused by the cancer experience and assumes that treatment effects are not identical for all people and will change over time.

This framework is particularly helpful when evaluating the importance of differences in meaning from a developmental perspective. The following example about the characteristics of pain (cause, source, intensity, and management) may help to illustrate these differences and their clinical importance. An adult may experience and interpret the characteristics of pain as pressure from a tumor (cause and source) that is quite painful (intensity) but manageable with morphine sulphate (management). Children of a certain developmental perspective experience and interpret pain as I did something for which I am being punished (cause) by powerful adults (source) who do things that cause more pain (intensity) from which I must escape or withdraw (management).

Substantive Models for Quality of Life Pediatric Oncology Patients

Although the construct of pediatric QOL is not yet clearly defined, factors that influence it are now being identified. Hinds (1990) used a combined deductive and inductive approach to develop a model of environmental sources of influences. The assumptions underlying this model are that QOL in children and adolescents with cancer is: (1) sensitive to input from external others; (2) highly changeable due to daily events and chronic problems; and (3) tempered by personality styles, cognitive abilities, and expectations and desires. The three levels of environment that may directly influence QOL (Figure 7-1) are the internal environment, which represents factors of the child or adolescent such as feelings about self; the immediate environment, which includes factors of significant others such as family members and health care providers and their ability to deal with the demands of the illness; and the institutional environment, or factors of the greater social system such as financial support

Figure 7-1. **Quality of life model depicting the direct influence of three levels of environment.**

from the public for cancer care and research. Additional examples of the components of each level of environment are shown in Figure 7-1. Two other methods of assessing QOL in adolescents exist that also propose interrelated multilevel influences on adolescents' health behavior (Lindstrom, 1994; Raphael, 1996), although the focus of those models is healthy adolescents.

A second substantive model that identifies factors that influence the QOL of adolescents with cancer is the Adolescent Resilience Model (ARM) (Haase, Heiney, Ruccione, & Stutzer,1999; Figure 7-2). This model, also developed from both deductive and inductive methods, helps to distinguish the influencing factors from the actual dimensions of QOL. The initial work in developing the ARM was a phenomenological study of courage in chronically ill adolescents. Since the initial study, the ARM has been tested and refined in two samples of adolescents (n = 73; n = 130) with chronic illness or cancer. The model is currently being examined longitudinally. The model indicates that individual (patient-specific), family, and social characteristics directly influence how the adolescent responds to an illness experience. That response, in turn, influences the adolescent's resilience to the experience. Ultimately, the adolescent's resilience directly influences his or her QOL (the greater the adolescent's resilience, the greater the QOL).

The third substantive model is the Self-Sustaining Model (Figure 7-3), which was developed inductively with adolescents who had cancer (Hinds & Martin, 1988). The model was developed to convey how adolescents help themselves to achieve and

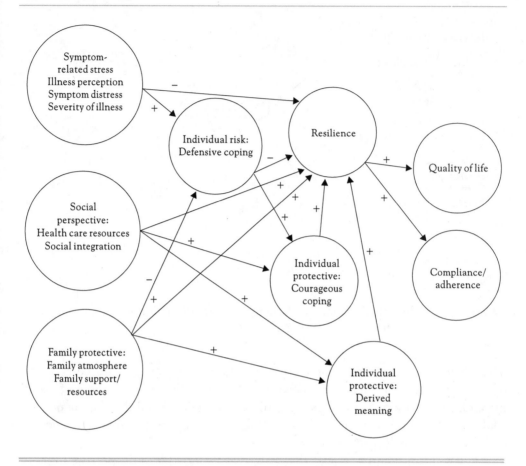

Figure 7-2.   **Depiction of the adolescent resilience model (ARM).**

maintain hopefulness during their cancer experience. The assumptions underlying the model were that hopefulness is crucial for adolescents with cancer because it helps them cope with a life-threatening illness, and that adolescents' ability to help themselves feel hopeful is a developmentally important accomplishment for them. The model was comprised of four sequential phases representing adolescents' efforts to comfort themselves during health-threatened periods by using certain behavioral and cognitive strategies (labeled "Self-Care Strategies" in Figure 7-3). Their efforts result in a sense of personal competence in resolving health threats. The model has been further developed and tested in a recent study of 78 adolescents newly diagnosed with cancer. Correlation findings provide moderate to strong support for all of the theorized linkages in the model (Hinds, 1995; Hinds, Quargnenti, Bush et al., 2000). The study findings for this model represent a test of the internal environment on selected dimensions of QOL.

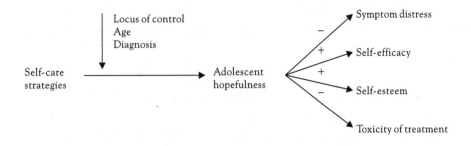

Figure 7-3. **Self-sustaining model of adolescents with cancer.**

None of the previously described models has been applied to dying children and adolescents. The fourth substantive model is based on a combination of inductive and deductive research studies and depicts QOL in pediatric oncology patients who are dying (see Figure 7-4). In this recently developed model, the underlying premises are that the focus is jointly on the child or adolescent and his or her family and that QOL is likely the ultimate outcome of interest in end-of-life care (Bradlyn, Varni, & Hinds, 2003). Because the formal study of QOL at end of life for children, adolescents, and

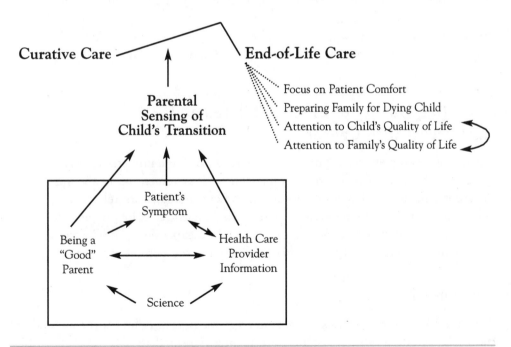

Figure 7-4. **Model of quality of life at end of life that emphasizes the dual focus on the dying child or adolescent and his family.**

their families has only recently begun, we do not yet know what exact type and number of domains might best represent these patients and their families. Dying children and adolescents commonly and repeatedly express intense concerns about the well-being of their family members (Hinds, Oakes, & Furman, 2001), as do family members about the dying child. This mutual concern is the basis for the joint focus in this model on the dying child and on his family. The presence of symptoms that are inadequately managed adversely affects the patients' and family members' QOL (Hinds, Bradshaw, Oakes, & Pritchard, in press). Other sources of influence include the parents' satisfaction with their ability to be "good parents" to their dying child, the ability of the family to maintain some degree of normalcy, and the influence of child development and culture (Goh et al., 1999; Rushton, 1994; Hinds, Oakes, & Furman et al., 2001). Both research findings and clinical observations suggest that a model of QOL at end of life for a child or adolescent and his family needs to reflect fluidity of the clinical situation.

Because they provide additional information about validity and generalizability, the conceptual and empirical similarities and differences among these substantive models are the focus of much interest. Careful comparison among the factors identified in each model helps to distinguish influencing factors from the outcome of QOL itself (and its components). Factors sometimes measured elsewhere as indicators of QOL are viewed in these models as contributing to, but not equating with, QOL in children and adolescents with cancer. The same comparison of the four substantive models also helps to identify the complex, multidimensional nature of the factors that influence QOL.

Measuring Quality of Life in Children and Adolescents with Cancer

Because of incomplete conceptual work, there is no single universally accepted way to measure the QOL of children and adolescents. Measurement issues abound and include concerns about premature closure in the conceptual work related to QOL in order to focus on measurement; self-report in the pediatric oncology population; shifting standards of comparison during the cancer care experience; the developmental, clinical, and cultural sensitivity of the measures; and the purpose for measurements.

Premature Closure

Due to the increasing requests to include QOL measures in clinical trials (Bradlyn, Harris, & Spieth, 1995), researchers are feeling pressured to abort the unfinished conceptual work in order to attempt to measure QOL. This haste has resulted in researchers selecting flawed measures or measurement approaches. Once a collaborative group or research team selects a definition of QOL, the goal frequently shifts to selecting a core set of measures or a single, multidimensional measure that can be used across clinical trials. Once the measures are selected, dialogue about the nature of QOL in children and adolescents will diminish and subsequent dialogue likely will focus on the psychometric strengths of the chosen measures. Premature closure could then lead to incomplete, incorrect, and misleading data being the basis for clinical interventions. Further, premature closure can occur as review articles summarize and draw conclusions from findings of several studies that are based on measures not sensitive enough to detect changes. One recent review indicated that many studies found no differences in outcomes of child cancer survivors, compared with healthy children. Yet, this same review strongly criticized the measures used in most of the studies reported (Eiser, Hill, & Vance, 2000).

Self-Report Measures

Measures that solicit subjective reports directly from children and adolescents help to ensure that these perspectives are considered. Multiple measures exist for evaluating one or more dimensions of QOL, but few are derived from the perspective of the child or adolescent. Children as young as 7 and adolescents are willing and able to respond to developmentally appropriate interview questions or questionnaires. However, they may provide bogus or incomplete responses if they lose interest or find the questions irrelevant or difficult to understand (Hinds, Quargnenti, & Wentz, 1992).

Because of that possibility, a serious commitment to developing sensitive measures for children and adolescents should begin with careful qualitative efforts to learn the pediatric perspective. Measures developed in this manner will reflect language and ideas understood by the child or adolescent and are more likely to result in greater receptiveness and increased participation (including fewer unanswered items) from the pediatric patient. For example, in a study by Haase and Rostad (1994), adolescents with cancer completed a lengthy interview about their cancer experience. Interview questions such as "In what way have your friendships changed since your diagnosis?" and "What helps you to get through treatments?" directly solicited the adolescents' perspectives and were positively received by the participants. The researchers received comments of appreciation from some adolescents, who expressed relief at being asked about what was important to them. An additional factor that contributes to a measure's developmental sensitivity is its administration. Allowing an adolescent to independently complete a self-report measure acknowledges his or her competence. However, the same measure may need to be adapted for a younger child to ensure valid responses.

Shifting Standards of Comparison

Usefulness in a repeated-measures design implies that the measure is able to capture real change in the dimensions of QOL, and brief enough that the child or adolescent will not object to completing it more than once during his or her cancer experience. Of concern here is the ability of the measure to determine whether the standard of comparison used by the child or adolescent changes over time. Hinds (1995) observed that adolescents based their subjective reports on a shifting standard of comparison. For example, newly diagnosed adolescents would provide ratings that compared present perceptions with those they had prior to diagnosis or any symptoms being noticed. Three months later, those same adolescents provided ratings that compared their present perceptions with what they imagined to be the experience of other patients in more serious health condition. One way to control for the effect of a shifting standard is to include a standard of comparison in the directions for the measure, so that true change over time can be determined.

Developmental Sensitivity of the Measures

A concern with QOL measures that are used over time with pediatric oncology patients is the developmental appropriateness of the measures. For example, Bradlyn and colleagues (personal communication, 1994) used the Rand questionnaires to measure QOL in pediatric patients, including pediatric oncology patients. The questionnaires were developed for specified age groups 0 through 4 years, 5 through 13 years, and 14 years and older. When these questionnaires are used over time with pediatric oncology patients, it is possible that more than three years may separate a child's or adolescent's diagnosis and the gathering of post-treatment QOL scores. Differences between these scores and those obtained at diagnosis may reflect true change in QOL measure or change in the value or expectations of the respondent to specific QOL dimensions. The measurement challenge here is to accurately determine change in QOL reports or scores when the patient moves to another age group with different desires and needs and is administered a different measure.

Clinical Sensitivity of Measures

Another concern is the need for measures that detect clinically significant changes in QOL. There is considerable evidence that interpretations of QOL in adults are a moving target. For example, the fatigue one experiences initially may be adapted to over time and subsequent measures will indicate a decrease in fatigue, when in reality the fatigue level is the same, but the ability to cope with it has changed. It is possible that such adjustments in reporting also occur with children and adults.

Cultural Sensitivity of the Measures

The cultural meanings associated with illness need to be reflected in measures of QOL for children and adolescents (Leininger, 1994; Marshall, 1990; Sartorius, 1987). Cultural concepts of collective rather than individualistic goal setting, acceptance of "what is" rather than prevention or cure, and time as passages of life rather than a linear progression are several of the distinguishing features that will need to be incorporated in measures of quality of life. Indeed, even perspectives on such concepts as pain and suffering, need to be studied within cultural contexts. For example, a qualitative theme identified in a group of Middle Eastern children as a strategy they use to deal with pain was labeled "learning to suffer well" but the predominate Western cultural perspective is to "alleviate suffering" (Voightman, 2001).

Purpose of Measurement: Statistical or Clinical Significance

The issue of clinical versus statistical significance addresses the change in score of a particular quality of life measure (e.g., outcome indicator in a clinical trial or an indicator for clinical management) that would be considered important. The degree to which a measure is statistically significant is important when QOL data are being collected, for example, to help determine the impact of a particular therapy on children. In contrast, measures need to have high clinical significance when the information gathered is to be used in decision making for one particular child. The scores and the size of the change in the scores over time would be weighed differently in these two situations.

General Guidelines for Measuring Quality of Life in Children and Adolescents

The following general principles of measurement may help clarify the issues that should be addressed when measuring quality of life.

1. The purpose of the study needs to be explicit, to guide decisions about which dimensions of quality of life to measure and which methods and measures to use. For example, comparing patients' functional status in two arms of a clinical trial differs considerably from describing their quality of life trajectories throughout their cancer experience. Consequently, different study purposes lead to the incorporation of different designs and measures.

2. Selection of measures needs to be based on a clearly identified theoretical or conceptual model in which quality of life and other included concepts are defined, model assumptions are specified, relationships are described and are logically

congruent, and a developmental perspective is incorporated. Without careful stipulation, we will be unable to build a coherent body of knowledge about QOL in children and adolescents. Equally serious, we could waste costly resources in studies that lack these characteristics.

3. In its current definition, QOL appears to be a latent variable, one that cannot be directly measured (Aaronson et al., 1987; Rudin, Martinson, & Gillis, 1988). Therefore, multiple measures or indicators of QOL are necessary. However, the quality of studies reported in the literature using multiple measures has been evaluated as poor (Eiser, 2001). This is likely a reflection of the lack of a sound theoretical perspective in selection of instruments and caution is advised in design of such studies as they often require a larger sample.

4. Concept analysis work and inductive development of concepts and measures need to continue, particularly when the components of a proposed model are unclear. The sources of influence and the components of QOL seem similar or related. Efforts to better identify the antecedents and consequences of quality of life in children and adolescents and the critical attributes of this concept need to continue.

5. Conceptualizations of QOL and their underlying assumptions should be examined for cultural relevance, especially when measures based on these conceptualizations are to be used in different cultures.

Measures Used to Index Quality of Life in Children and Adolescents

The number of generic and disease-specific QOL measures for children and adolescents is rapidly increasing, with over 40 instruments reported in the literature in various stages of development and testing (Eiser & Morse, 2001). Self-report measures are being used with children as young as 5 years of age (Varni, Seid, & Rode, 1999) as indicators of QOL dimensions in children and adolescents, but there remains a limited number of child-report measures. For many instruments, evidence of reliability as either stability or internal consistency is preliminary and only a few measures have sustained evidence of validity (Eiser & Morse, 2001).

The number of domains studied in any instrument ranges from one to 17 (Eiser & Morse, 2001). Most measures include WHO-identified components of QOL. Some instruments more clearly reflect the pediatric experience as indicated by the child-centered measurement approach or the domains represented. For example, Eiser's Perceived Illness Experience measures three unique domains reflective of child and adolescent concerns: disclosure, appearance, and peer rejection (Eiser, Havermans, Craft, & Kernahan, 1995).

Recommendations for Future Conceptual, Research, and Clinical Work with Quality of Life in Children and Adolescents

Future conceptual work needs to focus on reports solicited directly from children and adolescents that describe their definition and perception of QOL during the cancer experience. This focus will entail careful qualitative work to completely capture their language and meaning and the importance they place on quality of life. This conceptual work will be most beneficial if completed across the continuum of cancer care (from diagnosis to long-term survivorship or terminal care), so that the actual trajectory of QOL is documented. In addition, the conceptual work must include the perspectives of children and adolescents of different ages, and these perspectives should be analyzed for any differences associated with age or developmental level.

Conceptual work with parents needs to focus on their definition and experience of their quality of life (as parents and as a family) throughout the cancer care continuum. Their definition and experience of their diagnosed child's QOL also should be addressed; the comparison of their perspectives may lead to a better understanding of these two experiences. Conceptual models particular to QOL in children and adolescents should then be developed more fully.

Measures based on the conceptual work described earlier need to be developed. Those measures must be tested in multiple studies that have different purposes (e.g., clinical trials and clinical intervention studies). The resulting QOL scores should be examined for differences related to age, diagnosis, point on the care continuum, and other disease or patient variables. In addition, scores on QOL measures as reported by the patient, parent, and/or health care provider will need to be compared, and sources of agreement or difference identified and explained. Intervention studies that include measures of QOL prior to and following a nursing care intervention also should be completed. Finally, studies that measure the meaning of quality of life work for nurses in terms of their role meaning and satisfaction are necessary.

Even though the conceptual and research work with QOL in children and adolescents with cancer is incomplete, nurses will continue to incorporate such issues in their daily care of these patients. The following guidelines are offered to help nurses design general questions for assessing the QOL in the child or adolescent. Questions should be modified to ensure that they are developmentally appropriate for patients of different ages. Using the same general question over time and patients will help nurses recognize usual and unexpected responses. Questions that work best clinically include a built-in standard of comparison—for example, "When you think back on how things were for you during your first chemotherapy session, how are things going for you right now?" More specific questions designed to elicit the child or adolescent's perception of each of the dimensions of QOL might follow. Nurses will obtain a more comparable assessment standard if each patient is asked the same set of questions at key times throughout the cancer experience.

Nurses need to determine in advance the purpose of the clinical assessment of the child's QOL. Is it a general assessment question, an issue-specific question, or a protocol- or treatment-driven question? The purpose of the assessment will give direction to the manner in which the questions posed to the child are varied. Nurses can also provide valuable clinical observations by documenting (1) the responses offered by the child or adolescent, (2) the exact intervention initiated by the nurse, and (3) the patient outcomes of that intervention. These anecdotal reports will contribute to the future clinical care efforts for that child or adolescent, while also helping to build conceptual models of quality of life for children and adolescents with cancer.

CONCLUSION

The definition of QOL from the perspective of the child or adolescent with cancer is receiving renewed attention. Because of their considerable interest in this construct, nurses are likely to expend the efforts necessary for completely defining quality of life and identifying its attributes. As a result, QOL assessments derived from sound empirical research will become standard in the nursing care of children and adolescents with cancer.

REFERENCES

Aaronson, N., Bakker, W., Stewart, A., van Dam, F., van Zandwijk, N., Yarnold, J., & Kirkpatrick, A. (1987). Multidimensional approach to the measurement of quality of life in lung cancer clinical trials. In N. K. Aaronson & J. Beckman (Eds.), *The quality of life of cancer patients.* New York: Raven Press.

Baltes, P. B. (1979). Life-span developmental psychology: Some converging observations on history and theory. In P. B. Baltes & O. G. Brim (Eds.), *Life-span development and behavior* (pp. 225–279). San Diego, CA: Academic Press.

Barr, R., Chalmers, D., De Pauw, S., Furlong, W., Weitzman, S., & Feeny, D. (2000). Health-related quality of life in survivors of Wilms' tumors and advanced neuroblastoma: A cross-sectional study. *Journal of Clinical Oncology, 18*(18), 3280–3287.

Barr, R. D., Furlong, W., Dawson, S., Whitton, A. C., Strautmanis, I., Pai, M., Feeny, D., & Torrance, G. (1993). An assessment of global health status in survivors of acute lymphoblastic leukemia in childhood. *The American Journal of Pediatric Hematology/Oncology, 15*(4), 284–290.

Bradlyn, A. S., Harris, C., & Spieth, L. (1995). Quality of life assessment in pediatric oncology: A retrospective review of Phase III reports. *Social Science and Medicine, 41,* 1463–1465.

Bradlyn, A. S., Harris, C. V., Warner, J. E., Ritchey, A. K., & Zaboy, K. (1993). An investigation of the validity of the quality of well-being scale with pediatric oncology patients. *Health Psychology, 12*(3), 246–250.

Bradlyn, A. S., & Pollock, B. H. (1995). Quality of life research in the Pediatric Oncology Group: 1991–1995. Department of Behavioral Medicine and Psychiatry, Robert C. Byrd Health Sciences Center, Morgantown, WV.

Bradlyn, A. S., & Pollock, B. H. (1996). Quality-of-life research in the Pediatric Oncology Group: 1991–1995. *Journal of the National Cancer Institute* (Monographs 1996), 20, 49–53.

Bradlyn, A. S., Ritchey A. K., Harris, C. V., Moore, A. K., O'Brien, R. T., Parsons, S. K., Patterson, K., & Pollock, B. H. (1995). Quality of life research in pediatric oncology: Research methods and barriers. Department of Behavioral Medicine and Psychiatry, Robert C. Byrd Health Sciences Center, Morgantown, WV.

Bradlyn, A., Varni, J., & Hinds, P. (2003). Assessing health-related quality of life in end-of-life care for children and adolescents. In M. Field & R. Behrman (Eds.), *Care of dying children and their families.* Institute of Medicine.

Cadman, D., Goldsmith, C., Torrance, G. W., Boyle, B. H., & Furlong, W. (1986). *Development of a health status index for Ontario children.* Final report to the Ontario Ministry of Health on research grant DM 648 (00633). Hamilton, Ontario: McMaster University.

Costain, K., Hewison, J., & Howes, M. (1993). Comparison of a function-based model and a meaning-based model of quality of life in oncology: Multidimensionality examined. *Journal of Psychosocial Oncology, 11*(4), 17–37.

Czyzewski, D. I., Mariotto, M. J., Bartholomew, L. K., LeCompte, S. H., & Sockrider, M. M. (1994). Measurement of quality of well being in a child and adolescent cystic fibrosis population. *Medical Care, 32*(9), 965–972.

Eisen, M., Donald, C. A., Ware, J. E., Jr., & Brook, R. H. (1980). *Conceptualization and measurement of health for children in the Health Insurance Study.* Santa Monica, CA: RAND Corporation.

Eiser, C. (1997). Children's quality of life measures. *Archives of Disease in Childhood, 77*(4), 350–354.

Eiser, C. (1999). Health-related quality-of-life measures for children. *International Journal of Cancer—Supplement, 12,* 87–90.

Eiser, C. (2000). Examining the psychological consequences of surviving childhood cancer: Systemic review as a research method in pediatric psychology. *Journal of Pediatric Psychology, 25*(6), 449–460.

Eiser, C. (2001). The measurement of quality of life in children: Past and future perspectives. *Journal of Developmental & Behavioral Pediatrics, 22*(4), 248–256.

Eiser, C., Cotter, I., Oades, P., Seamark, D., & Smith, R. (1999). Health-related quality-of-life measures for children. *International Journal of Cancer Suppl., 12,* 87–90.

Eiser, C., Havermans, T., Craft, A., & Kernahan, J. (1995). Development of a measure to assess the perceived illness experience after treatment for cancer. *Archives of Disease in Childhood, 72,* 302–307.

Eiser, C., Havermans, T., & Eiser, J. R. (1995). Parents' attributions about childhood cancer: Implications for relationships with medical staff. *Child: Care, Health & Development, 21*(1), 31–42.

Eiser, C., Hill, J. J., & Vance, Y. H. (2000). Examining the psychological consequences of surviving childhood cancer: Systematic review as a research method in pediatric psychology. *Journal of Pediatric Psychology, 25*(6), 449–460.

Eiser, C., Kopel, S., Cool, P., & Grimer, R. (1999). The perceived illness experience scale (PIE): Reliability and validity revisited. *Child Care Health Development, 25*(3), 179–190.

Eiser, C., & Morse, R. (2001). Quality-of-life measures in chronic diseases of childhood. *Health Technology Assessment, 5*(4),1–110.

Feeny, D., Furlong, W., Barr, R., Torrance, G. W., Rosenbaum, P., & Weitzman, S. (1992). A comprehensive multiattribute system for classifying the health status of survivors of childhood cancer. *Journal of Clinical Oncology, 10*(6), 923–928.

Feeny, D., & Leiper, A. (1993). The comprehensive assessment of health status in survivors of childhood cancer: application to high-risk acute lymphoblastic leukaemia, *British Journal of Cancer, 67*(5), 1047–1052.

Goh, A. Y., Lum, L. C., Chan, P. W., Baker, F., & Chong, B. O. (1999). Withdrawal and limitation of life support in pediatric intensive care. *Archives of the Disabled Child, 80,* 424–428.

Goodwin, D. A., Boggs, S. R., & Graham-Pole, J. (1994). Development and validation of the pediatric oncology quality of life scale. *Psychological Assessment, 6*(4), 321–328.

Grant, M., Padilla, G., & Creimel, E. (1996). Survivorship and quality of life issues. In R. McCorkle, M. Grant, M. Frank-Stromborg, & S. Baird (Eds.), *Cancer nursing: A comprehensive textbook* (pp. 1312–1321). Philadelphia: W. B. Saunders.

Haase, J. (1987). The components of courage in chronically ill adolescents: A phenomenological study. *Advances in Nursing Sciences, 9*(2), 64–80.

Haase, J. (1991). Instrument and model development for the Becoming Courageous Model. (Abstract) Conference of the American Nurses Association, Council of Nurse Researchers, Los Angeles, CA.

Haase, J. (1994). Method triangulation to increase conceptual clarity and measurement sensitivity for quality of life assessment. Paper abstract. American Cancer Society Nursing Research Conference, Newport Beach, CA.

Haase, J. E., Heiney S. P., Ruccione, K. S., & Stutzer, C. (1999). Research triangulation to derive meaning-based quality-of-life theory: adolescent resilience model and instrument development. *International Journal of Cancer—Supplement, 12,* 125–131.

Haase, J., & Rostad, M. (1994). Experiences of completing cancer treatments: Child and adolescent perspectives. *Oncology Nursing Forum, 21,* 1483–1492.

Haase, J., & Rostad, M. (In press). Experiences of completing cancer therapy: Parents' perspectives contrasted with child perspectives. *Cancer Investigations.*

Haase, J., Stutzer, C., & Berry, D. (1993, June). Quality of life outcomes for chronically ill adolescents based on the adolescent resilience model. Paper abstract. Sigma Theta Tau Nursing Research Congress, Madrid, Spain.

Hinds, P., Quargnenti, A., & Wentz, T. (1992). Measuring symptom distress in adolescents with cancer. *Journal of Pediatric Oncology Nursing, 9,* 84–86.

Hinds, P. S. (1990). Quality of life in children and adolescents with cancer. Seminars in *Oncology Nursing, 6,* 285–291.

Hinds, P. S. (1995). *Self-care outcomes in adolescents with cancer.* Final report to the National Cancer Institute on research grant 1 R01 CA 48432. Memphis, TN: St. Jude Children's Research Hospital.

Hinds, P., Bradshaw, G., Oakes, L., Pritchard, M. (in press). Children and their rights in life and death situations. In R. Kastenbaum (Ed.), *Encyclopedia of Death and Dying.* Macmillan Reference Publishers.

Hinds, P. S., & Gattuso, J. S. (1991). Measuring hopefulness in adolescents. *Journal of Pediatric Oncology Nursing, 8*(2), 92–94.

Hinds, P. S., & Martin, J. (1988). Self-care outcomes in adolescents with cancer. *Nursing Research, 37*(6), 336–340.

Hinds, P. S., Oakes, L., & Furman, W. (2001). End-of-life decision making in pediatric oncology. In B. R. Ferrell & N. Coyle (Eds.), *Textbook of Palliative Nursing* (pp. 450–460). New York: Oxford University Press, Inc.

Hinds, P. S., Oakes, L., Furman, W., Quargnenti, A., Olson, M. S., Foppiano, P., & Srivastava, D. K. (2001). End-of-life decision making by adolescents, parents, and healthcare providers in pediatric oncology. *Cancer Nursing, 24,* 122–136.

Hinds, P., Quargnenti, A., Bush, A., Fairclough, D., Betcher, D., Rissmiller, G., Pratt, C., & Gilchrist G. (2000). An evaluation of the impact of a self-care coping intervention on psychological and clinical outcomes in adolescents with newly diagnosed cancer. *European Journal of Oncology Nursing, 4*(1),6–17.

Hinds, P. S., Quargnenti, A. G., Hickey, S. S., & Mangum, G. H. (1994). A comparison of the stress-response sequence in new and experienced pediatric oncology nurses. *Cancer Nursing, 17*(1), 61–71.

Hinds, P. S., & Varricchio, C. G. (1996). Quality of life: The nursing perspective. In B. Spilker (Ed.), *Quality of life and pharmacoeconomics in clinical trials* (2nd ed.) (pp. 529–533). Philadelphia: Lippincott-Raven.

Hockenberry-Eaton, M., & Hinds, P. S. (2000). Fatigue in children and adolescents with cancer: Evolution of a program of study. *Seminars in Oncology Nursing, 16*(4), 261–272.

Jones, C. (1990). Staff nurse turnover costs: Part II: Measurement and results. *Journal of Nursing Administration, 20*(5), 27–32.

Kanabar, D. J., Attard-Montalto, S., Saha V., Kingston, J. E., Malpas, J. E., & Eden, O. B. (1995). Quality of life in survivors of childhood cancer after megatherapy with autologous bone marrow rescue. *Pediatric Hematology and Oncology, 12*, 29–36.

Keith, K., & Schalock, R. (1994). The measurement of quality of life in adolescence: The Quality of Student Life Questionnaire. *The American Journal of Family Therapy, 22*(1), 83–87.

King, C., Hinds, P. S., Dow, K., Schum, L., & Lee, C. (2002). The nurses relationship-based perceptions of patient quality of life. *Oncology Nursing Forum, 29*(10), E118–E126.

Knafl, K., & Deatrick, J. (1993). Knowledge synthesis and concept development in nursing. In B. Rodgers & K. Knafl (Eds.), *Concept development in nursing: Foundations, techniques and applications* (pp. 35–50). Philadelphia: W. B. Saunders.

Lansky, S., List, M., Lansky, L., Ritter-Sterr, C., & Miller, D. (1987). The measurement of performance in childhood cancer patients. Cancer, 60, 1651–1656.

Leininger, M. (1994). Quality of life from a transcultural nursing perspective. *Nursing Science Quarterly, 7*, 22–28.

Lerner, R. M. (1986). *Concepts and theories of human development* (2nd ed.). New York: Random House.

Levi, R.B., & Drotar, D. (1999). Health-related quality of life in childhood cancer: discrepancy in parent-child reports. *International Journal of Cancer—Supplement, 12*, 58–64.

Lindstrom, B., & Kohler, L. (1991). Youth, disability and quality of life. *Pediatrician, 18*, 121–128.

Lindstrom, B. (1994). *The essence of existence: On the quality of life of children in the Nordic countries.* Goteborg, Sweden: Nordic School of Public Health.

Makipernaa, A. (1989). Long-term quality of life and psychosocial coping after treatment of solid tumours in childhood. *Acta Paediatrica Scandinavica, 78,* 728–735.

Marshall, P. (1990). Cultural influences on perceived quality of life. *Seminars in Oncology Nursing, 6,* 278–284.

Mulhern, R. K., Horozwitz, M. E., Ochs, J., Friedman, A. G., Armstrong, F. D., Copeland, D., & Kun, L. E. (1989). Assessment of quality of life among pediatric patients with cancer. *Psychological Assessment, 1,* 130–138.

Mulhern, R., Heideman, R. L., Khaib, Z. A., Kovnar, E. H., Sandord, R. A., & Kun, L. E. (1994). Quality of survival among children treated for brain stem glioma. *Pediatric Neurosurgery, 20,* 226–232.

Olson, M. S., Hinds, P. S., Euell, K., Quargnenti, A., Milligan, M., Foppiano, P., & Powell, B. (1998). Peak and nadir experiences and their consequences described by pediatric oncology nurses. *Journal of Pediatric Oncology Nursing, 15*(1), 13–24.

Parsons, S. K., Barlow, S. E., Levy, S. L., Supran, S. E., & Kaplans, H. (1999). Health-related quality of life in pediatric bone marrow transplant survivors: according to whom? *International Journal of Cancer-Supplement, 12,* 46–51.

Pediatric Oncology Group, Quality of Life Subcommittee. (1993). Guidelines for incorporaing quality of life measures into clinical trials.

Phipps, S., Dunavant, M., Jayawardene, D., & Srivastava, D. (1999). Assessment of health-related quality of life in acute in-patient settings: use of the BASES instrument in children undergoing bone marrow transplantation. *International Journal of Cancer—Supplement, 12,* 18–24.

Raphael, D. (1996). Quality of life and adolescent health. In R. Renwick, I. Brown, & M. Nagre (Eds.), *Quality of life in health promotion and rehability: Conceptual approaches, issues and applications* (pp. 307–324). Thousand Oaks, CA: Sage.

Rosenbaum, P., Cadman, D., & Kerpalani, H. (1990). Pediatrics: Assessing quality of life. In B. Spilker (Ed.), *Quality of life assessments in clinical trials* (pp. 205–215). New York: Raven Press.

Rudin, M., Martinson, I., & Gillis, C. (1988). Measurement of psychosocial concerns of adolescents with cancer. *Cancer Nursing, 11,* 144–149.

Rushton, C. (1994). Moral decision making by parents of infants who have life-threatening congenital disorders. Ph.D. dissertation, School of Nursing, Catholic University of America, Washington DC.

Sartorius, N. (1987). Cross-cultural comparisons of data abot quality of life: A sample of issues: In N. K. Aaronson & J. Beckman (Eds.), *The quality of life of cancer patients.* New York: Raven Press.

Seid, M., Varni, J. W., Rode, C. A., & Katz, E. R. (1999). The Pediatric Cancer Quality of Life Inventory: A modular approach to measuring health-related quality of life in children with cancer. *International Journal of Cancer Suppl.*, *12*, 71–76.

Starfied, B., Riley, A. W., Green, B. F., Ensminger, M. E., Ryan, S. A., Kelleher, K., Kim-Harris, S., Johnston, D., & Vogel, K. (1995). The adolescent child health and illness profile. A population-based measure of health. *Medical Care*, *33*(5), 553–566.

Vance, Y. H., Morse, R. C. Jenny, M. E., Eiser, C. (2001). Issues in measuring quality of life in childhood cancer: Measures, proxies, and parental mental health. *Journal of Child Psychology & Psychiatry & Allied Disciplines*, *42*(5), 661–667.

Varni, J. M., Seid M., & Rode, C. (1999). The PedsQL: Measurement model for the pediatric quality of life inventory. *Medical Care*, *37*(2), 126–139.

Vivier, P. M., Bernier, J. A., & Starfield, B. (1994). Current approaches to measuring health outcomes in pediatric research. *Current Opinions in Pediatrics*, *6*(5), 530–537.

Voigtman, J. (2002). "Learning to Suffer: Pain Response in a Community of Saudi Arab Children with Sickle Cell Disease," Dissertation, University of Arizona.

Wakefield, D., Curry, J., Price, J., Mueller, C., & McCloskey, J. (1988). Differences in unit outcomes: Job satisfaction, organizational commitment, and turnover among hospital nursing department employees. *Western Journal of Nursing Research*, *10*(1), 98–105.

Ware, J. E., & Sherbourne, C. D. (1992). The MOS 36-item short-form health survey. *Medical Care*, *30*(6), 473–483.

Weekes, D. (1991). Application of the life-span developmental perspective to nursing reserach with adolescents. *Journal of Pediatric Nursing*, *6*, 38–48.

World Health Organization (1947). The Constitution of the World Health Organization. WHO Chronicle.

Research

8

Quality of Life
Methodological and Measurement Issues

MEL R. HABERMAN • NIGEL BUSH

The construct of quality of life (QOL) offers oncology nursing an organizing framework for describing the caring behaviors of nurses. A QOL paradigm for practice is holistic, acknowledging important endpoints of care such as physical mobility, adherence to treatment regimens, self-care behaviors, psychosocial and cognitive functioning, and spirituality, to name a few. Oncology nurses systematically incorporate QOL endpoints into standards of care, guidelines for practice, and care pathways. Moreover, QOL outcomes are of value to all members of the multidisciplinary cancer team and appear to be relevant whether the goal of therapy is cure or palliation and comfort (Clinch & Schipper, 1993; Klee, King, Machin, & Hansen, 2000; McCahill et al., 2002).

Oncology nursing is challenged to conduct research and to build a systematic knowledge base for practice. The purpose of this chapter is to describe some of the conceptual and methodologic issues that influence the design of QOL studies, in an effort to promote QOL research. The chapter focuses on the measurement issues that pertain to research conducted on adults rather than those pertaining to pediatric, adolescent, or family-centered research.

Conceptual Issues That Guide QOL Measurement

Multidimensional Nature of QOL

Health care researchers agree that QOL is a multidimensional construct (Cella, 1993; Donnelly, Rybicki, & Walsh, 2001; Gotay, Korn, McCabe, Moore, & Cheson, 1992; Gotay & Muraoka, 1998; King et al., 1997). However, since no specific definition of

QOL is widely accepted among researchers, investigators have implicitly defined the concept by the operations used to measure it (Clinch & Schipper, 1993; Ganz, 1994; Holzner et al., 2001). This convention is contrary to the usual methods of quantitative science in which measurement is based on clearly defined concepts. Moreover, investigators have often neglected to base their measurement operations on an explanatory model or theoretical framework of QOL.

Some consensus exists among health researchers about the minimum components to include when measuring QOL. QOL measurement can be enhanced by including a minimum of four dimensions plus a global measure of perceived health status and QOL (Aaronson, 1990; Bush, Haberman, Donaldson, & Sullivan, 1995; Bush, Donaldson, Haberman, Dacaney, & Sullivan, 2000; Ganz, 1994; Moinpour & Hayden, 1990; Velikova, Stark, & Selby, 1999). The four dimensions include physical functioning, emotional and psychological functioning, social functioning, and disease/treatment-related symptoms. Table 8-1 identifies some of the components of each dimension of QOL.

In addition to the core set of QOL indicators listed in Table 8-1, many other health-related issues may be of interest to nurse scientists when measuring QOL. Some of these additional facets of QOL include vocational and insurance discrimination, the stigma of cancer, financial well-being, the demands or hardships of cancer survivorship, and patterns of growth following childhood cancer. In designing a QOL study, investigators must decide what they mean by QOL and identify the specific dimensions that are to be measured (Gill & Feinstein, 1994; Montazeri, Gillis, & McEwen, 1996). Moreover, some situational or disease characteristics of QOL may be time-limited and available for measurement only at specific windows of time in the continuum of cancer (Epstein, 2000). For instance, the disruptions caused by cancer recurrence would not be expected to influence QOL until the actual recurrence of disease.

QOL as a Research Outcome

QOL outcomes are now an integral component of many cancer clinical trials. In 1990 the National Cancer Institute (NCI) held a landmark workshop to identify guidelines for systematically assessing QOL outcomes (Nayfield, Ganz, Moinpour, Cella, & Hailey, 1992; Nayfield, Hailey, & McCabe, 1991). Several American, Canadian, and International cooperative research groups have standardized the measurement of QOL endpoints in Phase III clinical trials (de Haes et al., 2000; Lee & Chi, 2000; Moinpour & Hayden, 1990; Osoba, Dancey, Zee, Myles, & Pater, 1996).

QOL endpoints constitute a major study endpoint in addition to, or instead of, the limited information obtained from traditional cancer outcomes (e.g., the length of disease-free survival, relapse rates, disease progression, or tumor response) (Gotay

Table 8-1. **Dimensions of Quality of Life**

Physical Functioning
Activities of daily living
Physical mobility, independence, and ability to exercise
Ability to perform work, school, and recreation activities
Self-care and personal hygiene activities
Nutrition and dietary management activities

Psychological Functioning
Mood states: depression, anxiety, anger, joy
Cognitive or mental status: orientation, memory, concentration, attention, perception,
thinking, alertness, confusion
Perceptions of well-being: life satisfaction, happiness, positive attitude, life outlook, morale,
meaning and purpose, inner peace, personal success, perceived control, hope
Spirituality, self-transcendent experiences, altruism
Self-esteem, self-image, self-worth, self-mastery, self-efficacy

Social Role Functioning
Sexual functioning, intimacy, and warmth
Managing interpersonal, family, work, and school relationships
Managing relationships with health care providers
Negotiating health care organizations and bureaucracies
Participating in support groups or volunteer activities

Disease- and Treatment-Related Symptoms
Fatigue and energy levels
Physical stamina, strength, and endurance
Nausea, vomiting, diarrhea, constipation
Mucositis, dysphagia, dyspnea
Taste changes, pain, infections, dermatitis
Sleep alterations and rest
All regimen-related toxicities or side effects of therapy

et al., 1992). Phase III clinical trials are incorporating QOL outcomes to compare the efficacy of new unproven therapies against the current standard of care (Moinpour et al., 1989). QOL endpoints are recent adjuncts to studies on treatment cost-effectiveness (Reynolds, 1994) and survival analysis (Cole, Gelber, Gelber, Coates, & Goldhirsch, 2001). Popular in the oncology nursing literature are QOL instrumentation studies (Ferrans & Powers, 1985; Padilla & Grant, 1985), reviews of QOL measurement issues and instrumentation (King et al., 1997; Padilla, Grant, & Ferrell, 1992; Whedon & Ferrell, 1994; Zebrack, 2000), and studies that describe the human dimensions of cancer survivorship (Belec, 1992; Ferrell, Dow, Leigh, Ly, & Gulasekaram, 1995; Haberman, Bush, Young, & Sullivan, 1993; Hassey Dow, Ferrell, Haberman, & Eaton, 1999; Whedon, Stearns, & Mills, 1995).

The selection of QOL study endpoints should be limited to health-related outcomes. Health-related outcomes focus on the goals and objectives of cancer care and on issues directly under the influence of clinicians, rather than on aspects of life peripheral or distal to the goals of health care (Aaronson, 1990). For instance, although QOL may encompass such factors as a general outlook on life, sense of well-being, and life satisfaction, these outcomes would not be considered health-related unless they were linked to disease or treatment issues (e.g., satisfaction with care and psychological well-being following the diagnosis of cancer). However, some investigators argue in favor of obtaining a balanced assessment of overall QOL, one that combines health-related factors and the effects of nonmedical phenomena, such as employment and family relationships (Gill & Feinstein, 1994).

Identifying QOL outcomes requires a thorough understanding of disease characteristics, treatment-delivery schedules, types of treatment settings, and the phases of psychosocial adjustment to cancer (Epstein, 2000). For example, if the specific aim of the study is to compare the expenses associated with inpatient and ambulatory care, a variety of endpoints must be identified. These endpoints must have the potential to explain factors that influence cost differences, such as the types of cancer treated, therapies administered in both settings, average length of stay in the hospital, readmission rates, types of medical complications, the costs actually reimbursed by health insurance, and clients' out-of-pocket expenses.

Health-related QOL outcomes can be used to (a) predict survival rates, (b) document patterns of impairment and complete recovery, (c) compare the results of different types of therapy for the same disease, (d) establish norms of morbidity among diverse cultural groups and populations of cancer survivors, (e) document quality of care for the purpose of improving care and the outcomes of therapy, (f) compare the efficacy of traditional and nontraditional therapies, (g) screen persons at risk of developing psychosocial morbidity, (h) track the median survival and long-term recovery of cancer survivors, and (i) compare the incidence and severity of regimen-related toxicities among therapies that have similar disease outcomes but different toxicities (Aaronson, 1990; Bush et al., 2000; Clinch & Schipper, 1993; Ganz, 1994; Shapiro, et al., 2001).

Design and Measurement Issues

The science of QOL measurement has progressed sufficiently to provide investigators with guidelines for designing QOL studies and selecting reliable and valid measures. Table 8-2 provides a checklist of some of the most common design and measurement issues that pertain to the development of a QOL study. Some of these issues are unique to cancer-related QOL studies, while others pertain to the design of all

| Table 8-2. | **Design and Measurement Issues for QOL Research** |

- Describe the specific aims, purpose, and significance of the study.
- Provide a conceptual definition and theoretical framework for QOL.
- Link the theoretical framework to health-related QOL outcomes.
- Select a research design, e.g., descriptive or intervention trial.
- Select methods for data collection, e.g., qualitative and/or quantitative.
- Select a single QOL instrument or battery of questionnaires.
- Select a comprehensive, multidimensional assessment strategy.
- Select either generic or cancer-specific instruments.
- Examine the reliability and validity of all methods of data collection.
- Identify QOL measures suitable for use with diverse cultures.
- Obtain data at a single time point or on multiple occasions.
- Identify the appropriate time for obtaining baseline measurement.
- Standardize measurement procedures across sites and treatment groups.
- Obtain data from the perspective of the client.
- Evaluate the strengths and limitations of data obtained by self-report.
- Minimize responder burden and sources of measurement error.
- Conduct a pilot study of procedures and pretest of the instruments.
- Select a sampling plan and identify study entry and exclusion criteria.
- Identify a sampling plan and estimate sample size.
- Establish scoring procedures for all instruments.
- Develop an analysis plan for all forms of raw data.
- Conduct a data audit trail to monitor the reliability of all data operations.
- Ensure the self-determination and protection of human participants.
- Monitor the informed consent process and the ethical conduct of the study.

research studies in general. The design and methodologic issues that pertain to QOL studies are now discussed in detail.

Lack of a Gold Standard for Measurement

Health researchers have yet to reach agreement on a gold standard or best method of measuring QOL (Cella & Tulsky, 1990; King et al., 1997). There is simply no perfect way to measure QOL given the current state-of-the-science and the complex nature of the construct. Systematic advances in QOL measurement will occur in tandem with finding answers to other unresolved issues such as how to define QOL in the context of many different cultures, personal lifestyles, types of cancer, and alternative therapies. Because the majority of health-realted QOL questionnaires were developed in non-minority and well-educated groups, researchers are beginning to examine if these questionnaires are conceptually and methodologically equivalent across diverse subpopulations (Stewart & Napoles-Springer, 2000). In the absence of reaching some universal consensus on the ideal way to measure QOL, researchers should strive to define the concept clearly and to set some boundaries on a suitable theoretical framework. In addition, investigators should endeavor to establish the relevance of QOL measurement across the distribution of health issues that are potentially responsive to treatment (Testa, 2000).

Quantitative and Qualitative Measurement

Quantitative Measurement. A variety of methods exist for measuring QOL. Each method provides a different vantage point and type of outcome data. One method of QOL measurement is the use of standardized, fixed-item or forced-choice questionnaires (Velikova et al., 1999). Some examples of this type of QOL instrument include the 30-item European Organization for Research and Treatment of Cancer (EORTC) Quality of Life Questionnaire (Aaronson et al., 1993) and the Functional Assessment of Cancer Therapy (FACT) Scale (Cella et al., 1993).

There are several advantages to using standardized measures. Standardized tools usually have known reliability and validity, they ensure every participant is asked the same set of items, the questionnaires are often easy to administer and complete, the statistical analysis is generally straightforward, and the results can be compared across studies that use the same instruments. However, since fixed-item questionnaires limit responses only to the items contained on the questionnaire, many aspects of QOL may be overlooked. For instance, if the questionnaire focuses on physical functioning and activities of daily living, participants will not be asked to identify problems related to social, emotional, or cognitive functioning.

Qualitative Measurement. Qualitative inquiry is another form of systematic measurement that is becoming increasingly popular. Selecting a qualitative method may be as simple as including a few open-ended questions at the tail end of a forced-choice questionnaire or conducting a short semistructured interview. Some examples of open-ended questions include, "How would you describe your quality of life today?" "How does your quality of life today compare with your qualify of life before cancer?" Some additional qualitative methods include participant observation, storytelling, interviews with key informants, the systematic examination of archived records and artifacts, and the use of client diaries as a way to chronologically log symptoms or health behaviors.

More formal and methodologically rigorous approaches to qualitative inquiry include ethnography, phenomenology, grounded theory, and hermeneutics, to name a few (Haberman, 1995b; Haberman & Lewis, 1990). Each of these formal approaches is based on a unique worldview and philosophical stance as well as specific strategies for sampling, data collection, analysis, and write-up. Although rigorous forms of qualitative inquiry provide a rich source of empirical data, the methodologies are labor-intensive and require advanced research preparation to learn.

It is becoming common for investigators to use multiple types of data collection in one study, a strategy known as methodologic triangulation (Mitchell, 1986). A standardized instrument that obtains self-report information may be administered together with a semistructured interview. For instance, in a mailed survey to long-term cancer survivors, Hassey Dow and colleagues (1999) combined open-ended questions and standardized QOL questionnaires to obtain multidimensional perspective of QOL. Instrument development research often adds a qualitative component to complement the formal, psychometric testing of questionnaires. Respondents may be asked to complete both a forced-choice questionnaire that is under development and a brief set of open-ended items on the same topic. The open-ended data can be used to generate new items for the questionnaire and to revise the wording or clarity of existing items. Gill and Feinstein (1994) indicated that all QOL standardized questionnaires should be augmented with additional open-ended items that ask the client to identify missing factors. However, Padilla and Frank-Stromborg (1997) cautioned that multiple operationalism may not always be practical or even possible.

Obviously, the analysis plan will be different for qualitative forms of data collection than for quantitative measures. Simple forms of qualitative data can be analyzed using standard content analysis or thematic analytic techniques (Denzin & Lincoln, 1984; Miles & Huberman, 1994). Data obtained from the more sophisticated approaches to qualitative inquiry should be analyzed according to the methods developed for those particular approaches.

Unidimensional, Multidimensional, Modular, and Global Assessment of QOL

Unidimensional Assessment.   Historically, QOL measurement included the use of unidimensional, single-item scales, such as a simple five-point rating scale to measure fatigue or pain intensity. The use of unidimensional scales as the only measure of QOL in a study is falling out of vogue in favor of a more comprehensive assessment. In fact, some QOL proponents argue that unidimensional scales should not even be considered as QOL measures since they fail to provide a multidimensional assessment (Cella & Tulsky, 1990; Osoba, 1994).

The Karnofsky Performance Scale (KPS) is a popular unidimensional scale that measures physical functioning. Regrettably, some clinical researchers still consider it an adequate measure of QOL. The KPS (Karnofsky & Burchenal, 1949) is completed by clinicians or other proxies. Studies have shown that the scale suffers from poor interrater reliability and that clinician-based ratings of QOL universally correlate poorly with ratings provided by clients themselves (Aaronson, 1990). Osoba (1994) reported that emerging evidence suggests some multidimensional measures of QOL may be better predictors of survival than unidimensional scales such as the KPS.

Multidimensional Assessment.   Health-related QOL is a collective phenomenon representing many intertwining facets of life. Instruments that provide a comprehensive assessment of QOL are the current recommended standard. One option for multidimensional assessment is to select a group of instruments each of which only measures a single domain or component of QOL, for example, symptom side effects, cognitive functioning, self-esteem, and mood states. Another option is to select a single multidimensional instrument designed to measure many domains or components of QOL. Multidimensional questionnaires vary greatly in the content measured; consequently, it may be difficult to compare results across studies. Since multidimensional instruments are limited in focus; investigators often combine measures, adding one or more single-domain instruments to supplement the information obtained from a multidimensional scale (Bush et al., 2000; Mast, 1995). Jalowiec (1990) observed that it is exceptionally difficult for any single multidimensional instrument to identify the entire constellation of life changes that occur with a life-threatening illness such as cancer.

A battery approach combines several types of measures to obtain a comprehensive assessment of QOL, for example, unidimensional scales, global scales, and a combination of single-domain and multidimensional instruments (Ganz, 1994). Investigators can select a single scale or battery of questionnaires based on the specific aims of the study, characteristics of the client population, and desired study endpoints (Grant, Padilla, Ferrell, & Rhiner, 1990).

Selecting a battery of instruments for a comprehensive assessment of QOL creates its own special problems. Investigators must evaluate the equivalency of response formats to determine if the different formats will confuse respondents. For example, one questionnaire may use a five-point Likert-type scale while another may use a 100-mm visual analog scale. Other aspects to evaluate are the clarity of the instructions and the equivalency of the time period used to frame responses. One questionnaire may ask participants to recall events that occurred during the past week, and another, during the past month. Researchers must examine the content of different questionnaires on an item-by-item basis, while also examining the instruments' reliability, validity, and scoring instructions, the time needed to complete the entire battery, and the potential for substantial responder burden.

Modular Assessment.   Another recent trend in QOL measurement is the modular approach. A modular-type questionnaire is composed of two main sections. A core set of general items, applicable to many types of cancer, is combined with a disease- or treatment-specific module (Aaronson, Bullinger, & Ahmedzai, 1988). The core items are useful for comparing results across different cancer populations. However, due to their general nature, the core items may fail to capture disease- or treatment-specific issues, such as the body image changes that occur following surgical intervention for breast cancer. Modules have been developed for the late complications of bone marrow transplantation (Bush et al., 1995, 2000); lung cancer (Aaronson et al., 1993); and for breast, prostate, head and neck, and pancreatic cancer (Cella et al., 1993).

Global Scales to Measure QOL or Health Status.   Another current trend in QOL assessment is to use a single-item indicator that measures global perceptions of QOL and/or health status. Global scales should not be confused with the single-item, unidimensional scales that were described previously, such as the Karnofsky Performance Status Index. A typical global indicator may ask, "How would you rate your overall quality of life?" or "How would you rate your overall health?" Global items may be scaled using a 100-mm visual analog scale, in which responses range from 0 (worst imaginable QOL or health) to 100 (best imaginable QOL or health). Likert-type scales, with response options ranging from 1 (poor QOL or health) to 5 (excellent QOL or health) also are common.

A global item is sensitive enough to reflect the different values and preferences of clients (Gill & Feinstein, 1994). Global items also are useful for making comparisons between treatments and evaluating changes across times because they represent the summation of personal meaning and many factors that are often difficult to quantify (Bernard, Sullivan, Hurny, Coates, & Rudenstam, 2001). Oftentimes, QOL studies use different batteries of QOL instruments but the same global measure of health status or QOL, making it relatively easy to compare global ratings across studies. Since global ratings reflect a common-sense alternative or complementary approach to QOL measurement, some authors recommend the use of two global ratings in all studies, one that asks about nonillness QOL and another that asks about health-related QOL (Gill & Feinstein, 1994).

Generic and Cancer-Specific Instruments

Generic Instruments.   A distinction can be made between generic and cancer-specific questionnaires (Velikova, Stark, & Selby, 1999). Generic instruments measure health functioning across a wide variety of chronic illnesses and cancers and provide a common database for comparing results, allocating resources, and developing health policy (Aaronson, 1990). Some examples of this type of questionnaire include the Demands of Illness Inventory (Haberman, Woods, & Packard, 1990), the Sickness Impact Profile (Bergner, Bobbitt, Carter, & Gilson, 1981), the Medical Outcome Study Short Form General Health Survey (Stewart, Hays, & Ware, 1988), and the Functional Assessment of Cancer Therapy Scale (FACT-G) by Cella and colleagues (1993). The FACT-G is a general QOL scale. It can be used to measure QOL in other situations besides oncology, including heart disease, chronic obstructive pulmonary disease, renal disease, arthritis, or AIDS. Many generic instruments are lengthy and research oriented, making them of little use for routine clinical assessment. Although generic measures are commonly used in QOL research, they may not identify issues unique to the cancer experience.

Cancer-Specific Instruments.   Cancer-specific instruments are designed to focus on the QOL of various populations of persons with cancer. A cancer-specific measure must be sensitive enough to identify differences between treatments or types of cancer, for example, different patterns of symptoms experienced by people with leukemia undergoing chemotherapy versus those undergoing blood cell transplantation.

The nonequivalence of cancer-specific questionnaires may make it difficult, if not impossible, to compare results across studies. Some cancer-specific tools are applicable to a single type of cancer, while others are general and pertain to a variety of cancers and therapies. For instance, the Breast Cancer Chemotherapy Questionnaire (Levine et al., 1988) is limited to QOL issues associated with breast cancer while the Cancer Rehabilitation Evaluation System (CARES) is applicable to virtually all types of cancer (Ganz, Rofessart, Polinsky, Schag, & Heinrich, 1986). Table 8-3 lists many of the most commonly used generic and cancer-specific QOL questionnaires. The abbreviated versions of many of these questionnaires can be found in the May 1990 issue of the journal *Oncology* (Tchekmedyian & Cella, 1990). Moreover, the reliability and validity of many of these questionnaires are described by Dean (1997) and Padilla and Frank-Stromborg (1997) in a new book by Frank-Stromborg and Olsen (1997) entitled, *Instruments for Clinical Health-Care Research* (second edition).

Reliability and Validity of Measurement

Reliability refers to the reproducibility of data from one measurement occasion to another. Common forms of reliability are test-retest, internal consistency, alternate forms, and interrater reliability (Haberman, 1995a). Validity provides some assurance that the questionnaire actually measures what it claims to measure, such as physical functioning, regimen-related toxicities, or fatigue (Haberman, 1994). Establishing validity is a cumulative process that occurs over several research studies. The most popular types of validity are content, construct, and criterion-related validity, which includes both predictive and concurrent validity (Haberman, 1995a). A comprehen-

Table 8-3. **QOL Questionnaires**

Generic Questionnaires
  The Beck Depression Inventory (BDI)
  The Crumbaugh Purpose-in-Life Test (PIL)
  Demands of Illness Inventory (DOII)
  Functional Assessment of Cancer Therapy-General Scale (FACT-G)
  Global Adjustment to Illness Scale
  The Lewis Psychological Coherence Scale
  The McCorkle & Young Symptom Distress Scale
  The McGill Pain Questionnaire
  The McMaster Health Index Questionnaire
  Medical Outcome Study Short-Form General Health Survey (MOS)
  The Norbeck Social Support Scale
  The Nottingham Health Profile
  Profile of Mood States (POMS)
  Psychosocial Adjustment to Medical Illness (PAIS)
  Quality of Life Index by Padilla et al. (QLI)
  Quality of Life Index by Spitzer et al. (QL-Index)
  The Rosenberg Self-Esteem Scale
  Sickness Impact Profile (SIP)
  The Spielberger State-Trait Anxiety Inventory (STAI)
  The Ware Health Perceptions Questionnaire

Cancer-Specific Questionnaires
  Breast Cancer Chemotherapy Questionnaire
  The Bush Bone Marrow Transplant Symptom Inventory
  Cancer Rehabilitation Evaluation System (CARES)
  City of Hope, Quality of Life: Bone Marrow Transplant
  Demands of Bone Marrow Transplant Inventory (DBMT)
  European Organization for Research and Treatment of Cancer (EORTC) Quality of Life
    Questionnaire (QLQ-C30). Modules for lung cancer and bone marrow transplant symptoms
  Functional Assessment of Cancer Therapy Scale (FACT-G). Modules for head and neck,
    breast, prostate, lung, and colorectal cancer
  Functional Living Index: Cancer (FLIC)
  Linear Analog Self-Assessment (LASA): Breast Cancer
  Quality Adjusted Time Without Symptoms or Toxicity (Q-TWIST)
  Quality of Life Index: Cancer Version, by Ferrans and Powers
  The Rotterdam Symptom Checklist (QOL after breast cancer)
  Southwest Oncology Group Quality of Life Questionnaire
  Time Without Symptoms or Toxicity (TWIST)

sive discussion of reliability and validity can be found in several excellent references (Cella & Tulsky, 1990; Grant et al., 1990; Lewis, 1990; Haberman, 1995a).

QOL researchers continue to experience a dilemma when selecting instruments. Instruments with good reliability and validity are often designed for research purposes and may lack face validity and clinical relevance (Gill & Feinstein, 1994). Consequently, investigators often resort to developing a new QOL questionnaire that is pertinent to their clinical population, but with untested reliability and validity (Cella & Tulsky, 1990). The current trend is to use existing tools with established psychometric properties rather than develop another generation of new QOL questionnaires (Grant, 1995; King et al., 1997). Virtually all of the latest generation of QOL tools have published reliability and validity estimates, or these data can be obtained directly from the author(s) of the instrument.

Additional Measurement Issues

Consideration must be given to several other measurement issues when designing a QOL study. The design and methodologic issues now discussed include the use of a single-measure or repeated-measures design, obtaining a meaningful baseline measurement, the standardization of data collection procedures, and the use of self-report data. Additional issues discussed include the potential for responder burden, methods for scoring QOL questionnaires, the need to pilot procedures and pretest instruments, and factors that influence the selection of study entry criteria. Also described are treatment effectiveness designs, the concept of statistical power, and options for statistical analysis.

Single or Repeated Measurements. Investigators must determine if the data will be collected at one point in time or on multiple occasions. A cross-sectional design that gathers data on a single occasion is economical, places little burden on research participants, and often results in less missing data than a repeated-measures design. Since cross-sectional designs only provide a static, snapshot view, they do not capture the dynamic changes in QOL that occur over time.

Serial or repeated measurement presents many challenges for QOL research design, analysis, and interpretation (Gotay et al., 1992). Some of the methodological issues pertaining to a QOL instrument's sensitivity and responsiveness to detecting changes in clinical status over time are described in Epstein (2000). The advantage of using a repeated-measures design is that QOL outcomes can be examined longitudinally for fluctuations across time. QOL data are time dependent. Unlike survival rates and disease progression data, QOL data cannot be recovered once lost, or retrieved at some later time if initially overlooked (Clinch & Schipper, 1993; Gotay et al., 1992). The psychosocial morbidity that may occur during the acute phase of therapy, for instance, can easily be measured prospectively on a "real-time" basis, but not readily captured once the person moves to another phase of adjustment.

Some disadvantages of serial measurement are that it is labor intensive and prone to galloping measurement error. If a questionnaire has poor reliability, for example, any unreliability of measurement that occurs at the first measurement occasion will be repeated and magnified across subsequent measurement occasions. When using a serial measurement design, data collection intervals need to be chosen carefully so the effects of the treatment-delivery schedule and any anticipated changes in the client's QOL will be captured (Gotay et al., 1992). A fixed schedule of data collection that is not linked to disease- or therapy-specific issues and to clients' life circumstances is unlikely to yield any useful information (Epstein, 2000; Gotay et al., 1992; Moinpour et al., 1989). In an effort to standardize the serial collection of QOL data in clinical trials, the Southwest Oncology Group recommended obtaining data on a minimum of three occasions: a baseline measurement prior to the initiation of therapy, a second measurement that occurs sometime during the course of active treatment when symptoms are at their maximum intensity, and a final measurement at some point after the conclusion of therapy (Moinpour & Hayden, 1990).

Other measurement challenges occur with the use of repeated-measures designs. Prospective, longitudinal designs are prone to higher attrition rates than cross-sectional designs. Research participants may become bored when asked to complete the same questionnaires time after time. Moreover, individuals may become too sick to participate in the study or die while enrolled in a study that spans several months or years. Strategies for minimizing study attrition with repeated-measures designs include the use of one data collector who can establish a relationship with the participant; being flexible and collecting the data when it is convenient to the participant's treatment regimen or daily activities; and, if possible, collecting data in the participant's home or during a regularly scheduled clinic visit (Haberman, 1993).

Baseline Measurement. When to obtain entry-level or baseline data is a long-standing measurement issue that is not amenable to an easy solution (Clinch & Schipper, 1993; Gotay et al., 1992). QOL studies generally use participants as their own internal controls, and normative baseline data are often unavailable. The data obtained at the first data point must provide the anchor or point of comparison for all subsequent measurement (Bush et al., 2000; Clinch & Schipper, 1993).

The most meaningful baseline data point occurs prior to the onset and diagnosis of cancer. Obviously, a precancerous baseline is generally impractical if not impossible to obtain unless data are available from prospective, long-range cancer prevention trials or studies of healthy people that span many decades. In choosing the first data point, investigators must consider the emotional fluctuations that accompany the period of initial diagnosis and therapy; the demands of illness placed on newly diagnosed persons with cancer and their families; the treatment-delivery schedule; the intensity and duration of side effects; as well as patterns of disease progression, remission, and relapse. Selecting the first data point is often an ethical dilemma. Investigators must strive to balance the need to obtain meaningful baseline data with the realities of clinical practice and the need to protect the privacy, self-determination, and well-being of participants.

Standardized Data Collection Procedures.   It is imperative that data be collected systematically in a consistent manner. For instance, if the study has two groups or arms (experimental and treatment-as-usual), it is essential to collect the data at the identical time point in each arm of the study. Also, the consistency of data collection is critical if more than one person is gathering the data or if data collection is taking place at several research sites. Training sessions are needed to ensure that everyone involved with data collection can practice the full range of data gathering procedures and receive constructive feedback from the investigator on protocol breaches. Data collectors should undergo repeated training until a high degree of interrater reliability is achieved. Moreover, all procedures must be monitored for the entire life cycle of the study to ensure continuing adherence to the established data collection protocol.

Another strategy for standardizing data collection is the use of an audit trail. An audit trail is a systematic method of monitoring the reliability of data collection, management, and entry activities. Audit trails are one important component of monitoring the scientific integrity of clinical research. An audit trail may include the routine examination of all questionnaires and data collection sheets for missing or incorrect data entry. Additionally, data extracted from the medical record and forced into categories, such as ratings of symptom toxicities, must be audited by comparing the categorized ratings with the original raw data. Data entered into a statistical software program for data storage and management must be checked for accuracy to identify any errors in data entry. Similarly, transcribed interview data should be compared with the original audiotape recordings to check for reliable transcription.

The Use of Self-Report Data.   It is widely acknowledged that QOL data should be gathered from the perspective of the person with cancer rather than from proxies (health care professionals or family members) (Bush et al., 1995; King et al., 1997; Osoba, 1994). Assessment of QOL by an observer will be biased by the observer's own internal standards of what constitutes a desirable QOL (Osoba, 1994). Gill and Feinstein (1994) noted that QOL assessment is "aimed at the wrong target unless individual patients are given the opportunity to express their individual opinions and reactions" (p. 624). Evidence exists that self-report QOL data obtained from oncology patients is consistent with QOL-related information contained in the medical records (Velikova et al., 2001).

Self-report is the only direct method for obtaining appropriate information on the meaning of illness, the burden of therapy, deficits in functioning, and symptom distress, to name a few. Of course, there are exceptions to this viewpoint. When the purpose of the study is to compare different perspectives of QOL, or to investigate the QOL of children who are too young to complete questionnaires designed for adults, or when the health status of the client is waning, data must be obtained from family members, caregivers, parents of young children, or health care providers.

Investigators must evaluate the limitations of self-report data, namely, missing or inconsistent responses, misunderstood directions, and barriers due to language differences and cultural diversity (Cella & Tulsky, 1990). Other major limitations of self-assessment data are the effects of social desirability and problems with memory decay and the poor recall of distant events. Because it is difficult to obtain a reliable retrospective account of life events, the time frame for questionnaire responses should be limited to the past one or two weeks (Bush et al., 1995; Cella & Tulsky, 1990). A time frame greater than this will result in response biases due to memory loss, distortion, and the selective recall of events.

Responder Burden.   Investigators should try to minimize the burden placed on research participants, clinical staff, and institutional resources. Interestingly, many respondents in QOL studies view their participation as therapeutic rather than burdensome (Bush et al., 1995). Respondents are generally relieved and gratified when researchers are willing to listen to their personal stories and document any deficits in QOL.

Responder burden can be reduced in many ways. Generally speaking, the use of a single instrument or short packet of questionnaires is better than administering a taxing battery of tools. Some investigators compile a large packet of instruments because they fear they are going to miss a critical variable. However, large batteries of standardized tools are often redundant and measure the same thing, albeit somewhat differently. Participants become easily frustrated when they are asked to answer repeatedly either identical or similar questions. In an effort to ease responder burden and to test the feasibility of using new technology, Velikova and colleagues found good reliability, data quality, and acceptance when cancer patients were given QOL tools by paper and pencil and by automated computer touch-screen (Velikova et al., 1999).

Any fatigue or irritability that occurs during data collection can lead to measurement error, missing data, or study attrition. Investigators should watch for disease- and treatment-related symptoms that may contribute to measurement error or responder burden, such as disease progression, periods of active therapy, nausea, fatigue, confusion, or insomnia. Moreover, longitudinal or serial assessment requires more effort from participants than data collection at a single time point, especially if there are time-dependent changes in the respondents' health (disease progression, regimen-related toxicities, disease relapse, or a dying life course). In general, participants are more likely to decline initial participation in the study or drop out early if they are experiencing active symptoms. In designing a study, researchers should estimate the magnitude of attrition and either intentionally oversample or have a plan for the systematic replacement of study participants.

When QOL data are gathered during active treatment, responder burden can be kept within reasonable limits by staggering the administration of instruments. For instance, the full battery of questionnaires can be administered at baseline, a smaller subset can be given during active therapy, and the full packet can once again be given at the conclusion of therapy. Obviously, the data selected for exclusion during active therapy will result in a nonequivalent data set; some questionnaires will not be completed at all measurement occasions. Investigators must decide which facets of QOL are of core interest and then give priority to collecting this minimum data set at all data points. This minimum set of core data can be used to make statistical comparisons across all time points, while the data that are collected at baseline and again at the conclusion of therapy provide comparisons at only two time points.

Pilot and Pretesting.   Whenever possible, investigators should pilot the data collection procedures and pretest the questionnaires. A rigorous pilot study can identify problems with obtaining informed consent, accruing participants, and approaching participants during periods of active therapy. A pilot test also can identify sources of measurement error, the total time needed to complete a packet of questionnaires or interview, the potential for missing data, and projected rates of attrition. A pretest will provide information on questionnaire selection and construction, such as the clarity of items and instructions and the possible offensiveness of some questions.

Scoring QOL Questionnaires.   Most standardized instruments come with a scoring manual that identifies which items belong to each QOL domain or subscale, the possible range of scores for the subscales and instrument as a whole, the items that are reverse-scored, the weighing of items, and so forth.

The weight given to individual QOL items or subscales on a multidimensional questionnaire has been handled differently by various researchers. Some investigators advocate a summing of scores to obtain a total score for the entire instrument, while others argue in favor of reporting only the separate scores. Summing scores to obtain an aggregate score assumes that all domains of QOL are equally weighted and contribute equally to the overall QOL score. However, the number of items in a subscale can lead to the over- or underemphasis of specific domains of QOL if some dimensions have either a greater or fewer number of questions, respectively (Clinch & Schipper, 1993). In this case, a total score that is obtained by summing the individual items is implicitly weighted by the number of items that compose each subscale or dimension of QOL. For instance, if a physical-functioning subscale has 30 items and a spirituality subscale has only 5 items, the total subscale scores can give the false impression that physical functioning is a more important component of QOL than spirituality. Moreover, two people may have the same total score on the instrument as a whole, but one person may have poor physical functioning and excellent social functioning while the other person may have just the opposite pattern of scores.

From both a conceptual and psychometric perspective, it is more informative to report QOL scores on an item-by-item or subscale-by-subscale basis than to aggregate the results into a single composite score (Bush et al., 1995, 2000; Gill & Feinstein, 1994; Haberman, 1995b; Osoba, 1994). Summing subscale scores on a multidimensional questionnaire is akin to mixing apples and oranges, resulting in a summary statistic that is conceptually meaningless (Edwards, 1970; Haberman, 1995a). Aggregate scores reduce the many facets of QOL to a single, summary statistic that provides little information about individual differences in QOL. Clinicians do not plan their interventions based on an aggregate score of QOL but on discrete issues, for example, the intensity of symptoms such as pain and nausea (Haberman, 1995b). Although the aggregation of scores does not effectively characterize QOL, it often forces investigators to describe how they weigh constituent dimensions of QOL (Gill & Feinstein, 1994). In an effort to clarify how people weigh the individual facets of their lives, Ferrans and Powers (1985) developed a QOL Index that asks respondents not only to rate the frequency or occurrence of individual items, but also to weigh each item for its relative importance. Gill and Feinstein (1994) advocated that all QOL studies should obtain ratings of both the severity and perceived importance of a problem. A clearer understanding of how to weigh individual items and domains of QOL still requires further study (Osoba, 1994).

Entry Criteria.   Inclusion and exclusion criteria place parameters on the selection of a research sample. Common inclusion criteria may include the type of disease or therapy, disease staging, age, ability to read and write English or another language, cognitive or mental status, and Karnofsky Performance Status rating. Entry criteria, as a form of design control, attempt to minimize the effects of confounding factors that may potentially threaten statistical power.

If a selected entry characteristic is expected to be correlated with the study's QOL outcomes, it should be stratified and statistically controlled either as an independent variable or covariate (Cella & Tulsky, 1990). For example, several studies have found an inverse relationship between the variable "age at the time of bone marrow transplant" and long-term QOL; the higher the age, the poorer the QOL (Andrykowski, Henslee, & Farrall, 1989; Bush et al., 1995). Age can be used to stratify the sample when testing for group differences in QOL outcomes. Conversely, if there is no reason to suspect that an entry characteristic is associated in some fashion with the study's QOL endpoints, then participants should not be excluded from the study based on that particular inclusion characteristic (Cella & Tulsky, 1990).

Treatment Effectiveness Designs. Treatment effectiveness studies are often called clinical trials or intervention studies. For example, a nursing intervention study may use a quasi-experimental design to test if a new information packet on the self-management of cancer-related fatigue improves QOL outcomes better than a routine treatment that does not include the information packets.

Treatment effectiveness designs have several key design characteristics: the random selection and assignment of participants to an experimental and control condition, an intervention that is administered in the treatment group but not the control condition, the application of design strategies that control for threats to internal validity, and the measurement of selected QOL-dependent variables (Haberman, 1995a; Lipsey, 1990). Conducting statistical tests to determine if a significant difference exists between the means of the intervention and treatment-as-usual groups on each QOL-dependent measure is a central feature of treatment effectiveness research designs (Lipsey, 1990).

Statistical Power and Statistical Analysis Plan. An important part of statistical analysis is the concept of statistical power. Statistical power is the probability that a statistically significant difference will be detected, given that a treatment effect really exists (Lipsey, 1990). It is determined by four factors: the alpha level, the effect size, the sample size, and the statistical analysis plan. The alpha level is the probability that the null hypothesis of "no difference" is rejected when, in fact, it is actually true. In other words, the investigator concludes falsely that a difference actually exists between two treatments when, in fact, it does not—a false positive (Haberman, 1995a). Investigators strive to minimize this type of erroneous conclusion by choosing a stringent alpha or p-value such as $p \leq 0.05$. A larger alpha makes statistical significance easier to attain than a smaller alpha.

The effect size is the second factor that influences statistical power. The effect size is the magnitude of response or the degree to which there is some real prespecified difference between the therapeutic conditions (Cella & Tulsky, 1990; Lipsey, 1990). Lipsey (1990) notes that the larger the effect produced by the new therapy on a given outcome measure, the more likely it is that statistical significance will be attained, and the greater will be the statistical power.

The third factor that influences statistical power is the sample size. Since sampling error is greater for small samples and virtually negligible for very large samples, the size of the sample affects the probability of making erroneous statistical conclusions and, consequently, the statistical power (Lipsey, 1990). Selecting a sufficiently large sample is a critical issue when conducting nursing intervention or treatment effectiveness research. A sample size estimation tells the investigator the exact number of participants needed to detect a statistical difference between the treatment and control condition, if the hypothesized therapeutic effect actually exists (Haberman, 1995a). Ordinarily, the investigator selects the desired parameters and then refers to a chart or table to ascertain the required sample size. The criterion for statistical power is usually set between 0.80 and 0.95. Alpha is usually set at $p \leq 0.05$ and a suitable effect size will range from low (0.20), to moderate (0.50), to high (0.80). Several references provide charts and, if necessary, additional statistical techniques that precisely calculate the estimated sample size (Cohen, 1988; Lipsey, 1990; Julious, Campbell, Walker, George, & Machin, 2000).

The analysis plan is the last factor that affects statistical power. Various statistical tests will result in different levels of power when used for the same data set. Descriptive analysis, the most basic type of summary analysis, examines how QOL variables are distributed based on properties of symmetry, peakedness, central tendency, and dispersion (Statistical Navigator Professional, 1992). Descriptive statistics include frequencies; the mean, median, and mode; standard deviations; ranges; and skewness.

At a higher level of analysis, QOL variables can be examined for their degree of association. Variables are said to be associated to the extent that they covary. On the other hand, if two variables are highly interrelated, then one variable is a good predictor of the other (Statistical Navigator Professional, 1992). Some examples of measures of association are the bivariate regression coefficient, chi-square, Pearson product-moment correlation, point-biserial r, Spearman's *rho*, and Kendall's *tau*.

Hypothesis testing and tests of significance are other types of analyses commonly used in QOL research. Hypothesis testing involves some type of statistical comparison for differences within or between two or more groups. For instance, the means on a QOL questionnaire can be compared for persons receiving experimental therapy versus treatment-as-usual to determine which therapy results in a higher QOL. In addition to determining if there is a statistically significant difference within or between groups, measures of association can be added to examine the magnitude of the relationship (Statistical Navigator Professional, 1992). Depending on the level of data (nominal, ordinal, interval, or ratio-level data) the types of statistical tests most commonly used to examine group differences are the chi-square, analysis of variance (ANOVA), Fisher's test, Kruskal-Wallis test, McNemar test, *t*-test, repeated-measures ANOVA, and the Wilcoxon test.

Causal analysis is the highest form of statistical analysis. Causal modeling is used when the investigator is trying to explain, predict, or control for the effect of one or more independent variables on a single QOL-dependent variable (Statistical Navigator Professional, 1992). More complex types of causal modeling may add some intervening or mediating variables into the path analysis. For example, multivariate causal analysis examines the effects of a set of selected variables on the dependent variable while controlling for other intervening variables statistically (Statistical Navigator Professional, 1992). Examples of causal analyses are analysis of covariance, canonical correlation, discriminant analysis, regression analysis, path analysis, LISREL, stratified analysis, and log-linear model testing.

Directions for Future Research

The current state-of-the science of QOL measurement calls for a comprehensive, multidimensional assessment of health-related cancer outcomes, gathered from the perspective of the person with cancer, and with minimal burden to the respondent. Investigators may choose from a variety of generic or cancer-specific QOL questionnaires that report excellent reliability and validity.

Investigators are encouraged to use multiple methods of data collection depending on the endpoints of interest and available resources. Data gathered from qualitative inquiry may either augment or serve as a substitute for data obtained by standardized questionnaires. Qualitative inquiry offers an explanatory richness that is unattainable from quantitative approaches. Cancer survivors can tell their stories in their own words and give voice to the personal meaning of quality of life through qualitative methods (Hassey Dow et al., 1999).

Although nurse scientists now have many tools for documenting the QOL endpoints of nursing care, there remains a need to develop QOL tools that are suitable for routine clinical assessment and the long-term monitoring of cancer survivors. To aid the collection of clinically relevant outcome data, Klee et al. (2000) developed a clinical model for the routine assessment of QOL in persons receiving chemotherapy. Moreover, Detmar and Aaronson (1998) found routine QOL assessments in an outpatient oncology setting stimulated physicians to discuss specific issues related to the QOL of their patients. Despite the desire by many clinicians to fold QOL evaluation into daily practice, more research is needed to examine the competing expectations that exist between patients and clinicians as to who should initiate the discussion of QOL issues (Detmar, Aaronson, Wever, Muller, & Schornagel, 2000).

Grant (1995) indicated that QOL research is needed to examine the cost-efficacy of different models of delivery, such as managed care or case management, and the efficacy of nursing therapeutics from a holistic view of cancer survivorship. Research also is needed to determine whether some facets of QOL are trait-like and prone to stability or state-like and predisposed to fluctuations and instability (Haberman, 1995b).

Osoba (1994) identified several future research issues. He noted that studies are needed to find better methods for selecting the most appropriate QOL instrument for a given situation and to distinguish the effects of disease from the outcomes of therapy. Osoba also commented that instrumentation research is needed to examine how to assign weights to the various domains of QOL as well as to identify which finding is more relevant, a statistically significant difference in QOL or a difference that is meaningful to the person with cancer.

Ganz (1994) also identified several future trends in QOL research. She indicated that (a) it will become routine to ask clients to assess their QOL so they can decide between alternative therapies with equivalent survival outcomes but different toxicities, (b) normative data will become available for many of the existing QOL instruments, (c) new tools will be developed for clinical practice, and (d) the periodic assessment of QOL will be a routine aspect of the long-term follow-up of cancer survivors. For this to occur, QOL outcomes will need to become a required component of all Phase III clinical trials, prospective chemoprevention trials, and nursing intervention studies. For instance, additional research is needed to identify the acute and late effects of cancer therapy on persons with cancer and their families (National Institutes of Health Consensus Development Conference Statement, 2000). Nursing therapeutics designed to improve QOL and family functioning need further testing as to the feasibility of delivering family-focused care in a variety of clinical venues (Lewis & Zahlis, 1997).

Nurses can encourage persons with cancer to enroll in clinical trials and nursing studies that examine QOL outcomes. Clinical trials are needed to determine the prognostic value of pretreatment QOL indicators for predicting on-treatment QOL, median and long-term survival, and for assigning people to suitable treatments (Osoba, 1994). While the majority of extant QOL studies have examined symptoms, functional status, distress, and well-being, more studies are needed to address the relationships among QOL, treatment efficacy, phase specific and long-term treatment costs, years of life lost from cancer, and the allocation of health care resources (Brown, Lipscomb, & Snyder, 2001; Owen, Klapow, Hicken, & Tucker, 2001).

The future will bring the increasing use of QOL outcomes by consumer advocates, insurance companies, and health policy makers to determine insurance benefits and to allocate limited cancer care resources (Ganz, 1994). However, because there is a potential to abuse QOL information and employ it as a form of discrimination, clinical trials are needed to determine how to protect persons with cancer from the unethical use of QOL information (Osoba, 1994).

Conclusion

In summary, oncology nurses are strategically positioned in the health care system to transfer the findings of QOL research into daily practice, to augment the existing scientific foundation for a QOL theory-based practice, and to resolve many of the design and methodologic challenges that confront QOL researchers.

References

Aaronson, N. K. (1990). Quality of life research in cancer clinical trials: A need for common rules and language. *Oncology, 4*(5), 59–66.

Aaronson, N. K., Ahmedzai, S., Bergman, B., Bullinger, M., Cull, A., Duez, N. J., Filiberti, A., Flechtner, H., Fleishman, S. B., & de Haes, J. C. (1993). The European Organization for Research and Treatment of Cancer QLQ-C30: A quality-of-life instrument for use in international clinical trials in oncology. *Journal of the National Cancer Institute, 85*(5), 365–376.

Aaronson, N. K., Bullinger, M., & Ahmedzai, S. (1988). A modular approach to quality-of-life assessment in cancer clinical trials. *Recent Results Cancer Research, 111,* 231–244.

Andrykowski, M. A., Henslee, P. J., & Farrall, M. G. (1989). Physical and psychosocial functioning of adult survivors of allogeneic bone marrow transplantation. *Bone Marrow Transplantation, 4,* 75–81.

Belec, R. (1992). Quality of life: Perceptions of long-term survivors of bone marrow transplantation. *Oncology Nursing Forum, 19*(1), 31–37.

Bergner, M., Bobbitt, R. A., Carter, W. B., & Gilson, B. S. (1981). The sickness impact profile: Development and final revision of a health status measure. *Medical Care, 19,* 787–806.

Bernhard, J., Sullivan, M., Hurny, C., Coates, A. S., & Rudenstam, C. M. (2001). Clinical relevance of single item quality of life indicators in cancer clinical trials. *British Journal of Cancer, 84*(9), 1156–1165.

Brown, M. L., Lipscomb, J., & Snyder, C. (2001). The burden of illness of cancer; Economic cost and quality of life. *Annu. Rev. Public Health, 22,* 91–113.

Bush, N. E., Donaldson, G. W., Haberman, M. H., Dacanay, R., & Sullivan, K. M. (2000). Conditional and unconditional estimation of multidimensional quality of life after hematopoietic stem cell transplantation: A longitudinal follow-up of 415 patients. *Biology of Blood and Marrow Transplantation, 6,* 576–591.

Bush, N. E., Haberman, M., Donaldson, G., & Sullivan, K. M. (1995). Quality of life of 125 adults surviving 6–18 years after bone marrow transplantation. *Social Science and Medicine, 40*(4), 479–490.

Cella, D. F. (1993). Quality of life as an outcome of cancer treatment. In S. L. Groenwald, M. Goodman, M. H. Frogge, & C. H. Yarbro (Eds.), *Cancer nursing: Principles and practice* (3rd ed.) (pp. 197–207). Boston: Jones and Bartlett.

Cella, D. F., & Tulsky, D. S. (1990). Measuring quality of life today: Methodological aspects. *Oncology, 4*(5), 29–38.

Cella, D. F., Tulsky, D. S., Gray, G., Sarafian, B., Linn, E., Bonomi, A., Silberman, M., Yellen, S. B., Winicour, P., Brannon, J., Eckberg, K., Lloyd, S., Purl, S., Blenowski, C., Goodman, M., Barnicle, M., Stewart, I., McHale, M., Bonomi, P., Kaplan, E., Taylor, S., IV, Thomas, C. R., Jr., & Harris, J. (1993). The Functional Assessment of Cancer Therapy scale: Development and validation of the general measure. *Journal of Clinical Oncology, 11*(3), 570–579.

Clinch, J. J., & Schipper, H. (1993). Quality of life assessment in palliative care. In D. Doyle, G. W. C. Hanks, & N. MacDonald (Eds.), *Oxford textbook of palliative medicine* (pp. 61–70). Oxford, England: Oxford University Press.

Cohen, J. (1988). *Statistical power analysis for the behavioral sciences* (2nd ed.). Hillsdale, NJ: Lawrence Erlbaum Associates.

Cole, B. F., Gelber, R. D., Gelber, S., Coates, A. S., & Goldhirsch, A. (2001). Polychemotherapy for early breast cancer: An overview of the randomised clinical trials with quality-adjusted survival analysis. *Lancet,* Jul 28, *358*(9278), 277–286.

Dean, H. (1997). Multiple instruments for measuring quality of life. In M. Frank-Stromborg & S. Olsen (Eds.), *Instruments for clinical health-care research* (2nd ed.) (pp. 135–148). Boston: Jones and Bartlett.

de Haes, J., Curran, D., Young, T., Bottomley, A., Flechtner, H., Aaronson, N., Blazeby, J., Bjordal, K., Brandberg, Y., Greimel, E., Maher, J., Sprangers, M., & Cull, A. (2000). Quality of life evaluation in oncological clinical trials—the EORTC model. *European Journal of Cancer, 36,* 821–825.

Denzin, N. K., & Lincoln, Y. S. (Eds.). (1984). *Handbook of qualitative research*. Thousand Oaks, CA: Sage.

Detmar, S. B., & Aaronson, N. K. (1998). Quality of life assessment in daily clinical oncology practice: A feasibility study. *European Journal of Cancer, 34*(8), 1181–1186.

Detmar, S. B., Aaronson, N. K., Wever, L. D. V., Muller, M., & Schornagel, J. H. (2000). How are you feeling? Who wants to know? Patients' and oncologists' preferences for discussing health-related quality of life issues. *Journal of Clinical Oncology, 18*(18)(September 15), 3295–3301.

Donnelly, S., Rybicki, L., & Walsh, D. (2001). Quality of life measurement in the palliative management of advanced cancer. *Support Care Cancer, 9,* 361–365.

Edwards, A. L. (1970). *The measurement of personality traits by scales and inventories*. New York: Holt, Rhinehart and Winston.

Epstein, R. S. (2000). Responsiveness in quality-of-life assessment: Nomenclature, determinants, and clinical applications. *Medical Care, 38*(9), (Suppl. II), 91–94.

Ferrans, C. E., & Powers, M. J. (1985). Quality of life index: Development and psychometric properties. *Advances in Nursing Science, 8*(1), 15–24.

Ferrell, B. R., Dow, K. H., Leigh, S., Ly, J., & Gulasekaram, P. (1995). Quality of life in long-term cancer survivors. *Oncology Nursing Forum, 22*(6), 915–922.

Frank-Stromborg, M., & Olsen, S. J. (Eds.). (1997). *Instruments for clinical health-care research* (2nd ed.). Boston: Jones and Bartlett.

Ganz, P. A. (1994). Quality of life and the patient with cancer: Individual and policy complications. *Cancer, 74*(Suppl. 4), 1445–1452.

Ganz, P. A., Rofessart, J., Polinsky, M. L., Schag, C. C., & Heinrich, R. L. (1986). A comprehensive approach to the assessment of cancer patients' rehabilitation needs: The cancer inventory of problem situations and a companion interview. *Journal of Psychosocial Oncology, 4*(3), 27–42.

Gill, T. M., & Feinstein, A. R. (1994). A critical appraisal of the quality of quality-of-life measurements. *Journal of the American Medical Association, 272*(8), 619–631.

Gotay, C. C., Korn, E. L., McCabe, M. S., Moore, T. D., & Cheson, B. D. (1992). Quality-of-life assessment in cancer treatment protocols: Research issues in protocol development. *Journal of the National Cancer Institute, 84*(8), 575–579.

Gotay, C. C., & Muraoka, M. Y. (1998). Quality of life in long-term survivors of adult-onset cancers. *Journal of the National Cancer Institute, 90*(9), May 6, 656–667.

Grant, M. (1995). Quality of life research: Where we are, where we need to go. *Nurse Investigator, 2*(1), 1–2.

Grant, M., Padilla, G. V., Ferrell, B. R., & Rhiner, M. (1990). Assessment of quality of life with a single instrument. *Seminars in Oncology Nursing, 6*(4), 260–270.

Haberman, M. (1993). Commentary. In C. Jansen, P. Halliburton, S. Dibble, & M. J. Dodd. Family problems during cancer chemotherapy. *Oncology Nursing Forum, 20*(4), 689–696.

Haberman, M. (1994). Quality of life as an outcome for oncology nursing. In P. T. Rieger (Ed.), *Fighting fatigue: Resolving issues for the cancer patient* (pp. 30–36). Continuing Medical Education Monograph. Beachwood, OH: Pro ED.

Haberman, M. (1995a). Nursing Research. In P. C. Buchsel & M. B. Whedon (Eds.), *Bone marrow transplantation: Administrative and clinical strategies* (pp. 365–402). Boston: Jones and Bartlett.

Haberman, M. R. (1995b). Commentary. In M. Whedon, D. Stearns, & L. E. Mills. Quality of life of long-term adult survivors of autologous bone marrow transplantation. *Oncology Nursing Forum, 22*(10), 1527–1537.

Haberman, M. R., Bush, N., Young, K., & Sullivan, K. M. (1993). Quality of life of adult long-term survivors of bone marrow transplantation: A qualitative analysis of narrative data. *Oncology Nursing Forum, 20*(10), 1545–1553.

Haberman, M. R., & Lewis, F. M. (1990). Selection of research designs. Section I: Qualitative paradigms. In M. M. Grant & G. V. Padilla (Eds.), *Cancer nursing research: A practical approach* (pp. 77–83). Norwalk, CT: Appleton & Lange.

Haberman, M. R., Woods, N. F., & Packard, N. J. (1990). Demands of chronic illness: Reliability and validity assessment of a demands-of-illness inventory. *Holistic Nurse Practitioner, 5*(1), 25–35.

Hassey Dow, K., Ferrell, B. R., Haberman, M. R., & Eaton, L. (1999). The meaning of quality of life in cancer survivorship. *Oncology Nursing Forum, 26*(3), 519–528.

Holzner, B., Kemmler, G., Sperner-Unterweger, B., Kopp, M., Dunser, M., Margreiter, R., Marschitz, I., Nachbaur, D., Fleischhacker, W. W., & Greil, R. (2001). Quality of life measurement in oncology—a matter of assessment instrument? *European Journal of Cancer, 37,* 2349–2356.

Jalowiec, A. (1990). Issues in using multiple measures of quality of life. *Seminars in Oncology Nursing, 6*(4), 271–277.

Julious, S. A., Campbell, M. J., Walker, S. J., George, S. L., & Machin, D. (2000). Sample sizes for cancer trials where health related quality of life is the primary outcome. *British Journal of Cancer, 83*(7), 959–963.

Karnofsky, D. S., & Burchenal, J. H. (1949). The clinical evaluation of chemotherapeutic agents in cancer. In C. M. MacLeod (Ed.), *Evaluation of chemotherapeutic agents.* New York: Columbia University Press.

King, C. R., Haberman, M., Berry, D. L., Bush, N., Butler, L., Dow, K. H., Ferrell, B., Grant, M., Gue, D., Hinds, P., Kreuer, J., Padilla, G., & Underwood, S. (1997). Quality of life and the cancer experience: The state-of-the-knowledge. *Oncology Nursing Forum, 24*(1), 27–41.

Klee, M. C., King, M. T., Machin, D., & Hansen, H. H. (2000). A clinical model for quality of life assessment in cancer patients receiving chemotherapy. *Annals of Oncology, 11,* 23–30.

Lee, C. W., & Chi, K. N. (2000). The standard of reporting of health-related quality of life in clinical cancer trials. *Journal of Clinical Epidemiology, 53,* 451–458.

Levine, M. N., Guyatt, G. H., Gent, M., De Pauw, S., Goodyear, M. D., Hryniuk, W. M., Arnold, A., Findlay, B., Skillings, J. R., & Bramwell, V. H. (1988). Quality of life in stage II breast cancer: An instrument for clinical trials. *Journal of Clinical Oncology, 6*(12), 1798–1810.

Lewis, F. M. (1990). Selection of the research designs. Section II: Experimental and quasi-experimental designs. In M. Grant & G. Padilla (Eds.), *Cancer nursing research: A practical approach* (pp. 83–100). Norwalk, CT: Appleton & Lange.

Lewis, F. M., & Zahlis, E. H. (1997). The nurse as coach: A conceptual framework for clinical practice. *Oncology Nursing Forum, 24*(10), 1695–1702.

Lipsey, M. W. (1990). *Design sensitivity: Statistical power for experimental research.* Newbury Park, CA: Sage.

Mast, M. E. (1995). Definition and measurement of quality of life in oncology nursing research: Review and theoretical implications. *Oncology Nursing Forum, 22*(6), 957–964.

McCahill, L. E., Krouse, R., Chu, D., Juarez, G., Uman, G. C., Ferrell, B., & Wagman, L. D. (2002). Indications and use of palliative surgery-results of Society of Surgical Oncology survey. *Annals Surgical Oncology, 9*(1), 104–112.

Miles, M. B., & Huberman, A. M. (1994). *Qualitative data analysis: An expanded sourcebook.* Thousand Oaks, CA: Sage.

Mitchell, E. S. (1986). Multiple triangulation: A methodology for nursing science. *Advances in Nursing Science, 8*(3), 18–26.

Moinpour, C. M., Feigl, P., Metch, B., Hayden, K. A., Meyskens, F. L., Jr., & Crowley, J. (1989). Quality of life end points in cancer clinical trials: Review and recommendations. *Journal of the National Cancer Institute, 81*(7), 485–495.

Moinpour, C. M., & Hayden, K. A. (1990). Quality of life assessment in Southwest Oncology Group Trials. *Oncology, 4*(5), 79–84, 89.

Montazeri, A., Gillis, C. R., & McEwen, J. (1996). Measuring quality of life in oncology: Is it worthwhile? I. Meaning, purposes and controversies. *European Journal of Cancer Care, 5*, 159–167.

National Institutes of Health Consensus Development Conference Statement: Adjuvant Therapy for Breast Cancer, November 1–3, 2000. *Journal of the National Cancer Institute, 93*(13), 979–989.

Nayfield, S. G., Ganz, P. A., Moinpour, C. M., Cella, D. F., & Hailey, B. J. (1992). Report from a national cancer institute (USA) workshop on quality of life assessment in cancer clinical trials. *Quality of Life Research, 1*, 203–210.

Nayfield, S. G., Hailey, B. J., & McCabe, M. (1991). *Quality of life assessment in cancer clinical trials.* Report of the Workshop on Quality of Life Research in Cancer Clinical Trials, July 16–17, 1990. Bethesda, MD: U.S. Department of Health and Human Services.

Osoba, D. (1994). Lessons learned from measuring health-related quality of life in oncology. *Journal of Clinical Oncology, 12*(3), 608–616.

Osoba, D., Dancey, J., Zee, B., Myles, J., & Pater, J. (1996). Health-related quality of life studies of the National Cancer Institute of Canada clinical trials group [Monograph]. *Journal National Cancer Institute, 20*, 107–111.

Owen, J. E., Klapow, J. C., Hicken, B., & Tucker, D. C. (2001). Psychosocial interventions for cancer: Review and analysis using a three-tiered outcomes model. *Psycho-oncology. 10*, 218–230.

Padilla, G., & Frank-Stromborg, M. (1997). Single instruments for measuring quality of life. In M. Frank-Stromborg, & S. Olsen (Eds.), *Instruments for clinical health-care research* (2nd ed.) (pp. 114–134). Boston: Jones and Bartlett.

Padilla, G. V., & Grant, M. M. (1985). Quality of life as a cancer nursing outcome variable. *Advances in Nursing Science, 8*(1), 45–60.

Padilla, G. V., Grant, M. M., & Ferrell, B. (1992). Nursing research into quality of life. *Quality of Life Research, 1*, 341–348.

Reynolds, T. (1994). Quality of life adds a human dimension to studies on treatment cost-effectiveness. *Journal of the National Cancer Institute, 86*(9), 661–662.

Shapiro, S. L., Lopez, A. M., Schwartz, G. E., Bootzin, R., Figueredo, A. J., Braden, C. J., & Kurker, S. F. (2001). Quality of life and breast cancer: Relationship to psychosocial variables. *Journal of Clinical Psychology, 57*(4), 501–519.

Statistical Navigator Professional, Version 2.0. (1992). Columbia, MO: The Idea Works, Inc.

Stewart, A. L., Hays, R. D., & Ware, J. E. (1988). The MOS Short-form General Health Survey: Reliability and validity in a patient population. *Medical Care, 26*, 724–735.

Stewart, A. L. & Napoles-Springer, A. (2000). Health-related quality of life assessments in diverse population groups in the United States. *Medical Care. 38*(9), (Suppl. II), 102–124.

Tchekmedyian, N. S., & Cella, D. F. (Eds.). (1990, May 5). Quality of life in current oncology practice and research [Special issue]. *Oncology, 4.*

Testa, M. A. (2000). Interpretation of quality of life outcomes: Issues that affect magnitude and meaning. *Medical Care. 38*(9), (Suppl. II), 166–174.

Velikova, G., Stark, D., & Selby, P. (1999). Quality of life instruments in oncology. *European Journal of Cancer, 35*(11), 1571–1580.

Velikova, G., Wright, E. P., Smith, A. B., Cull, A., Gould, A., Forman, D., Perren, T., Stead, M., Brown, J., & Selby, P. J. (1999). Automated collection of quality of life data: A comparison of paper and computer touch-screen questionnaires. *Journal of Clinical Oncology, 17*(3), 998–1007.

Velikova, G., Wright, P., Smith, A. B., Stark, D., Perren, T., Brown, J., & Selby, P. (2001). Self-reported quality of life of individual cancer patients: Concordance of results with disease course and medical records. *Journal of Clinical Oncology, 19*(7), 2064–2073.

Whedon, M., & Ferrell, B. R. (1994). Quality of life in adult bone marrow transplant patients: Beyond the first year. *Seminars in Oncology Nursing, 10*(1), 42–57.

Whedon, M., Stearns, D., & Mills, L. E. (1995). Quality of life of long-term adult survivors of autologous bone marrow transplantation. *Oncology Nursing Forum, 22*(10), 1527–1535.

Zebrack, B. (2000). Cancer survivors and quality of life: A critical review of the literature. *Oncology Nursing Forum, 27*(9), 1395–1401.

9

Quality of Life and Symptoms

BETTY R. FERRELL • MARCIA M. GRANT

A number of factors have been identified as impacting the physical well-being of the client with cancer. Many of these factors are associated with the disease itself, while others are associated with the various treatments for the disease (John, 2001; Vallerand, 1997). A major component of physical well-being is the area of symptom control. A number of symptoms have been identified as impacting physical well-being and quality of life (QOL) in general for the person with cancer (Padilla, Ferrell, Grant, & Rhiner, 1990). These include appetite disturbance, difficulty swallowing, nausea, vomiting, constipation, and diarrhea. In addition to these symptoms, other common areas of symptom control include dyspnea, fatigue, insomnia, changes in strength, and numbness. Pain is identified as another symptom with major implications for QOL (Barsevick et al., 2001).

Oncology nurses have been largely responsible for the increased priority given to symptom management. Cancer care is often focused on medical aspects such as tumor pathology, chemotherapy, surgical interventions, and laboratory data. Less priority is given to the patient's experience of the illness and resultant physical and psychological symptoms. Nursing attention to symptoms associated with treatment, such as nausea or pain, improves the quality of life (QOL) for patients and their families.

Nurses have recently extended the focus on symptoms to include their impact on QOL. Symptoms once viewed only as physical problems, such as fatigue, are increasingly examined for their impact on overall QOL. Table 9-1, an example of such research conducted by Dean and colleagues (1995), is a summary of patient comments regarding the experience of fatigue. This table illustrates that the physical experience of fatigue has multiple dimensions and impacts QOL (Wu & McSweeney, 2001; Barsevick, Whitmer, & Walker, 2001).

Table 9-1. **Descriptions of Fatigue by Patients Receiving Interferon Alpha**

Piper Fatigue Scale Dimension	Patients' Descriptions
Affective	"I can't understand why some days are normal and others I want to forget." "It (fatigue) is apparent for 24 hours after each injection while my temperature hovers around 100° . . . next day am nearly normal." "I feel quite well and very normal." "I have a lot going on in my body—killing cancer cells. So to me it's positive." ". . . makes me unable to be assertive."
Sensory	"Affects my ability to concentrate and seems to cause anxiety and edginess." "Had trouble concentrating giving lectures." "I feel physical fatigue more now when running. But my daily energy level seems okay." ". . . sometimes I feel like a wet wash cloth that has been wrung out and am so drained and exhausted. But it passes in a few hours." "Seem to be sleeping a lot, but maybe out of boredom and lack of active things to do." "Localized, constant muscle pains. Pain in joints." "General tiredness that is not localized in any one area." "Short tempered, fatigued, nauseated half the time; aggravates old pain—intensifies." "I never really felt tired or distressed that much before I started the program." "Sore muscles and no strength . . ." "My body has become very weakened and I feel a need to regain some strength. In this weakened condition, my body cannot heal itself." "It's great on Saturday or Sunday because there are more days between the (treatments) and I can get my strength and my appetite back for a while." "Further, it would be great to have my appetite back and some stamina for our vacation in March. Of course, I don't want to jeopardize my health, but I'm really feeling beat down."
Severity	"I am on vacation for 4 weeks and I do not know how to manage idle time. I spend more time than usual worrying about myself." "I don't feel like doing anything, including eating or any activity: reading, TV, or other activities." "Too tired to eat, nothing looks good or sounds good. I was on the verge of malnutrition and more. I'm tired of feeling (bad)." "This drug has really thrown my life off-key. I never have energy to do things. Never any social plans can be kept, due to never knowing how I feel." "(I) worry about my ability to work next week." ". . . I can't miss much more or I will lose my position. How clear can I be!" "My fatigue isn't intense, except after my (treatment) for a day or two."

continues

Table 9-1.   **continued**

Piper Fatigue Scale Dimension	Patients' Descriptions
Temporal	"The fatigue occurs primarily on Monday, about six hours after the (treatment) . . . lasts about eight hours. Generally when it hits, you can break through the fatigue if you push it for about two hours."
	"After (treatment) very fatigued . . . one to two days. Periods of relief though."
	"To sit down for an hour or so until it passes, and it usually passes in that time . . ."
	"(It) tires me . . . I change every day . . . (I) feel weak the first day of (treatment) . . . (My) breathing is not good when I walk (but) okay when I lay down."
	"Predictability of fatigue seems to vary with time following (treatments) or change in pain medications."

Source: Adapted from Dean, Spears, Ferrell, Quan, Groshon, & Mitchell, 1995. Used with permission of *Cancer Practice*.

Impact of Symptoms on Quality of Life

The major domains of QOL include physical well-being, psychological well-being, social concerns, and spiritual well-being (Figure 9-1). While these domains can be isolated and discussed as separate entities, a dynamic interaction exists among them. Disturbances in physical status and the occurrence of physical symptoms have a direct and profound impact on all aspects of QOL. Physical concerns such as uncontrolled symptoms or decreased function impact psychological well-being by creating tremendous anxiety, depression, and frustration in the client. Case examples are included in Figure 9-2.

Physical symptoms pose a very direct threat to the client's social concerns, as any limitation in the physical well-being of the client is almost certain to create a domino effect on family and friends who must assume care activities or symptom management duties (Andrews, 2001). Physical well-being also has a direct impact on spirituality. Studies have documented that declining physical status creates an increased awareness of personal mortality and often heightens the individual's spiritual needs (Baldacchino & Draper, 2001; Highfield, 1992). Clients struggle with the meaning of illness and issues of religiosity as they confront the deterioration of the body and multiple symptoms. Figure 9-1 illustrates the dynamic process of the impact of physical well-being on other dimensions of QOL. This model is derived from our recent research in cancer survivorship, which has demonstrated continued symptom

Figure 9-1. **Quality of life model applied to cancer survivors.**

Source: Ferrell, Hassey Dow et al., 1995. Used with permission of Oncology Nursing Press.

management concerns in long-term survival (Ferrell, Hassey Dow, Leigh, Ly, & Gulasekaram, 1995).

Symptom Management Defined

Some beginning definitions are in order. Symptoms as related to disease have been previously differentiated from signs of disease. This differentiation was identified long ago in the medical literature. In 1869, diseases were distinguished from each other by alterations in the organs as can be ascertained by an observer (physical signs) or by changes in the function of the effected parts (symptoms) (Fenwick, 1869). This differentiation is related to whether the clinician observed it (a sign) or the client experienced it (a symptom). For example, Musser and Krumbhaar (1922) reported

---

Case 1—Pain and Quality of Life

Max is a 62-year-old barber who was diagnosed with colon cancer and has recently completed his treatment, which included bowel resection followed by chemotherapy. He has recovered well from his initial treatment but experiences pain of a 5–6 on a scale of 0 = no pain to 10 = severe pain. His wife Carol says that Max doesn't sleep well because of the pain, has become constipated from the medications, and seems to be exhausted. Max is eager to return to his customers at the barber shop and visit with his grandchildren. Carol tells the social worker that Max seems increasingly depressed and anxious and says he can't understand why God wants him to suffer so much.

Case 2—Nausea and Quality of Life

Olivia is a 55-year-old music teacher diagnosed with advanced-stage ovarian cancer. Despite her declining condition, Olivia's pain has been well managed but she has developed moderate to severe nausea related to tumor growth and subsequent gastrointestinal symptoms including reflux, pressure, and constipation. The nausea and vomiting have resulted in extreme fatigue, cachexia, and insomnia. Her children describe Oliva as increasingly anxious and withdrawn and she expresses fear about "what's next."

Figure 9-2.   **Case Examples**

that the first sign noticed in a client was cyanosis and the first symptom experienced was shortness of breath. Since this early recognition of the importance of symptoms in illness, increased attention has been focused on symptom assessment and management. Table 9-2 presents a summary of symptoms commonly cited in oncology literature.

One of the first researchers in oncology nursing to focus on symptoms was Jeanne Quint Benoliel (1963). Early in her research career, Dr. Benoliel focused on clients with breast cancer and recognized the importance of symptoms and QOL concerns. At that time, it was believed that individuals with breast cancer were content to have survived even if there were serious side effects of the radical mastectomy. Dr. Benoliel's research revealed many ongoing symptoms of breast cancer and treatment that influenced QOL. Benoliel pioneered oncology nursing research in the area of physical symptoms as well as psychosocial effects of cancer and its treatment. She also advocated scientifically sound nursing practice.

In 1987, Rhodes and Watson edited an edition of *Seminars in Oncology Nursing* that focused on symptom distress. This volume of the journal examined, defined, and discussed symptom occurrence and symptom distress and explored a broad spectrum of symptoms including fatigue, insomnia, depression, anxiety, nausea, vomiting, anorexia, elimination problems, and breathing difficulty. The authors emphasized that symptoms should be defined in terms of frequency, duration, and severity and that each of these aspects may require a different measurement or scale.

Table 9-2. **Symptoms Cited in the Oncology Literature Impacting QOL**

Alopecia	Insomnia
Anorexia	Memory loss
Anxiety	Menopausal symptoms
Bleeding problems	Mouth dryness
Concentration disturbances	Mucositis/stomatitis
Confusion	Nausea
Constipation	Numbness
Delirium	Pain
Depression	Sexual dysfunction
Diarrhea	Shivering
Dysphagia	Skin problems
Dyspnea	Strength
Fatigue	Taste changes
Fear	Urinary symptoms
Fever	Visual changes
Gas/flatus	Vomiting
Hearing change	Weight loss/gain
Immobility	

Equally important is the need to define symptom distress. Rhodes and Watson (1987) defined symptom distress as the "physical or mental anguish or suffering that results from the experience of symptom occurrence" (p. 242). Symptom distress has previously been distinguished in the work of Johnson (1973), who in the 1960s differentiated the amount of pain clients were experiencing from the distresses associated with the pain. In her work on decreasing distress following surgery, diagnostic tests, and other potentially painful clinical experiences, Johnson asked clients to rate not only the pain or discomfort they were experiencing, but also the associated distress.

The importance of symptom distress is that it is directly related to the impact of symptoms on the client and, thus, on QOL. Symptom distress is also what causes the client to seek medical help for the diagnosis of disease or for relief. Symptom distress, when alleviated, may promote recovery in the client. Alleviating symptom distress may also allow the chronically ill client to maintain function and improve QOL.

Clinical Issues in Symptom Management and QOL

Oncology patients, in fact, do experience multiple symptoms, most of which cannot be eliminated but may be reduced or controlled. While the goal in some instances may be elimination of symptoms, such as pain or nausea, most often the clinical goal is reduction of symptom intensity and distress while preserving QOL.

Dyspnea is an example of a symptom that many patients with respiratory disease, such as lung cancer, experience as a chronic burden. Several nurse investigators have focused research programs on helping clients to control this symptom (Dudgeon, Kristjanson, Lertzman, & Clement, 2001). Dyspnea is also an example of a physical symptom with significant impact on psychological well-being and on overall QOL. Additional research is needed in this area.

Symptoms, then, are subjective phenomena that indicate a departure from normal functioning, sensation, or appearance and are frequently used to diagnose disease. Because they are subjective, they are difficult to evaluate. When experiencing a symptom, individuals can frequently differentiate the intensity of the symptom from the amount of distress, both of which need careful measurement. Work is needed on both symptom alleviation and control (Dooks, 2001).

Symptom management fits well with nursing, and specifically oncology nursing. The American Nurses' Association (ANA) Council of Nurse Researchers' statement, *Directions for Nursing Research: Toward the Twenty-First Century* (1985, p. 1), stated that "nursing research focuses on the entire spectrum of human responses to actual and potential health problems across the life span." These responses are frequently seen in the form of physical or psychological symptoms.

Another reason symptom management fits so well with nursing is that most symptoms are multidimensional in nature and parallel the multidimensional models of care used to shape clinical nursing care and research. For example, Roy's Adaptation Model includes bio-psycho-social dimensions (Andrews & Roy, 1991). Roy's Adaptation Model has been used as the theoretical foundation of nursing research in concert with our QOL model to represent targeted areas of QOL concern for cancer patients.

An illustration of the importance of a multidimensional view when studying a particular symptom is that of pain. McGuire (1992) described the dimensions of the pain experience and defined physiological, sensory, behavioral, cognitive, affective, and sociocultural dimensions. Each of these is an important dimension of patient care, and each dimension may be approached differently. The physiological component includes such aspects as location, onset, duration, etiology, and associated symptoms. The sensory component includes the intensity, quality, and pattern of the pain. The behavioral component includes communication about pain, interpersonal aspects, physical activity, pain behaviors, medications, interventions, and sleep. The cognitive component includes the meaning of pain, the view of pain, coping strategies, previous therapy, attitudes and beliefs, influencing factors, and prior experience of pain. The affective component refers to the mood state and includes anxiety, depression, anger, and feelings of powerlessness. The sociocultural component of pain includes the ethnic component, family and social life, work and home roles, recreation and leisure factors, social behaviors, and activities.

Symptom management is also an important QOL concern across settings of cancer care. For example, nursing care in the acute setting, where 24-hour surveillance of patients' responses occurs, is often focused on symptom management. The expertise of the advanced practice nurse or expert clinician is critical, as expert assessment is required to be more sensitive to the subtle changes in patients' symptoms that require intervention. This area fits well with Benner's (1984) work on the novice to expert nurse and illustrates the value of clinical experience coupled with expanding clinical scientific knowledge in symptom management.

The home care setting also requires extensive attention to symptoms across the trajectory of care by the client, the nurse, and frequently the family caregiver. Many questions persist regarding scientific nursing care in this setting. Our research in home care has emphasized the importance of symptom control to family caregivers. Symptoms are the major source of family concern. The presence of uncontrolled symptoms effects QOL for both patient and family caregiver (Ferrell, Grant, Chan, Ahn, & Ferrell, 1995; Ferrell & Borneman, 1999; Ferrell & Borneman, 2000).

Symptom management also fits with the current focus in health care on outpatient care and on early discharge from the hospital. Implications for nursing include teaching the client self-care or teaching the family to provide care for the client. Family caregiver responsibilities may include assessing symptoms that are present and reporting new symptoms that may herald reportable complications. Follow-up contact with clients is important through telephone calls to clients and families and monitoring symptoms in outpatient clinics. The trend of increased home care management requires a focus on symptom management. The nurse is often the key person evaluating this system, implementing a plan of care, and providing symptom management and appropriate support for a family caregiver.

Another aspect of symptom management that underlines its importance is its impact on health care costs. For example, undertreatment of pain is very costly. Pain interrupts sleep (Grant, Rivera, Alisangco, & Francisco, 1999; McClement, Woordgate, & Degner, 1997), eating (Grant & Kravits, 2000), mobilization (Sarna & Conde, 2001), and functional status (Dodd, Miaskowski, & Paul, 2001).

The actual costs of pain to society are difficult to estimate. In one report, approximately 500 million days per year were estimated as sick days involving pain for full-time employees in the United States (Sternbach, 1986). Additionally, about 40 percent of individuals who contact a physician receive a prescription for pain medication and 20 percent, an over-the-counter analgesic. Readmissions for unmanaged pain also produce a cost that may or may not be reimbursable from the client's insurance. Many insurance companies will not reimburse for hospitalization that occurs within two weeks of discharge, unless that readmission is a planned event (e.g., for chemotherapy administration). Unreimbursed readmissions are costly to the individual, the institution, and to society (Ferrell & Griffith, 1994; Grant, Ferrell, Rivera, & Lee, 1995).

Barriers to Symptom Management

An important barrier to overcome in order to improve symptom management is a lack of basic research in describing symptoms, symptom distress, and associated pathology. For example, deficits in our understanding of the physiology of the gastrointestinal tract impede our understanding of the full impact of interruptions in food intake during disease or treatment. The differences in patients' responses to total parenteral versus enteral nutrition are beginning to identify functions in the gastrointestinal tract not previously known. Other areas of symptom management also deserve studying.

Another important barrier is a lack of adequate instrumentation to measure symptoms and symptom distress. Nursing scientists have begun to address this problem area through the development of texts, workshops, presentations, and publications focusing on instrumentation (Frank-Stromborg & Olsen, 1997; Vallerand, 1997). However, much needs to be done to develop instruments that are valid, reliable, sensitive, and easy to use clinically. Additionally, methods for clinical implementation of assessment instruments need to be developed and tested. If no assessment tools exist that can be used clinically, scientific evidence on the impact of interventions for clinical management will be difficult to demonstrate.

An additional barrier is the lack of descriptive research on the usual patterns of occurrence for various symptoms—that is, when do they occur, for how long, in relation to what other events, and what is the nature of the symptom?

The lack of intervention research is an additional barrier. Most of clinical practice is based on clinical nursing judgment backed by empirical knowledge not validated through research. For symptom management, nurses often rely on their best clinical judgment. This judgment needs to be subjected to scientific testing.

As interventions are identified and validated through research, it is possible that many of the interventions applicable to one area of symptom management may be applicable to others as well. For example, teaching clients imagery, relaxation, or distraction for use during chemotherapy may also be useful later in the course of disease in coping with pain. In some areas of symptom management, clinical practice guidelines are available and not fully utilized. Guidelines on cancer pain management such as those published by the Agency for Health Care Policy and Research (AHCPR) (1994); and the American Cancer Society/National Comprehensive Cancer Network (2001) are available and need to be applied to practice.

Barriers may also be found within nursing. In a recent course designed to prepare staff nurses to better manage pain, nurse participants reported opposition and resistance from physicians and also from nurse colleagues. Nurses reported reluctance on the part of their colleagues to implement pain management strategies and difficulty in getting other nurses to make symptom management a priority (Ferrell, Grant, Ritchey, Ropchan, & Rivera, 1993; McGuire, 1994).

Barriers may be related to professional "turf" issues. Symptom management is probably best viewed as a multidisciplinary endeavor involving nurses, physicians, physical therapists, social workers, and other health care professionals. Relief of symptoms requires ongoing communication between health care providers. When anticipated, barriers can become evident and can be overcome.

Research Issues in Symptom Management and QOL

There are at least two important dimensions in the assessment of symptoms and function. Research has shown that it is very helpful to assess not only the *intensity* of symptoms but also the distress associated with them. For example, in measuring pain, the patient is asked first, "How much pain do you have?" in order to assess intensity on a scale of 0 to 10, with 0 being no pain and 10 being severe pain. This tells us the intensity of the pain. The patient is then asked, "How distressing is the pain to you?" This technique enables the patient to express how bothersome or distressing that particular symptom may be. This technique also assists health care professionals to appreciate the importance of individual problems to the patient. For example, patients may rate their pain as fairly mild, but describe it as extremely distressing because it limits them from participating in important activities.

The second measurement issue relates to the timing of physical well-being assessments. Many of the symptoms that patients experience are in fact intermittent problems. It may sometimes be misleading to ask a patient a simple question such as, "Do you have any nausea?" Patients may be inclined to report their status only at that moment, rather than providing a sense of their usual patterns or their problems over recent days or weeks. It is important for the clinician or researcher to establish the time frame of the measurement.

We also favor scales that follow a symptom over time. Rather than asking questions with a simple "yes/no" response, more precise measures (i.e., 0 to 10 ordinal scales or visual analog scales) enable nurses to measure changes in a particular symptom over time or to evaluate the effectiveness of a nursing intervention.

Table 9-3 presents examples of symptom items in seven frequently used QOL instruments. Symptom items are commonly included in these instruments. Many symptoms, such as pain and nausea, are universal items, while assessment of other symptoms varies across instruments.

Table 9-3. **Examples of Symptom Items in Select QOL Tools**

Physical	CARES	FLIC	FACT-G	QOL-BMT	QOL-BR	SDS
Pain	X	X	X	X	X	X
Nausea/Vomiting	X	X	X	X	X	X
Fatigue	X		X	X	X	X
Function Ability	X	X	X			
Weight Changes	X				X	
Sleep Differences	X		X	X	X	X
Bowel/Bladder	X			X	X	X
Appetite	X			X	X	X
Concentration	X			X	X	X
Memory	X			X	X	
Vision				X		
Skin Changes				X		
Bleeding Problems				X		
Mouth Dryness				X		
Hearing Loss				X		
Ringing in Ears				X		
SOB/Breathing Difficulty				X		X
Fertility/Menopausal Symptoms				X	X	
State of Health/ Perceived Wellness		X	X	X	X	
Cough						
Strength	X			X		
Anxiety	X		X	X	X	
Depression	X	X		X	X	
Fear of Metastases	X			X	X	
Fear of Recurrence	X			X	X	
Fear of Second Cancer				X	X	
Sexual Function	X	X	X	X	X	

CARES—Cancer Rehabilitation Evaluation System (Schag, Heinrich, Aadland, & Ganz, 1990).
FLIC—Functional Living Index of Cancer (Schipper, Clinch, McMurray, & Levitt, 1984).
FACT-G—Functional Assessment of Cancer Therapy-General Version (Cella et al., 1993).
QOL-BMT—Quality of Life, Bone Marrow Transplant Version, City of Hope (Grant, Ferrell, Schmidt, Fonbuena, Niland, & Forman, 1992).
QOL-BR—Quality of Life, Breast Version, City of Hope (Ferrell, Hassey Dow, & Grant, 1995).
SDS—Symptom Distress Scale (McCorkle & Young, 1978).

Table 9-4. **The Impact of Symptoms on QOL in Breast Cancer**

Pain	". . . If you could have seen me a few weeks ago where it was difficult to get up out of the chair . . . that's not me! That's not me. And I have a hard time handling that . . . If I could just learn how to deal with it (the pain). You see, I just haven't accepted it. I just fight it. Why do I have to do this?"
Fatigue	". . . It seems like just last week, I was really, really tired . . . I'd take a nap and then I'd wake up and I'd do things around the house, and then I'd feel tired again."
	"Fatigue has affected my life because when I'm tired I can't, especially with the kids, or today I'm not going to cook. Let's have a pizza or order McDonald's or something like that."
Menopause	"It's the hot flashes . . . me, I'll have it maybe ten times a day. And it doesn't leave me. It will take minutes. I mean ten to fifteen minutes. I can't work outside because I'll be dripping, dripping, dripping."
	". . . It was really months before I could have intercourse because I was just so sore and sensitive there . . . It was a situation of when you're menopausal it takes longer to become aroused. It's a little harder to have orgasms. It justs affects your sex life. You have less desire overall . . ."
Fertility	". . . And I do have scars on my breast and my stomach that I see everyday, but I'm getting used to that. So, it's the menopause and the emotional part (that) you'll never have children . . ."
Weight Gain	". . . And that's why I'm having problems. I can't lose it. I'm starving myself."
	"Honestly, I don't know what to do. No dresses fit, how many clothes do I have? Nothing's fitting me. Nothing. I gained so much weight . . . that's the other worse thing."

Source: Ferrell, Grant, Funk, Otis-Green, & Garcia (1997). Used with permission.

Another method to assess physical well-being is the use of qualitative methods. Qualitative research methods can provide a mechanism for understanding the patient's experience of symptoms and physical status in a way not achievable through quantitative scales or methods. Most of the nursing studies conducted at the City of Hope Medical Center have combined quantitative and qualitative methods to obtain the most complete descriptions of QOL from cancer patients.

Table 9-4 is an example of descriptions of symptoms experienced by women with breast cancer. These examples illustrate the valuable information gained from qualitative reports of symptom experiences. The comments from these participants in breast cancer research also reinforce the importance of symptom control to overall QOL.

Another important area of future research is intervention studies in symptom control. Anxiety generally occurs at some time during a cancer patient's care. This anxiety may not be completely eliminated; however, interventions clinically known to diminish anxiety should be tested in future research. Improving the environment in which we treat patients and the formal and informal support provided, and providing educational strategies are some of the ways to help patients control their anxiety. Such approaches need to be standardized and tested for effectiveness.

CONCLUSION

Symptom management is a critical mandate for oncology nurses. Failure to manage symptoms adequately has a direct and profound influence on the QOL of clients. Cancer involves physical and psychological symptoms in response to the disease and treatment. As with many aspects of cancer care, nursing interventions in symptom management also have a profound influence on family members whose experiences are greatly influenced by the symptoms they observe in those they love. Table 9-5 is a summary of comments from family caregivers of children with cancer experiencing uncontrolled pain. These powerful comments are a reminder to us that the treatment of symptoms, such as alleviating pain, is more than a short-term intervention, but rather will create long-term memories for patients and family members.

Table 9-5. **What Is It Like Having a Child with Pain?**

Theme 1: Unendurable Pain
"So how long do you sit there and watch that child in excruciating pain before you start becoming either irate, demanding, or confronting somebody individually to see exactly what's being done? So, I mean, it's a helpless feeling. I mean, obviously I like to see him just like any parent would want to see their kid, you know, acting normally without pain. But, I felt as if I had it, and it was almost like seeing him dangle from the end of a rope."

Theme 2: Helplessness
"You can't do nothing for him, you know. He's your son. You love him. You want to help him in every way you can, but when he's in that kind of pain, you're helpless in a sense. You can't do nothing for him; to help that pain; and you're his daddy. I'm his daddy. It was—what was I suppose to do for him? I felt, you know, helpless."

Theme 3: Total Commitment
"I won't even leave. I will not. Before when she was hospitalized, I would leave, you know, go walk around the block or something. But, this time I won't leave. I refuse to leave because I know you never know when their pain's going to come."

continues

Table 9-5. **continued**

Theme 4: Feels the Pain Physically

"Sometimes I feel it. The other night she had pains in her chest. She felt like she couldn't breathe. Then I started getting pains over here in my right side of my chest, and even when her stomach started hurting a whole lot, next thing I know I got a pain in my stomach. I hurt all around here and on my ribs, and then the strangest thing was I was waiting in the line of McDonald's, and it (my leg) was hurting. It was really hurting, right? It was hurting so much I wanted to take the weight off of it. And, then I realized I was standing on one leg." [Daughter has phantom pains after hemipelvectomy.]

Theme 5: Unprepared

"When he was in pain in the hospital, I sort of felt confident that his pain would be taken care of in a very professional way, more so than at home. At home it was like, we're really not doctors and nurses here; we don't want to drug our kid up; what do we do? But, we knew we want to keep him at home. But, we saw that he was in pain, and you just have to stop what you're doing and just bring him into the hospital. So from that point of view, really there was no difference other than the fact that in the hospital, probably if he did have the pain, we felt more comfortable there because we knew that there were people who were trained to handle it, whereas we were not trained to handle it at home. We were just like neophytes opening up a *Reader's Digest* medical book."

Theme 6: Horrible/Frightening

"I don't know. I mean, the whole word [pain] is so scary. It brings you to your knees. It's scary."

"It's like amputating your arm without putting you under. That's the way killing cancer is without pain medicine. It's like, oh, they're killing everything, but they're also making you in agony, and we would never have made it. There's no way he would have made it this far without medicine."

Theme 7: Child's Faith in God

"He [God] told her that if she came to heaven where He is, she wouldn't have the pain, and she wanted to know if that was true. You know, she asked me if that was true, and I said, 'Well, yes.' Then she asked me if I could go with her, and I told her not then."

Theme 8: Wish for Death

"I'm confused, they can't give me any better hope than this, but I know that's what happens with this disease. When she's in pain, I just want it to go away. I also want—if she's not going to get better—I don't want her to go through any more pain. So, I mean, if she's going to die, then have her die."

Source: Adapted from Ferrell, Rhiner, Shapiro, & Dierkes, 1994. Used with permission of the *Journal of Pediatric Nursing*.

Symptoms are an integral part of the cancer experience. Our research in the area of cancer pain has revealed that the pain experience transcends physical care and extends to cause clients to question the meaning of life. Table 9-6 summarizes the ultimate meaning attributed to pain as expressed by patients, family caregivers, and home care nurses. Clearly, the physical symptom of pain is all inclusive and alters the existential meanings attributed to illness.

Oncology nursing has helped to humanize the experience of cancer by addressing symptom management as a primary component of care. Aggressive treatment of symptoms, combined with genuine caring for the family experiencing cancer, is a cornerstone of quality of life.

Table 9-6. **Meanings Regarding the Ultimate Cause of Pain**

I. **Fate or Determinism**

"In my opinion, there's a built-in time clock for every one of us from the day we're born, the minute we're born till the day we leave this Earth, and there's not anything we can do to change it." (*Patient*)

"I know you have to go through a certain amount of suffering and, we all have to . . . There comes a time for everybody." (*Caregiver*)

II. **Probability or Randomness**

"I know that a lot of people go through pain, and it's a part of life that some people have to face, and unfortunately, my mom was chosen." (*Caregiver*)

"It can happen to anyone." (*Nurse*)

"I usually try to reassure them that it isn't something that they got because they were bad; I try to explain to them that cancer is arbitrary. I mean it's nonselective. It just picks whoever." (*Nurse*)

III. **God's Will**

"I put a lot of my faith in God. I know He takes care of things. It's in His hands. We get anxious and we wonder, well, why this and why that, but then you stop and think about it, you know, there's a plan for all of us." (*Patient*)

God's Beneficence

"My belief of God is that He is a loving God and that He does respond, if He can, and either He can't sometimes because of something that's happening, . . . or He chooses not to, because of the results of what it's going to be, you know. I have a little bit of a problem with that, that He chooses not to when He could solve pain, but I don't always, . . . I mean if He has made a decision not to interact, . . . He'd have to like stop everything, but I mean if He's going to stop pain for one person He'd have to stop it for someone else." (*Nurse*)

God's Maleficence

"None of my patients that I've ever worked with could have been that bad to deserve that—to be punished like that. I don't know." (*Nurse*)

Table 9-6. **continued**

"God chooses not to intervene." (*Caretaker*)

"I figure because I ate good, never drank, never smoked, so I figured it was just that God felt I was one that He picked out to go. . . . In a way I think God uses this as a way of keeping the Earth in balance so that we don't get overpopulated." (*Patient*)

Meanings from Religious Belief

"The only thing that I can think of that makes any sense to me is that God gives each person the ability to handle the pain that they have." (*Nurse*)

"I believe that there's sin in the world, and because we live in the imperfect world, there is pain and suffering since the beginning of time." (*Nurse*)

IV. **Heredity**

"It's in my genes." (*Patient*)

V. **Pain Serves a Positive Purpose**

"We go through the fiery test and remain true, then I mean I have them times here! But it says for every time I stay true or stay with Him, that I will have a seat at the marriage feast, and I can expect another jewel in my crown and . . . this is an example of hell, and I'm going through it here, and I'm not going to have to go through it later on." (*Patient*)

"We're here to learn." (*Caregiver*)

Source: Adapted from Ferrell, Johnston Taylor, Sattler, Fowler, & Cheyney, 1993. Used with permission of *Cancer Practice*.

REFERENCES

Agency for Health Care Policy and Research. (1994). *Management of cancer pain. Clinical practice guidelines* (AHCPR Pub. No. 94-0592). Rockville, MD: Agency for Health Care Policy and Research, Public Health Service, U.S. Department of Health and Human Services.

American Cancer Society, National Comprehensive Cancer Network. *Cancer pain treatment guidelines. Version 1.* January 2001.

American Nurses' Association Cabinet on Nursing Research. (1985). *Directions for nursing research: Toward the twenty-first century.* Kansas City, MO: American Nurses' Association.

Andrews, H. A., & Roy, S. C. (1991). *The Roy Adaptation Model: The definitive statement.* Norwalk, CT: Appleton & Lange.

Andrews, S. C. (2001). Caregiver Burden and Symptom Distress in People with Cancer Receiving Hospice Care. *Oncology Nursing Forum, 28*(9), 1469–1474.

Baldacchino, D., & Draper, P. (2001). Spiritual coping strategies: A review of the nursing research literature. *Journal of Advanced Nursing, 34*(6), 833–841.

Barsevick, A., Whitmer, K., & Walker, L. (2001). In their own words: Using the common sense model to analyze patient descriptions of cancer-related fatigue. *Oncology Nursing Forum, 28*(9), 1363–1369.

Benner, P. (1984). *From novice to expert.* Menlo Park, CA: Addison-Wesley.

Benoliel, J. C. Q. (1963). Impact of mastectomy. *American Journal of Nursing, 63,* 88–92.

Cella, D. F., Tulsky, D. S., Gray, G., Sarafian, B., Linn, E., Bonomi, A., Silberman, M., Yellen, S. B., Winicour, P., Brannon, J., Eckberg, K., Lloyd, S., Purl, S., Blenowski, C., Goodman, M., Barnicle, M., Stewart, I., McHale, M., Bonomi, P., Kaplan, E., Taylor, S., IV, Thomas, C. R., Jr., & Harris, J. (1993). The functional assessment of cancer therapy scale: Development and validation of the general measure. *Journal of Clinical Oncology, 11*(3), 570–579.

Dean, G. E., Spears, L., Ferrell, B. R., Quan, W. D. Y., Groshon, S., & Mitchell, M. S. (1995). Fatigue in patients with cancer receiving interferon alpha. *Cancer Practice, 3*(3), 164–172.

Dodd, M. J., Janson, J., Facione, N., Faucett, J., Froelicher, E., Humphreys, J., Lee, K., Miaskowski, C., Puntillo, K., Rankin, S., & Taylor, D. (2001). Advancing the science of symptom management. *Journal of Advanced Nursing, 33*(5), 668–676.

Fenwick, S. (1869). *Medical Diagnosis* (Ed. 1). London: Churchill.

Dodd, M. J., Miaskowski, C., & Paul, S. M. (2001). Symptom Clusters and their effect on the functional status of patients with cancer. *Oncology Nursing Forum, 28*(3), 365–470.

Dooks, P. (2001). Diffusion of Pain Management Research Into Nursing Practice. *Cancer Nursing, 24*(2), 99–103.

Dudgeon, D. J., Kristjanson, J. A., Lertzman, M., & Clement, K. (2001). Dyspnea in cancer patients: Prevalence and associated factors. *Journal of Pain and Symptom Management, 21*(2), 95–102.

Ferrell, B. R., & Borneman, T. (1999). Hospice home management of pain and symptoms. *Primary Care & Cancer, 19*(7): 8–10.

Ferrell, B. R., & Borneman, T. (2000). Maintaining quality of life in the home. *Principles and Practice of Supportive Oncology Updates, 3*(5), 1–8.

Ferrell, B. R., Grant, M., Chan, J., Ahn, C., & Ferrell, B. A. (1995). The impact of cancer pain education on family caregivers of elderly patients. *Oncology Nursing Forum, 22*(8), 1211–1218.

Ferrell, B. R., Grant, M., Funk, B., Otis-Green, S., & Garcia, N. (1997). Quality of life in breast cancer. Part I: Physical and social well being. *Cancer Nursing, 20*(6), 398–408.

Ferrell, B. R., Grant, M., Ritchey, K. J., Ropchan, R., & Rivera, L. (1993). The pain resource training program: A unique approach to pain management. *Journal of Pain and Symptom Management, 8,* 549–556.

Ferrell, B. R., & Griffith, H. (1994). Cost issues related to pain management: Report from the cancer pain panel of the Agency for Health Care Policy and Research. *Journal of Pain and Symptom Management, 9*(4), 221–234.

Ferrell, B. R., Hassey Dow, K., & Grant, M. (1995). Measurement of the quality of life in cancer survivors. *Quality of Life Research, 4,* 523–531.

Ferrell, B. R., Hassey Dow, K., Leigh, S., Ly, J., & Gulasekaram, P. (1995). Quality of life in long-term cancer survivors. *Oncology Nursing Forum, 22*(6), 915–922.

Ferrell, B. R., Johnston Taylor, E., Sattler, G. R., Fowler, M., & Cheyney, B. L. (1993). Searching for the meaning of pain. *Cancer Practice, 1*(3), 185–194.

Ferrell, B. R., Rhiner, M., Shapiro, B., & Dierkes, M. (1994). The experience of pediatric cancer pain. Part I: Impact of pain on the family. *Journal of Pediatric Nursing, 9*(6), 368–379.

Frank-Stromborg, M., & Olsen, S. J. (1997). *Instruments for clinical health-care research* (2nd ed.). Boston: Jones and Bartlett.

Ganz, P. A. (2001). Late effects of cancer and its treatment. *Seminars in Oncology Nursing, 17*(4), 241–248.

Grant, M., Ferrell, B. R., Rivera, L. M., & Lee, J. (1995). Unscheduled readmissions for uncontrolled symptoms: A health care challenge for nurses. *Nursing Clinics of North America, 30*(4), 673–682.

Grant, M., Ferrell, B., Schmidt, G. M., Fonbuena, P., Niland, J. C., & Forman, S. J. (1992). Measurement of quality of life in bone marrow transplantation survivors. *Quality of Life Research, 1,* 375–384.

Grant, M., & Kravits, K. (2000). Symptoms and their impact on nutrition. *Seminars in Oncology Nursing, 16*(2), 113–121.

Grant, M., Rivera, L. M., Alisangco, J., & Francisco, L. (1999). Improving cancer pain management using a performance improvement framework. *Journal of Nursing Care Quality, 13*(4), 60–72.

Highfield, M. F. (1992). Spiritual health of oncology patients. Nurse and patient perspectives. *Cancer Nursing, 15*(1), 1–8.

John, L. D. (2001). Quality of life in patients receiving radiation therapy for non-small cell lung cancer. *Oncology Nursing Forum, 28*(5), 807–813.

Johnson, J. E. (1973). The effects of accurate expectations about sensations on the sensory and distress components of pain. *Journal of Personality and Social Psychology, 27,* 261–275.

Loseth, D. B. (1991). *Changes in spirituality of the dying: A longitudinal study.* (1991). Unpublished thesis, New Haven, CT: Yale University.

Marks, R. M., & Sachar, E. J. (1973). Undertreatment of medical inpatients with narcotic analgesics. *Annals of Internal Medicine, 78,* 173–181.

McClement, S. E., Woordgate, R., & Degner, L. (1997). Symptom Distress in adults with cancer. *Cancer Nursing, 20*(4), 236–243.

McCorkle, R., & Young, K. (1978). Development of a symptom distress scale. *Cancer Nursing, 1*, 373–378.

McGuire, D. (1992). Comprehensive and multidimensional assessment and measurement of pain. *Journal of Pain and Symptom Management, 7*, 312–319.

McGuire, D. (1994). The nurse's role in pain relief. *Medical Surgical Nursing 3*(2), 94–98 .

Musser, J. H., & Krumbhaar, E. B. (Eds.). (1922). *The American Journal of the Medical Sciences.* Philadelphia: Lea & Febiger.

Padilla, G. V., Ferrell, B., Grant, M. M., & Rhiner, M. (1990). Defining the content domain of quality of life for cancer patients with pain. *Cancer Nursing, 13*(2), 108–115.

Rhodes, V. A., & Watson, P. M. (Eds.). (1987). Symptom distress. *Seminars in Oncology Nursing, 3*(4), 242–247.

Sarna, L., & Conde, F. (2001). Physical activity and fatigue during radiation therapy: A pilot study using actigraph monitors. *Oncology Nursing Forum, 28*(7), 1043–1046.

Schag, C. A., Heinrich, R. L., Aadland, R., & Ganz, P. A. (1990). Assessing problems of cancer patients: Psychometric properties of the Cancer Inventory of Problem Situations. *Health Psychology, 9*(1), 83–102.

Schipper, H., Clinch, J., McMurray, A., & Levitt, M. (1984). Measuring the quality of life of cancer patients: The Functional Living Index-Cancer: Development and validation. *Journal of Clinical Oncology, 2*(5), 472–483.

Sternbach, R. A. (1986). Survey of pain in the United States: The Nuprin Pain Report. *Clinics in Pain, 2*, 49–53.

Vallerand, A. H. (1997). Measurement issues in the comprehensive assessment of cancer pain. *Seminars in Oncology Nursing, 13*(1), 16–24.

Wu H., & McSweeney M. (2001). Measurement of Fatigue in People with Cancer. *Oncology Nursing Forum, 28*(9), 1371–1384.

Quality of Life
in Families Experiencing Cancer

KATHLEEN M. STETZ

Research literature to date on the impact of cancer on the family suggests that the family plays a large role in the psychological adjustment of its ill family members (Gotcher, 1992; Laizner, Yost, Barg, & McCorkle, 1993). In this chapter the theoretical perspectives on the family, the family as caregiver for a member with cancer, quality of life (QOL) and the family, research on indicators of QOL for families, and clinical practice issues will be discussed.

Theoretical Perspectives on Families and the Cancer Experience: Systems Theory, Developmental Theory, and Caregiver Stress and Coping Theory

Overview of the Three Theories

Theoretical frameworks provide a map for how to organize thinking as well as aspects of a thorough assessment. While each framework has its own significant contributions to understanding a phenomenon, such as family adjustment to a chronic illness, rarely is one framework sufficiently comprehensive to tap all areas of importance in an assessment of how families are coping. Systems theory provides a way of understanding how a family functions. Inherent in this theory are two assumptions: that the family unit functions differently from individual members, and that the behavior of one family member influences other members of the family unit. Developmental theory personalizes an assessment; it assists the clinician to look at the stage of the family unit as well as of its individual members. That stage-related knowledge helps a clinician to understand the complementary or conflictual issues that may arise in a family simply because of where individual members and/or the family as a whole is in the life course. In order to understand how families respond to the strain of living with a member who has a chronic illness, attention must be given to how families label their experiences (i.e., strain versus opportunity) and how they cope with and adapt to their situation. The caregiver stress and coping theory provides a way to understand the family's coping response to chronic illness. Together, these three theoretical frameworks provide a comprehensive approach for understanding and working with families who are experiencing cancer.

Systems Theory

Systems theory suggests that the family be considered as a unit and not as individuals (Broderick & Smith, 1979). A family system can be defined as a dyad or group of individuals with a shared history and a future. Five principles of a systems framework as identified by Wright and Leahy (1994) are useful in understanding this approach as it applies to families: (1) a family system is part of a larger suprasystem and is also composed of many subsystems; (2) the family as a whole is greater that the sum of its parts; (3) a change in one family member affects all family members; (4) the family is available to create a balance between change and stability; and (5) family member behaviors are better understood from a perspective of circular causality than that of linear causality. Linear causality refers to situations in which event A (alarm rings at 7:00 A.M.) impacts behavior B (family wakes up and eats breakfast). Circular causality refers to event A (wife has pain) affecting behavior B (husband gives her pain medication), followed by anticipation of and planning for event A in the future (husband gives his wife round-the-clock medication). In this way, the family experiencing cancer in one of its members is itself altered. Systems theory suggests that a diagnosis of cancer in a family member affects each family member and the functioning of the family as a unit. Family systems (the entire system or subsystems) also have a structure and function. The structure of a family includes its composition, gender, subsystems, extended family, ethnicity, race, social class, and religion (Wright & Leahy, 1994). In terms of function, the family must meet the everyday needs of its members as well as communicate to each other (through verbal and nonverbal communication, by problem solving, by enacting roles, and by sharing beliefs) (Wright & Leahy, 1994). Family structure is affected in a number of ways when a family member is being treated for cancer; care needs of the ill person may result in additional family members residing in the home to provide care or in children being located with other family members while a parent receives intensive treatment. Family functioning can be dramatically affected; patterns of communication may no longer be sufficient to maintain the operations of the family, and roles may be altered. For example, elder children may need to care for younger ones, or middle-aged daughters may need to care for their own children as well as their ill parent. The diagnosis of cancer in a family member can, therefore, be expected to affect every aspect of family life (Sales, Schulz, & Biegel, 1992).

Developmental Theory

The developmental stage of the family greatly influences the family's cancer experience and their perceptions of demands placed on them (Hileman & Lackey, 1990; Kristjanson, 1989; Kristjanson & Ashcroft, 1994). Developmental theory is useful for assessing the family as it exists over time. Each developmental stage introduces new tasks and responsibilities (Carter & McGoldrick, 1980; Duvall, 1977). Eight developmental stages are frequently described. These stages, along with the primary developmental task of each stage, are described as follows: Marital (establishing a marriage); Childbearing (adjusting to parenthood); Preschool (nurturing children); School-Age (socializing and educating children); Teenage (balancing teenagers' freedom and responsibility); Launching (releasing children as young adults; developing postparental interests); Middle-Aged (reestablishing the marital dyad; maintaining links with older and younger generations); and Aging (adjusting to retirement, aging, loneliness, and death) (Wright & Leahy, 1994). For most families these stages do not occur in isolation; for instance, the family with a school-age child may also have teenagers. When a member of the household (child or adult) is diagnosed with cancer, the family is challenged to continue to meet the developmental needs of its members.

At the current time, research findings present a conflicting picture regarding the impact a cancer diagnosis has on the family's ability to engage in developmentally appropriate tasks. Armsden and Lewis (1994) report on the behavioral adjustment and self-esteem of school-age (6–12 years) children of women with breast cancer (two or more years postdiagnosis and no evidence of disease), diabetes, or fibrocystic breast disease. On both mother and nurse observer ratings, children of women with breast cancer scored higher on behavioral adjustment than the noncancer groups. The children's self-reported self-esteem, however, was statistically significantly lower than that of children of the noncancer groups. In contrast to the findings of the Armsden and Lewis study, Siegel and colleagues (1992) reported that children of parents with cancer, when compared to a matched community sample, had more mood disturbances (depression and anxiety). In a study of 32 children of women with breast cancer, Howes and associates (1994) found that these children's behavior scores (Total Problem Scale) did not differ from normative samples. However, their mothers rated them as having more emotional and behavioral problems than were reported in a community sample (Howes, Hoke, Winterbottom, & Delafield, 1994). In terms of the assistance or resource that children can be to a couple experiencing cancer, Stommel and Kingry (1991) found that households with children under age 19 reported less help than households with children over age 19. However, families with children only under age 10 reported receiving additional assistance from outside family members.

Very few studies have focused on adult children of persons with cancer. In a descriptive study of 38 adult children, Germino and Funk (1993) found that role concerns and relationship issues with parents were the major themes described. Role concerns included role changes and difficulty meeting one's own needs. Relationship issues included the desire for closeness with the ill parent, unresolved relationship issues with the ill parent, and relationship issues with the non-ill parent.

In summary, the literature to date does convey that individual and family development may be affected by the presence of cancer in a family member. It is important, therefore, to take into account the developmental stage of families experiencing cancer.

Caregiver Stress and Coping

Stress and coping theory has its origins in the work of Lazarus and colleagues (Lazarus, Averill, & Opton, 1974). This framework suggests that stressors influence how a person copes. Coping is defined in terms of actions/behaviors and cognitions that one engages in when responding to stressors. A model for understanding stress and coping in terms of family caregiving has been offered by Pearlin, Mullan, Semple, and Skaff (1990). Rather than the general notion of stressors, they suggest that two types of caregiver strain exist: primary and secondary. Primary strains can result directly from the actual demands of physically caring for another person as well as from certain intrapsychic processes such as identification with the ill family member and the multiple losses that occur as a result of an illness, for example, losing the person as he or she once was. Secondary strains result from the problems that are created in other important areas of life due to being a caregiver, such as difficulties in relationships with noncaregiving relatives, employment, and finances.

The most salient stressors for the family serving as a caregiver are providing the physical care and managing uncertainty. Both of these affect a family's QOL. This is because these stressors are relatively persistent and enduring for the family. The continuing presence and the cumulative effect of these strains make them particularly stressful and ultimately affects the QOL of individual members and the family unit.

Two types of primary strain that have a large impact on the family with cancer are physical care and loss. Physical care includes how much care the family member must provide because the ill person is unable to provide it for him/herself. The expectation is that the greater the range and number is of such dependencies, the greater will be the strain experienced by the caregiving family member. For the caregiver, the primary responsibilities include managing functional abilities (i.e., bathing, eating, dressing) and symptoms of both cancer and its treatment (pain, fatigue, and nausea) (Stetz, 1987).

Loss is a far less visible primary strain. Family members typically experience three distinct types of loss: the loss of joint social leisure activities, the loss of affectional exchange, and the loss of the ill person's former self (Rando, 1986). The loss of joint social and leisure activities is usually quite profound. Although some shared activities are usually maintained, such as watching television and eating meals together, there is typically a dramatic constriction in the number and range of activities that were once enjoyed together. This can be even more poignantly true in the second type of loss, affective exchanges. Here the spouse or partner may be called upon to give continuously to a person who (depending on the stage of the treatment or illness) may not be able to reciprocate, to be a source of affection without being a love object, or to be no longer cared about by the one who is cared for. The expressions of love and affection are lost as well as the reciprocity on which the relationship with the patient was, at one time, developed. These are painful losses and powerful sources of strain. Along with what is lost in shared activities and affective exchange, the family member is commonly in a position of having to take care of someone in whom there are but few traces of the former person. Those attributes that previously were distinctly characteristic of the person with cancer are no longer in evidence. That the family member is required to continue to devote him/herself to someone who, in large measure, is now a stranger only serves to accentuate the awareness that the former person no longer exists.

Secondary strains can be observed in the roles and social relations that are inherently interconnected with providing care. For example, it has been noted (Niederehe & Fruge, 1984) that family conflict is a familiar concomitant of caregiving. One family member may feel that another is not attentive to the ill person or sufficiently helpful to the principal caregiver. There may be differences of opinion with regard to maintaining the ill person at home or institutionalizing her or him; some might even display impatience with, or a lack of compassion for, the family caregiver.

For those family caregivers who have employment outside of the household, there may also be conflicts between the demands of caregiving and those of the job. Employed caregivers report that they are more tired on the job since the onset of the illness, less able to concentrate, more often absent, and as a result of these problems, experience more insecurity about their occupational futures (Stommel et al., 1993). Interestingly, however, even among those exposed to these job pressures, there may be a reluctance to give up work. As difficult as it may be, the work setting is a place in which some family caregivers find relief from the day-to-day tedium of caregiving. Also, taking care of a physically or cognitively impaired family member can be costly (Stommel et al., 1993). In addition to the expenses of health care and related services, there may be a severe loss of income resulting from the inability of the ill person or family member to work.

Some families, however, appear to function quite well under very adverse conditions. Pearlin and associates (1990) suggested in their model of family caregiving that family members cope through three mechanisms: (1) coping to manage the situation, (2) coping to manage meaning, and (3) coping to manage symptoms of stress.

Coping to Manage the Situation.   The ultimate way to manage the difficulties involved in caring for a family member with cancer would be for the person to be cured of the disease. Since this is not always possible, family members must settle for making a difficult situation bearable. The types of management strategies family members use to manage their situations include: enforcing a prescribed medication regimen; establishing priorities when it is not possible to meet all the demands that exist; modifying the living environment for the comfort or safety of the ill person; and engaging in anticipatory planning for the future. Although caregivers may be efficient and effective in management skills, it is unlikely that they are ever able to lower the demand to a point at which it no longer exists. This is not to say that these strategies are pointless, but rather that they make the situation more bearable. By reducing the demands of the situation, time and energy can be conserved.

Coping to Manage Meaning. When people face stressful situations they cannot change, their coping strategies will largely be directed toward functions other than the management of the situation. Giving care to a family member who suffers from a severe and potentially progressive impairment, such as cancer, represents such a situation. In these situations, it can be expected that a major amount of energy is directed toward constructing meaning in the situation, which in turn reduces its threat (Pearlin et al., 1990). Essentially, if people cannot change a difficult situation, they will search for ways they can live with it. This search motivates caregivers to perceive the caregiving role and its associated demands in ways that help them to survive and continue in the role. Types of strategies to manage meaning include positive comparisons, present-oriented thinking, holding onto the past (recreate the past or part of it; spend time reflecting about the "good times"), use of prayer or spirituality, and involvement in organizations related to the diagnosis or treatment of the cancer. Some families report that this latter activity, involvement in a cause or organization, provides an avenue whereby personal tragedy can be converted into a social cause (Stetz & Brown, 1997).

Coping to Manage Symptoms of Stress. A third set of coping strategies include those activities that serve to lessen or control symptoms of stress experienced by family members. Among the behaviors that family caregivers identify as making them feel better are drinking alcohol, eating more, smoking, sleeping, exercising, or reading. These behaviors can be useful in that they keep people from being immobilized and allow them to bring other coping repertoires into play. If used exclusively, however, they create problems that do not compensate for the benefits that they yield in the short run.

The three theoretical frameworks share a focus on the family as a unit but differ from each other in terms of underlying assumptions, clinical assessment focus, and type of theoretically derived research questions. A listing of these differences is included in Table 10-1.

The Family as Caregiver

The family as a source of caregiving is an area of interest as well as concern for health care providers. The reliance on the family as caregiver in the future will increase because of advances in medical technology and increasing cancer survival rates. Additionally, shorter hospital stays and the shift of procedures and treatments from the hospital to outpatient

Table 10-1.   Comparison of Three Theoretical Frameworks for Working with Families Experiencing Cancer

Theoretical Framework	Assumptions	Clinical Focus	Research Questions
Systems Theory	The family as a whole is greater than the sum of its parts. A change in one family member affects all family members. The family is capable of creating a balance between stability and change.	Focus on all members of the family as well as family environment/tone. Identify family strengths.	Measure all family members on QOL outcome variables (e.g., physical and emotional functioning). Utilize family-level measurement (e.g., family functioning, family satisfaction).
Developmental Theory	Families move through stages that have unique tasks. Families may be in multiple stages at a given time (e.g., Preschool and Launching).	Determine family stages. Assess family for engagement in developmentally appropriate tasks.	Measure developmentally appropriate family adaptation.
Caregiver Stress and Coping	Providing care to an ill member results in primary and secondary strains. Coping strategies include managing the situation, managing the meaning of the situation (e.g., lack of appetite means ill member is dying), and managing one's symptoms of stress.	Assess family caregiver for multiple types of strain (e.g., physical, emotional, role, financial). Assess coping patterns of family members. Facilitate discussion of types of losses experienced.	Measure caregiving strain multidimensionally (e.g., physical effort, role adjustment, emotional distress, economic impact). Determine the relationship between coping strategies and QOL indicators.

and home settings suggest increased family involvement in the care of ill relatives. Available literature commonly refers to the family as a caregiving system, but research literature indicates that, more typically, one family member assumes the role of primary caregiver (Kahana, Kahana, Johnson, Hammond, & Kerchner, 1994). It has been estimated that families provide the majority of home care to persons with cancer (Given & Given, 1991; Siegel, Raveis, More, & Houts, 1991). The identity of the primary family caregiver for ill adults follows a hierarchical pattern with the primary provider being the spouse, followed by a child. If there is not a spouse or a child available, then other relatives, such as siblings, grandchildren, nieces, and nephews, emerge in this role (Aldous, 1994).

Bowers (1987), in her grounded theory research on intergeneration caregiving, conceptualized caregiving by the meaning or purpose the caregiver attributes to behaviors, rather than by the nature or the demands of the behavior itself. A dimensional analysis of her data revealed five distinct but empirically overlapping categories of family caregiving: (1) Anticipatory Caregiving, which includes behaviors or decisions based on anticipated or possible needs of a care recipient; (2) Preventive Caregiving, in which activities are engaged in for the purpose of preventing illness, injury, complications, and physical or mental deterioration; (3) Supervisory Caregiving, which involves checking to be sure that certain care-related tasks have been completed such as taking prescribed medicines; (4) Instrumental Caregiving, which involves assisting the care recipient with physical tasks; and (5) Protective Caregiving, which attempts to minimize the consequences of the disease for the care recipient. These five dimensions are useful for expanding the way health care providers think about the family as care provider. Frequently, only physical or instrumental caregiving is considered, when in fact, family caregivers provide a much wider range of care activities.

Defining Quality of Life for Families

The concept of QOL has been used and referred to in a variety of ways in the clinical and research literature. In its more generic or global sense it refers to a subjective experience of well-being (Baker & Intagliata, 1982; de Haes, 1988), although it has evolved into a multidimensional construct (Aaronson, 1988; Ganz, 1994). The domains of quality of life typically include a combination of the following: physical functioning, mental/emotional functioning, symptoms, social functioning/interaction, and spirituality. Extending present conceptualization of QOL to the family requires that attention be given to these domains as they relate to family members. Thus, assessing the families' social interactions or emotional functioning requires that information on family-level issues be collected from each member. In addition, since a primary role of the family is to provide financially for its members, economic functioning needs to be added to this list of domains. These domains of quality of life will be considered in the following selective literature review which describes the quality of life of families across the cancer experience.

Research on Quality of Life of Families across the Cancer Experience

The research literature to date on the family's experience with cancer focuses on specific stages of the cancer experiences, particularly those of diagnosis, initial treatment, and late or terminal stages of the illness. Only a limited number of studies have followed the family's experience over time (Woods, Lewis, & Ellison, 1989) or have focused on the family's experience with recurrence (Schumacher, Dodd, & Paul, 1993). In the next section, certain phases of the family cancer experience are reviewed in terms of the research that has been done on emotional and physical functioning, symptomatology, and social and financial functioning. The phases included are diagnosis and treatment, follow-up/rehabilitation, recurrence, and end of life/terminal. Research studies described here are limited to research done on adults with cancer and their families.

Diagnosis and Treatment Phase

Research studies on the impact of newly diagnosed cancer on family functioning repeatedly conclude that family members' greatest needs are emotional/psychological in nature (Hileman & Lackey, 1990). Research by Oberst and James (1985) and Oberst and Scott (1988) indicated that spouses of persons with cancer experience increased emotional distress as the time since diagnosis increases, and that distress peaks at two months posthospitalization. Northouse (1988) documented the psychosocial adjustment of male spouses of women with breast cancer and found that this adjustment was related to both the woman's and husband's levels of social support. Northouse (1992), in a study of women newly diagnosed with breast cancer and their spouses, reported that the spouses perceived significantly less support from family and friends than did their wives. In a study of 150 persons with cancer and their caregivers, Kurtz, Kurtz, Given, and Given (1995) found that caregivers who had a high degree of optimism had lower depression and tended to view caring as having a smaller impact on their own health. This study also found that depression in the person with cancer was correlated with family caregiver depression. Forty mothers recently diagnosed with breast cancer and their 40 male partners and school-age children were studied by Lewis, Hammond, and Woods (1993). They found that higher levels of experienced illness demands increased both the mother's and partner's depressed mood, both of which negatively impacted the marriage. Less well adjusted marriages were found to negatively affect the family's ability to reflect on their interactions in response to each other or to alter responses as needed. Children were found to function better when their non-ill parent more frequently interacted with them and when their family coped with problems that arose.

In 1993 Schott-Baer studied 113 spouse caregivers of persons receiving radiation or chemotherapy in terms of the relationship between self-care agency (or the ability to take care of self) and caregiver burden. This investigator found that self-care agency was nega-tively related to subjective burden, indicating that persons with high self-care agency (more able to do for themselves) perceived themselves to experience fewer negative emotional reactions to the caregiving experience.

Carey, Oberst, McCubbin, and Hughes (1991), in a study of 49 family caregivers of persons receiving chemotherapy, found that the emotional mood state of caregivers was related to the difficulty the caregivers experienced in providing emotional support to their ill relatives. Caregivers who appraised their own health as poor were more likely to view the caregiving role negatively. These caregivers, in turn, had greater mood disturbance.

The impact and treatment of pain on the person with cancer and their family care-giver were studied in 1991 by Ferrell, Rhiner, Cohen, and Grant. They found that pain serves as a metaphor for progressive illness and ultimate death. A major theme from the qualitative data analysis was the feeling of helplessness experienced by the family mem-bers, resulting in personal/emotional pain and distress. Suffering experienced by family members who accompany their ill member through the cancer experience was described by Hinds (1992) in a study of 83 family caregivers of persons with cancer. Emotional responses indicative/reflective of suffering included feelings of abandonment, helplessness, and despair.

A study by Blood, Simpson, Dineen, Kauffman, and Raimondik (1994) of 75 spouses of individuals with laryngectomies found that caregiver strain and burden were highest in those most recently diagnosed (within six months). Significant differences were found in gender, with female caregivers reporting higher stress than male caregivers. Neither care-giver strain nor burden was found, however, to be related to physical health status. In con-trast to the gender-specific findings of Blood and associates, Schumacher and colleagues (1993) found that male caregivers reported higher strain with respect to their role in a study of family members of persons receiving current treatment for cancer. Most studies to date include more women than men as family caregivers; thus, this discrepancy may be due in part to the small number of men included in the research.

The financial and economic impact of caring for a family member with cancer, if not felt during the time of diagnosis, is felt during the treatment phase. Stommel, Given, and Given (1993) have documented how shortened hospital stays and increased outpatient care have had economic consequences for the family. The informal costs of providing care can go unrecognized. Given, Given, and Stommel (1994) have found that families face out-of-pocket expenses (for transportation, clothing, and phone calls) as well as family labor costs (time spent providing care). Researchers have reported that many caregivers have difficulty maintaining their work roles (Perry & Roades de Meneses, 1989) and may actually lose work hours, which result in reduced earnings (Given & Given, 1991). Stommel, Given, and Given (1993) reported on the financial impact on families when a member is receiving treatment for cancer. They considered costs in four ways: direct costs (out-of-pocket cash); indirect costs (forgone earnings due to illness); labor costs of caregiver services; and labor costs of other family members. Findings from this study indicate that cancer home care costs for a three-month period average $4,563.

Follow-Up/Rehabilitation

Cancer continues to impact families even when the disease is held in check (Lewis, Woods, Bensley, & Hough, 1989). Zahlis and Shands (1993) reported that in families 18 months past diagnosis and with women considered to be disease-free, 27 percent of husbands reported negative feelings about the experience and the effect their wife's cancer had on their life. Lewis and Hammond's (1992) study of families with mothers experiencing breast cancer found that the mother's mood, as reflected by her level of depression, was related to poorer marital adjustment and consequently less active coping on the part of the family. Ptacek, Ptacek, and Dodge (1994) found that husbands and wives coped differently, although both are affected by cancer.

Recurrence

There is a paucity of literature on the impact of cancer recurrence on the family. Those studies that do exist identify the significance of the recurrence for the couple experiencing cancer (Chekryn, 1984; Given, 1990; Given & Given, 1992). Many studies have included families with cancer recurrence in their samples, but have not specifically addressed the unique demands that these families may experience. Kurtz, Given, Kurtz, and Given (1994) reported in a study of 208 cancer patient–caregiver dyads that as the stage of the illness progressed, caregivers reported higher levels of depression. In a study of 75 persons with cancer and their family caregivers, recurrence resulted in an increased level of depression for the caregivers in the family (Schumacher, Dodd, & Paul, 1993). In a study of 15 couples in which the wife had breast cancer, Lewis and Deal (1995) observed that although the couples found ways to manage their situation through the process of "balancing our lives," the majority experienced depression and marital adjustment issues. Further research is needed on the QOL of families experiencing recurrence.

End of Life/Terminal

A substantial body of literature exists regarding the experiences of families during the end stage of cancer. In a study of 65 spouse caregivers caring for a partner with advanced cancer, Stetz (1987) found that the most challenging aspects of being a spouse caregiver included managing the physical care and treatment, managing the household and finances, and standing by and observing the spouse's slow deterioration without being able to stop it. The experience of "standing by" reflects the psychological/emotional distress experienced by family members of persons who are terminally ill. Spouses also reported that their own well-being and patterns of living were altered as a result of being a caregiver. Additionally, Stetz (1989) found that the caregivers' uncertainty about their spouses' health status and future was a predictor of their perceptions of their physical health. The more uncertain they were about their spouses' health, the more negatively they perceived their own health.

Hull (1992) studied stressors and coping strategies identified by hospice families caring for a dying relative at home. The three areas of stress that caregivers dealt with most frequently were (1) the overall caregiving experience, (2) uncertainty, and (3) changes in the ill relative's mental status. How families coped with these stressors in order to maintain their quality of life included social comparison, cognitive reformulation, avoidance, taking a day at a time, acceptance and resignation, and utilization of resources such as other family and hospice services.

In a study of families with terminally ill members, Reimer, Davis, and Martens (1991) found that these families faced two major tasks. The first is a process of redefining family roles and who comprises the family in light of the actual or pending loss of the ill family member. The second task is coping with new role related burdens and the loss of the original family due to the death of a family member. Families were found to experience challenges, deal with feelings of emptiness, struggle with paradox, contend with change, and search for meaning.

Herth (1993) found that as the length of time being a caregiver increased and as the death of the ill member approached, caregivers reported more fatigue, more difficulty sleeping, less personal time, and more role responsibilities. In a study of the needs of rural families with cancer, Buehler and Lee (1992) found that the greater the deterioration of the person with cancer, the greater the caregiver burden (e.g., taking on few or expanded roles, and experiencing inadequate resources).

Nursing Interventions to Enhance Quality of Life in Families

The research to date on the QOL of families experiencing cancer reveals that these families are primarily affected in terms of their emotional well-being, roles and social interactions, and finances. Alterations in the physical functioning of "well" members was not found to be a significant issue for families. Nursing interventions need to be directed toward a comprehensive approach in order to meet the needs of families with a member diagnosed with cancer. This approach must include assessment and the design and implementation of family-specific interventions. Table 10-2 provides suggestions of theoretically based assessment strategies.

Table 10-2. **Guidelines for Family Assessment**

Area of Assessment	Tools or Questions to Be Used
Family System	*Structural Assessment:* Genogram (Wright & Leahy, 1994). Draw a two- or three-generation genogram for the family as you interview them about family composition and household membership. *Functional Assessment:* Communication patterns ("Who do you go to to talk about what it's like to care for your husband?" "When there is an issue/situation impacting the family, who typically initiates discussion about it?") Roles ("Who is responsible for child care arrangements?" "Who does the liaison relationship with the school?" "Who is responsible for household chores?") Problem solving ("Describe a challenge your family recently experienced and how your family handled it.")
Developmental Stage	Ask family members questions that elicit information related to developmental tasks. ("You have both grade-school children and a teenager in the house; describe what it is like for you to address your children's different needs." "What adjustments have occurred in your family since 'Sam' left for college?")
Caregiver Stress and Coping	Ask family member about the demands they experience. ("Tell me what issues are of greatest concern for you.") Draw an Ecomap (Wright & Leahy, 1994). Have the family describe their network outside of the household family and the extent to which it is supportive, neutral, or conflictual.

Assessment

Utilization of a family systems approach to assess the family will result in an accurate picture of who constitutes the family. For example, the nurse needs to determine who makes up the family system; one technique that is useful for this purpose is a family genogram (Wright & Leahy, 1994). The process of this assessment will reveal who is in the household family and which family members are available outside of the family to help. In addition, the genogram provides information about the developmental stage of the family. The caregiver stress and coping model provides direction for assessing how the family is adapting to its caregiving role. Areas for assessment include primary strains (problems in providing care and the experience of uncertainty and loss) and secondary strains (symptoms of stress and financial impact). In addition, how the family has responded to the challenges, such as the coping strategies used (sources of support, personal and interpersonal resources), is a component of this assessment.

An assessment of the impact of the physical caring done by family members must take into account the amount and type of care provided, and how the demands are subjectively experienced. Frequent reference by family members to elements of overload, such as being "completely exhausted" and "having to do the work of two people," are examples of experienced strain. This can be determined directly and objectively by assessing the daily and instrumental activities for which the ill person depends on the caregiver. It can be determined subjectively by asking how difficult the tasks are for the family. Assessing the family for their experience of uncertainty and loss is critical. Simply asking family members what worries them most will reveal their greatest fears.

Determining how the family copes can be accomplished by asking the family to reflect on how they have handled problems (coping to manage the situation) in the past (Stetz, Lewis, & Primomo, 1986). The nurse can also effectively assess coping strategies by asking how families have handled situations in which they were not able to reach the solution desired (coping to manage meaning). Lastly, the nurse can assess for both the presence of symptoms of stress (e.g., insomnia, anorexia, or overeating) and the strategies families have used to manage those symptoms. See Table 10-2 for a summary of assessment strategies associated with each of the theoretical models.

Interventions

The three theoretical frameworks described earlier (systems, developmental, and caregiver coping and stress theories) also provide direction for the development of nursing interventions. Interventions need to be geared toward the family as a unit as well as toward individual members. Also, interventions must consider family structure and functional changes and be developmentally appropriate. Of paramount importance, however, is that interventions be focused on what *the family perceives* is their greatest challenge or issue. Following are strategies nurses can use with families in order to improve their QOL:

1. Provide information with respect to the type and purpose of diagnostic tests, what to expect as side effects, and how to manage symptoms associated with the disease and treatment.

2. Encourage the family to take time for themselves (personal and recreational) as well as for the family as a system. This will mean building in respite time. The nurse can suggest that the family consider establishing "windows of time" in which they are free from the suffering associated with the cancer. This is particularly important in families with school-age children. Children need to know that it is important and fitting that they have activities that keep them engaged with their social network and planning for their future even though the parent may not be part of it.

3. Facilitate the mobilization of resources. The research literature repeatedly indicates (Hull, 1992; Stetz, 1987) that families frequently wait until "things really get tough" before asking for help or assistance. The problem with this strategy is that by this point the caregivers are so exhausted that they risk ill health and needing to relinquish their roles as caregivers. In terms of professional services, families typically are not aware of community-based programs and need to be educated about available resources such as the American Cancer Society, support groups, and home health care services. We Can Weekends or similar group formats in which families can spend time with other families while striving to improve communication have also been found to be helpful to families (Walsch-Burke, 1992). With respect to lay help, family caregivers often do not know what to say when asked by friends or other family how they can be of assistance. Encourage the family to keep a list on the refrigerator or by the phone of those things that need to be done and that could be done by someone other than themselves. They may need assistance developing this list.

4. Be sensitive to the family's losses. A number of strategies have been identified by Rando that assist people to deal with loss and grief (Rando, 1986). Example strategies include having family members give themselves time and permission to grieve the losses they feel; encouraging the family to reminisce with their ill member and with each other; and facilitating efforts to finish unfinished business (e.g., suggest looking through photo albums or creating them and/or memory books if they don't currently exist). Many times what family members need most is someone to listen and be sensitive to their concerns. The nurse can engage in this by listening for cues and participating in reflective listening. Raudonis (1993) found that the establishment of an empathetic relationship, one that meant being acknowledged as an individual and as a person of value, had a positive impact on emotional well-being.

5. Families with a terminally ill member need assistance preparing for the death of their member. Encourage the use of hospice services. Many families and persons with cancer continue to equate "hospice" with death and are thus reluctant to accept services when they would be beneficial to family coping.

For additional strategies to assist families, Lewis (1990) and Northouse and Peters-Golden (1993) offered further suggestions. Lewis suggested that support services for families focus on informational, anticipatory, interpretive, skill-based, problem-focused, and physical services. Northouse and Peters-Golden suggested that nurses anticipate what information family members need and provide that information specific to the phase of the illness. In addition, Northouse and Peters-Golden recommended that support services (emotional and physical) be made available to these families.

SUMMARY AND FUTURE DIRECTIONS

The literature on the QOL of families experiencing cancer indicates that families are most affected in the domains of emotional, social, and financial functioning and, to a lesser extent, physical functioning and symptoms (other than anxiety and depression). Nursing interventions based on a combined theoretical approach (systems, developmental, and caregiver stress and coping) will be most effective in meeting family needs. Further directions for nursing research should include longitudinal research with families during and after caring for ill members to better understand the effect caregiving has on the QOL of survivors. Also, intervention research should be created that targets the family as well as the ill person. Lastly, studies of outcome indicators for people being treated for cancer should include QOL measures of their family members to better understand how cancer impacts the entire family and not just the ill person.

REFERENCES

Aaronson, N. K. (1988). Quality of life: What is it? How should it be measured? *Oncology, 2*, 69–74.

Aldous, J. (1994). Someone to watch over me. In E. Kahana, D. E. Biegel, & M. L. Wykle (Eds.), *Family caregiving across the lifespan* (pp. 42–68). Thousand Oaks, CA: Sage.

Armsden, G. C., & Lewis, F. M. (1994). Behavioral adjustment and self-esteem of school aged children of women with breast cancer. *Oncology Nursing Forum, 21*(1), 39–45.

Baker, F., & Itagliata, J. (1982). Quality of life in the evaluation of community support systems. *Evaluation and Program Planning, 5*, 69–75.

Blood, G. W., Simpson, K. C., Dineen, M., Kauffman, S. M., & Raimondik, S. C. (1994). Spouses of individuals with laryngeal cancer: Caregiver strain & burden. *Journal of Communication Disorder, 27*, 19–35.

Bowers, B. (1987). Intergenerational caregiving: Adult caregivers and their aging parents. *Advances in Nursing Science, 9*(2), 20–31.

Broderick, C., & Smith, J. (1979). The general systems approach to the family. In W. Burr, R. Hill, F. Nye, & I. Reiss (Eds.), *Contemporary theories about the family* (pp. 112–129). New York: The Free Press.

Buehler, J. A., & Lee, H. J. (1992). Exploration of homecare resources for rural families with cancer. *Cancer Nursing, 15*(4), 299–308.

Carey, P. J., Oberst, M. T., McCubbin, M. A., & Hughes, S. H. (1991). Appraisal and caregiver burden in family members caring for patients receiving chemotherapy. *Oncology Nursing Forum, 18*(8), 1341–1348.

Carter, E. A., & McGoldrick, M. (1980). *The family life cycle*. New York: Gardner.

Chekryn, J. (1984). Cancer recurrence: Personal meaning, communication, and marital adjustment. *Cancer Nursing, 7,* 491–498.

de Haes, J. C. (1988). Quality of life: Concepts and theoretical consideration. In M. Watson, S. Greer, & C. Thomas (Eds.), *Psychosocial oncology* (pp. 61–70). Oxford, England: Pergamon Press.

Duvall, E. (1977). *Marriage and family development.* Philadelphia: Lippincott.

Ferrell, B. R., Rhiner, M., Cohen, M. Z., & Grant, M. (1991). Pain as a metaphor for illness. Part 1: Impact of cancer pain on family caregivers. *Oncology Nursing Forum, 18*(8), 1303–1309.

Ganz, P. (1994). Quality of life and the patient with cancer, *Cancer, 74,* 1445–1452.

Germino, B. B., & Funk, S. G. (1993). Impact of parent's cancer on adult children: Role and relationship issues. *Seminars in Oncology Nursing, 9*(2), 101–106.

Given, B. (1990). Study critique. Psychosocial adjustment to recurrent cancer. *Oncology Nursing Forum, 17*(Suppl. 3), 53–54.

Given, B., & Given, C. W. (1991). Family caregivers of cancer patients, In S. Hubbard, P. Greene, & M. Knobf (Eds.), *Current issues in cancer nursing practice* (pp. 1–9). Philadelphia: W. B. Saunders.

Given, B., & Given, C. W. (1992). Patient and family caregiver reaction to new and recurrent breast cancer. *Journal of the American Medical Women's Association, 47*(5), 201–206.

Given, C. W., Given, B., & Stommel, M. (1994). Family and out-of-pocket costs for women with breast cancer. *Cancer Practice, 2*(3), 187–193.

Gotcher, J. M. (1992). Interpersonal communication and psychosocial adjustment. *Journal of Psychosocial Oncology, 10*(3), 21–39.

Herth, K. (1993). Hope in the family caregiver of terminally ill people. *Journal of Advanced Nursing, 18,* 538–548.

Hileman, J. W., & Lackey, N. R. (1990). Identifying the needs of home caregivers of patients with cancer. *Oncology Nursing Forum, 19*(5), 771–777.

Hinds, C. (1992). Suffering: A relatively unexplored phenomenon among family caregivers of noninstitutionalized patients with cancer. *Journal of Advanced Nursing, 17,* 918–925.

Howes, M. J., Hoke, L., Winterbottom, M., & Delafield, D. (1994). Psychosocial effects of breast cancer on the patient's children. *Journal of Psychosocial Oncology, 12*(4), 1–21.

Hull, M. M. (1992). Coping strategies of family caregivers in hospice and homecare. *Oncology Nursing Forum, 19*(8), 1179–1187.

Kahana, E., Kahana, B., Johnson, J., Hammond, R., & Kercher, K. (1994). Developmental challenges and family caregiving. In E. Kahana, D. E. Biegel, & M. L. Wykle (Eds.), *Family caregiving across the lifespan* (pp. 3–41). Thousand Oaks, CA: Sage.

Kristjanson, L. J. (1989). Quality of terminal care: Salient indicators identified by families. *Journal of Palliative Care, 5*(1), 21–30.

Kristjanson, L. J., & Ashcroft, T. (1994). The family's cancer journey: A literature review. *Cancer Nursing, 17*(1), 1–17.

Kurtz, M. E., Given, B., Kurtz, J., & Given, C. W. (1994). The interaction of age, symptoms and survival status on physical and mental health of patients with cancer and their families. *Cancer, 74*, 2071–2078.

Kurtz, M. E., Kurtz, J., Given, C. W., & Given, B. (1995). Relationship of caregiver reactions and depression to cancer patients' symptoms, functional states and depression—a longitudinal view. *Social Science in Medicine, 40*(6), 837–846.

Laizner, A. M., Yost, L. M., Barg, F. K., & McCorkle, R. (1993). Needs of family caregivers of persons with cancer: A review. *Seminars in Oncology Nursing, 9*(2), 114–120.

Lazarus, R. S., Averill, J., & Opton, E. (1974). The psychology of coping: Isssues of research and assessment. In G. V. Coehlo, D. A. Hamburg, & J. E. Adams (Eds.), *Coping and adaptation* (pp. 249–315). New York: Basic Books.

Lewis, F. M. (1990). Strengthening family supports. *Cancer, 65*(3), 752–759.

Lewis, F. M., & Deal, L. W. (1995). Balancing our lives: A study of the married couple's experience with breast cancer recurrence. *Oncology Nursing Forum, 22*(6), 943–953.

Lewis, F. M., & Hammond, M. A. (1992). Psychosocial adjustment of the family to breast cancer: A longitudinal analysis. *Journal of the American Medical Women's Association, 47*(5), 194–200.

Lewis, F. M., Hammond, M. A., & Woods, N. F. (1993). The family's functioning with newly diagnosed breast cancer in the mother: The development of an explanatory model. *Journal of Behavioral Medicine, 16*(4), 351–370.

Lewis, F. M., Woods, N. F., Bensley, L., & Hough, E. (1989). Family functioning in chronic illness: The spouse's perspective. *Social Science in Medicine, 29*(11), 1261–1269.

Niederehe, G., & Fruge, E. (1984). Dementia and family dynamics: Clinical research issues. *Journal of Geriatric Psychiatry, 17*, 21–56.

Northouse, L. L. (1988). Social support in patients' and husbands' adjustment to breast cancer. *Nursing Research, 37*(2), 91–95.

Northouse, L. L. (1992). Psychological impact of the diagnosis of breast cancer on the patient and her family. *Journal of the American Medical Women's Association, 47*(5), 161–164.

Northouse, L. L., & Peters-Golden, H. (1993). Cancer and the family: Strategies to assist spouses. *Seminars in Oncology Nursing, 9*(2), 74–82.

Oberst, M. T., & James, R. H. (1985). Going home: Patient and spouse adjustment following cancer surgery. *Topics in Clinical Nursing, 7*, 46–57.

Oberst, M. T., & Scott, D. W. (1988). Post discharge distress in surgically treated cancer patients and their spouses. *Research in Nursing and Health, 11*(4), 223–233.

Pearlin, L., Mullan, J. T., Semple, A. J., & Skaff, M. M. (1990). Caregiving and the stress process: An overview of concepts and their measures. *The Gerontologist, 30,* 583–594.

Perry, G. R., & Roades de Meneses, M. (1989). Cancer patients at home: Needs and coping styles of primary caregivers. *Home Healthcare Nurse, 7*(6), 27–30.

Ptacek, J. T., Ptacek, J. J., & Dodge, K. L. (1994). Coping with breast cancer from the perspectives of husbands and wives. *Journal of Psychosocial Oncology, 12*(3), 47–70.

Rando, T. A. (1986). *Loss and anticipatory grief.* Lexington, MA: Lexington Books.

Raudonis, B. M. (1993). The meaning and impact of empathetic relationships in hospice nursing. *Cancer Nursing, 16*(4), 304–309.

Reimer, J. C., Davis, B., & Martens, N. (1991). Palliative care: The nurse's role in helping families through the transition of fading away. *Cancer Nursing, 14*(6), 321–327.

Sales, E., Schulz, R., & Biegel, D. (1992). Predictors of strain in families of cancer patients: A review of the literature. *Journal of Psychosocial Oncology, 10*(2), 1–26.

Schott-Baer, D. (1993). Dependent care, caregiver burden, and self-care agency of spouse caregivers. *Cancer Nursing, 16*(3), 230–236.

Schumacher, K. L., Dodd, M. J., & Paul, S. M. (1993). The stress process in family caregivers of persons receiving chemotherapy. *Research in Nursing & Health, 16,* 395–404.

Siegel, K., Mesegno, F. P., Karus, D., Christ, G., Banks, K., & Moynihan, R. (1992). Psychosocial adjustment of children with a terminally ill parent. *Journal of the American Academy of Child and Adolescent Psychiatry, 31,* 327–333.

Siegel, K., Raveis, V. H., More, V., & Houts, P. (1991). The relationship of spousal caregiver burden to patient disease and treatment-related conditions. *Annals of Oncology, 2,* 511.

Stetz, K. M. (1987). Caregiving demands during advanced cancer: The spouses's needs. *Cancer Nursing, 10*(5), 260–268.

Stetz, K. M. (1989). The relationship among background characteristics, purpose in life and caregiving demands on perceived health of spouse caregivers. *Scholarly Inquiry for Nursing Practice, 3*(2), 133–153.

Stetz, K. M., & Brown, M. (1997). Taking care: Caregiving to persons with cancer and AIDS. *Cancer Nursing, 20*(1), 12–22.

Stetz, K. M., Lewis, F. M., & Primomo, J. (1986). Family coping strategies and chronic illness in the mother. *Family Relations, 35,* 515–522.

Stommel, M., Given, C. W., & Given, B. (1993). The cost of cancer home care to families. *Cancer, 71*(5), 1867–1874.

Stommel, M., & Kingry, M. (1991). Support patterns for spouse caregivers of cancer patients. The effect of the presence of minor children. *Cancer, 14*(4), 200–205.

Walsch-Burke, L. (1992). Family communication and coping with cancer: Impact of the We Can weekend. *Journal of Psychosocial Oncology, 10*(1), 63–81.

Woods, N. F., Lewis, F. M., & Ellison, E. S. (1989). Living with cancer: Family experiences. *Cancer Nursing, 7,* 371–374.

Wright, L. M., & Leahy, M. (1994). *Nurses and families.* Philadelphia: F. A. Davis.

Zahlis, E. H., & Shands, M. E. (1993). The impact of breast cancer on the partner 18 months after diagnosis. *Seminars in Oncology Nursing, 9*(2), 83–87.

Practice

Chapter

11

Quality of Life
Issues in Breast Cancer

DEANNA KUHN • KAREN HASSEY DOW

Introduction and Background

One out of every eight American women will develop breast cancer during her life-time. In 2002, about 200,000 women are expected to be diagnosed with invasive breast cancer (Jemal, Thomas, Murray, & Thun, 2002). Breast cancer is primarily a disease occurring with advancing age. However, the incidence in younger women rose in the early nineties due to improved technology and earlier screening. With the aging of the baby boom generation however, the incidence in women under 45 is declining once again (Jemal et al., 2002).

While the incidence of breast cancer has risen, improvements in screening, early detection, and treatment have led to a decline in mortality. It is estimated 39,600 women will die of breast cancer in 2002 (American Cancer Society, 2002). Five-year survival rates for localized tumors have increased from 72% in the 1940s to 96% today (American Cancer Society, 2002). Eighty-six percent of all women diagnosed with breast cancer will survive five years. Moreover, unlike survival for other cancers, which levels off after 5 years, 76% of women diagnosed with breast cancer survive 10 years and 58% survive 15 years (American Cancer Society, 2001). Thus, more women with a history of breast cancer are living longer and their quality of life (QOL) concerns have become a major focus, particularly in research.

The purpose of this chapter is to: (a) describe current trends in breast cancer treatment and their influence on QOL; (b) identify research related to high inci-dence QOL problem areas; (c) describe QOL tools used in breast cancer research; and (d) explore future QOL issues for research.

Changes in Treatment and Approach to Breast Cancer

Advances in our understanding about the biologic and molecular changes occurring in the development and progression of breast cancer have opened up new areas of QOL evaluation. For example, clinical trials evaluating Tamoxifen™ as a chemo-preventive agent have led to more focus on decision making about clinical trials. QOL issues in treatment have moved from symptom management to evaluation of long-term effects of therapy. The Consensus Statement on Adjuvant Therapy for Breast Cancer (2000) published by the National Institutes of Health (NIH) advo-cated further evaluation of QOL by randomized clinical trials to evaluate the acute and long-term effects of adjuvant treatments. The main areas of focus recommended by the NIH include premature menopause, weight gain, mild memory loss, and fatigue. They also support the use of newly developed methods for shared decision making between patients and their physicians that take into account QOL issues. With longer-term survival, women may live with advanced disease. QOL issues relat-ing to targeted therapy and hormonal therapy are also now beginning to be evaluated.

Research in QOL and Breast Cancer

Quality of life is defined as a multidimensional construct depicting the interrelation-ship among four domains of well-being: physical, psychological, social, and spiritual (King et al. 1997). The following discussion of selected research studies focuses on specific problems affecting women with breast cancer across each QOL domain. These problem areas include physical well-being (i.e., ovarian dysfunction, meno-pausal symptoms, fertility issues, fatigue, weight gain, and lymphedema); psychologi-cal well-being (i.e., changes in body image and sexuality); social well-being (i.e., interpersonal and family relationship issues); and spiritual well-being (i.e., uncer-tainty, hope).

Physical Well-being

Traditionally, the majority of QOL studies reported in the literature investigate the effect of breast cancer treatment on functional status. The QOL instruments used in-clude standard symptom management and toxicity scales. These studies, while using the term QOL, have generally limited their focus on specific symptoms or adverse physical effects on QOL. Moreover, QOL assessment relied on proxy ratings by health professionals rather than defining QOL as a multidimensional and subjective con-struct. In their study on the perception of QOL by patients, partners, and treating physicians, Wilson, Dowling, Abdolell, & Tannock (2000) found that physicians systematically underestimated QOL particularly in regard to the social and role functions of breast cancer survivors.

Several studies have shifted their focus from documented symptoms occurring during treatment to long-term, interrelated concerns affecting QOL (Broeckel et al., 1998; Dow, Ferrell, Leigh, Ly, & Gulasekaran, 1996; Wang, Cosby, Harris, & Liu 1999). In a descriptive study of QOL among 294 long-term survivors of breast cancer, Dow and colleagues (1996) found that menopausal and fertility concerns, fatigue, aches/pains, and sleep disturbance were the major physical changes influencing QOL. These findings were further verified by Ferrell and colleagues (1997) who identified weight gain and hair and breast loss as additional concerns related to physical well-being.

Ovarian Failure. Studies indicate that chemotherapy-induced premature ovarian failure occurs in approximately 63–85% of women with breast cancer (Reichman & Green, 1994; Shapiro & Recht, 1994). The alkylating agents are the primary cause of ovarian failure due to a decrease in estradiol and progesterone levels and an increase in pituitary gonadotropins similar to levels observed in postmenopausal women (Averette, Mirhashemi, & Moffat, 1999; Moore, 2000; Shapiro & Recht, 1994).

Koyama and colleagues (1977) indicate that the cumulative dose range for development of permanent amenorrhea was 5.2 grams of cyclophosphamide. Age is the major determining factor in the development of premature ovarian failure. Women younger than 35 years are able to tolerate larger cumulative doses of chemotherapy before developing permanent amenorrhea. Older women, on the other hand, have depleted numbers of follicles and, thus, are more susceptible to the effects of chemotherapy. In general, 30–50% of women under age 40 develop ovarian failure. This figure rises to 90% in women over age 40. Reversible amenorrhea has been observed in women under age 35 (Sutton, Buzdar, & Hortobagyi, 1990). Ovarian failure can lead to significant changes in QOL. Younger women may experience the effects of menopausal symptoms or changes in fertility while older women may experience menopausal symptoms prematurely.

Menopausal Symptoms. In a study on health-related QOL issues and sexual functioning, Ganz and colleagues (2000) found that breast cancer survivors reported more menopausal symptoms than healthy women, but in general did not find an associated decrease in their QOL or sexual functioning. The major menopausal symptoms associated with breast cancer treatment include vasomotor instability (hot flashes, insomnia, and night sweats), genitourinary effects (vaginal dryness, atrophy, severe discomfort, and dyspareunia), skeletal effects (osteoporosis), and cardiovascular disease (Swain, Santen, Burger, & Pritchard, 1999). In general, vasomotor instability is the most troublesome, affecting up to 65% of breast cancer survivors (Carpenter &

Andrykowski,1999; Couzi, Helzlsouer, & Fetting, 1995). Stein and colleagues (2000) found vasomotor symptoms such as hot flashes to be associated with increased fatigue, sleep problems, depression, and anxiety in breast cancer survivors. They also found that younger pre-menopausal women experience symptoms that are more disrupting to their QOL than those who have already experienced menopause.

Ovarian failure is also related to the increased risk of osteoporosis and cardiovascular disease. In the general population, one third of women over the age of 65 are at risk of developing spinal fractures. By extreme old age, an additional one third of women are at risk of developing hip fractures. The increased risk of developing heart disease increases significantly after menopause, putting postmenopausal women at a greater risk of developing heart disease than men. Women in general are six times more likely to die of cardiovascular disease than breast cancer.

Estrogen replacement therapy (ERT) has been shown effective in decreasing vasomotor symptoms of menopause as well as mitigating the effects of osteoporosis. Although recent studies do not show a similar decrease in cardiac morbidity, ERT is still often prescribed to lower a patient's cardiac risk. However, the use of ERT in women with a history of breast cancer is considered controversial (Stein et al., 2000; Cobleigh, et al., 1994). The concern with using ERT in women with a history of breast cancer is the possibility of added morbidity and mortality from activation or growth acceleration of micrometastasis, or the development of second primaries (Theriault & Vasilipoulou-Sellin, 1994).

While the debate rages about the use of ERT in women with breast cancer, there are nonhormonal alternatives available in the management of menopause (Bachmann, 1994; Cobleigh, 2000). Sedatives such as phenobarbital, progestins, and clonidine in the form of transdermal patches, and venlafaxine (Loprinzi et al., 2000) have all been used to treat hot flashes. The use of herbal remedies and dietary supplements with phytoestrogens has been suggested to decrease vasomotor symptoms (Moschen et al., 2001). While many women claim they are effective, their efficacy has not been closely studied and the safety of their use in breast cancer patients has not been established.

Genitourinary and atrophic conditions are often treated with low dose locally applied estrogen to the urogenital area. Nonestrogen lubricants and moisturizers, nonhormonal vaginal preparations, kegel exercises, and vaginal dilators are also recommended to decrease urovaginal symptoms.

While ERT is the most effective treatment for the prevention of osteoporosis, there are other pharmacological alternatives such as bisphosphonates (i.e., Alendronate®), raloxifene (Evista®), and Calcitonin® nasal spray. Additional nonpharmacological measures such as weight-bearing exercises (i.e., walking) and a well-balanced, moderate protein diet with calcium (1,500 mg/day) and vitamin D (400–1,000 mg/day) supplementation can also be utilized to prevent osteoporosis.

To address some of the cardiovascular effects, health care professionals have prescribed exercise, a low-fat diet, low-dose aspirin, and cholesterol lowering medications (as needed). The nonhormonal management of menopausal symptoms is increasingly being used to address QOL issues among women who are undecided about the use of hormones after breast cancer.

Fertility Concerns. Although the incidence of breast cancer in premenopausal women is less than 20%, the impact of treatment on fertility is a major stressor among young breast cancer survivors. Age and alkylating agents are known risk factors that influence fertility. In addition, taxanes, hormonal therapy, and use of assisted reproductive technologies (ART) are additional concerns that may influence fertility and pregnancy outcomes.

No epidemiologic studies have suggested an adverse effect of pregnancy on survival. Several retrospective institutional reports published between 1940–1979 show accumulating evidence that do not support the theoretical concern that women having children after breast cancer are an increased risk of developing recurrent disease (Danforth, 1991; Donegan, 1977; Dow, Harris, & Roy, 1994; Harrington, 1937). These studies have several methodological problems (retrospective designs, small numbers, and differential sampling techniques [historical outcomes, case matching]). Yet, the majority of evidence supports the notion that women having children are at no greater risk of recurrent breast cancer than women who do not have subsequent pregnancy. In fact, five case-control studies, between 1990 and 1997, using newer treatment regimens (Dow, 1994; Kroman et al., 1997; Sutton, Buzdar, & Hortobagyi, 1990; Valagussa, De Candis, & Antonelli, 1996; von Schoultz, Johansson, Wilking, & Rutquist, 1995) did not show evidence that pregnancy adversely affected breast cancer outcome.

Four large, population-based studies conducted between 1994 and 1999, (Kroman et al., 1998; Sankila, Heinavaara, & Hakulinen, 1994; Velentgas et al., 1999; von Schoultz et al., 1995) have not shown an adverse effect on survival after pregnancy. A form of bias called "healthy mother effect" could explain why women who become pregnant may be more likely free of disease at the time of pregnancy compared with women who do not have subsequent pregnancy.

Fatigue. Fatigue has long been recognized as one of the most common side effects of cancer treatment. Ninety nine percent of breast cancer patients report feeling fatigue during the course of radiation and/or chemotherapy, and more than 60% rate the fatigue as moderate to severe (Bower et al., 2000). Some studies have found breast cancer survivors experience significantly more fatigue than age-matched healthy women (Andrykowski, Curran, & Lighner, 1998; Broekel et al., 1998). However, in a survey of 1957 breast cancer survivors, Bower and colleagues (2000) found that the majority of breast cancer survivors did not experience heightened levels of fatigue when compared to an age-matched group of healthy peers. A portion of the survivors, however, did report severe and persistent fatigue. Through logistic regression they found that depression ($p < 0.0001$) and pain ($p < 0.0001$) were the most highly predictive variables of fatigue followed by age ($p = 0.02$). The difference between these findings and previous studies possibly could be related to the populations studied. Bower et al. included women who were between one and five years post diagnosis (mean 3.0), while Andrykowski's and Broekel's populations averaged 2.3 and 1.3 years post treatment, respectively. These results may indicate that, while fatigue is a common problem during and immediately after breast cancer treatment, its effects may diminish over time for the majority of women.

In an attempt to diminish the effects of fatigue, Mock and colleagues (1997) conducted a study of the effects of a walking exercise program on 46 women beginning during radiation therapy for breast cancer. They found significant differences between the exercise and control groups ($p < 0.001$). The exercise group reported better physical function and lower symptom intensity, particularly fatigue ($p = 0.018$), anxiety ($p = 0.029$), and difficulty sleeping ($p = 0.027$). These results were supported by Schwartz (1999) who found low to moderate exercise significantly reduced fatigue, while lack of exercise and high intensity exercise worsened fatigue. These findings suggest that there may be an optimal dose of exercise to reduce fatigue.

Weight Gain. Anecdotally there have been reports of weight gain associated with certain hormonal therapies. While weight gains of 5–10 % have been documented in clinical trials of patients receiving megestrol acetate (Buzdar et al., 1996; Buzdar et al., 1997). In a clinical trial of over 10,000 women receiving tamoxifen for breast cancer prevention there was no significant weight gain noted (Day et al., 1999).

Lymphedema. Lymphedema is gaining increased clinical and research attention. Although fewer than 10% of breast cancer patients have reported lymphedema (Velanovich and Szymanski, 1999), it can have a severe and long-lasting effect on QOL. Underreporting of the incidence of lymphedema may be related to the fact that there is no uniform definition of lymphedema or standard measure or assessment (Petrek, Pressman, and Smith, 2000).

In a study of long-term (8 years post treatment) breast cancer survivors, Dorval and associates (1998) found arm problems and sexuality issues were the only two QOL factors that were significantly different when compared with controls. The most troubling aspects of lymphedema are the increased weight and physical disfigurement of the affected limb that affect both functioning and psychological factors. (Passik and McDonald, 1998).

In a series of interviews, Carter (1997) reports that while most women with lymphedema are able to continue living their normal lives, some women experience depression, anxiety, and impairments related to their work, social, and intimate relationships. Due to these effects on QOL, many patients are instructed on the importance of lymphedema prevention. Unfortunately, physician recommendations are often based on anecdotal reports as opposed to clinical trials, are seemingly contradictory (i.e., lose weight and don't exercise), and can impose significant lifestyle changes (i.e., avoid air travel, exercise). It is with this in mind that further research on the benefits of specific lymphedema preventative activities is recommended so patients can be educated on the actual risks and benefits of each activity (Passik and McDonald, 1998).

Psychological Well-being

The major psychological concerns affecting QOL in breast cancer include depression, anxiety, body image changes, fear of recurrent cancer, and uncertainty over the future (Ferrell et al., 1998). The diagnosis of breast cancer at any age triggers fears about losing desirability or capacity for sexual pleasure (Schover, 1994). Generally, the younger the woman, the greater the potential impact of cancer treatment on sexuality and body image. The research studies of the impact of breast cancer and treatment indicate three major moderating variables in assessing its impact on sexuality: (1) age, (2) choice of primary treatment, and (3) breast reconstruction.

Sexuality Changes. In a study of breast cancer survivors from two metropolitan areas, Ganz and associates (1998) found that in general, while breast cancer survivors report more physical and menopausal symptoms than age-matched women without cancer, they do not experience a diminished subjective quality of life. Nonmenstruating survivors younger than 50 years old and chemotherapy patients of all ages did however, experience significantly worse sexual functioning. These data support the earlier findings of Schover (1994), which suggest that younger women are generally more distressed psychologically by changes in sexuality than are older women.

Yet, when younger women have their sexuality concerns addressed or when the dysfunction is treated, they adjust better than older women. The influence of age on sexual function makes sense given the many developmental tasks younger women must attend to. For example, Schover (1994) indicated that the many assaults that women experience, such as loss of the breast, surgical scar, and chemotherapy, may be extremely difficult for a young woman who has not yet dealt with impact of premature aging on her body. Younger women may fear rejection by a potential mate that is related to the fear of physical imperfection and recurrent disease.

Despite the many problems with methodological flaws, small sample size, non-random assignment, use of untested assessment tools, inconsistent follow up, and lack of specification about menopausal status in research studies comparing the differences in sexual function between women having mastectomy versus breast-conserving surgery, the conclusions are remarkably similar and psychological adjustment (whether measured by psychiatric disorders or emotional distress) does not vary significantly between the two groups (Ganz et al., 2000; Schover, 1994). Age was the only factor having an influence on sexual functioning. Younger women were more distressed in both mastectomy and breast-conserving surgery groups.

Body Image Changes.   Body image changes are more apparent in women having mastectomy compared with breast-conserving surgery (Pusic et al., 1999). Women with mastectomy report feeling less attractive and less sexually desirable than those with breast conserving surgery.

Wapnir, Cody, and Greco (1999) compared the effect of mastectomy and lumpectomy with axillary lymph node dissection (LAD) on QOL. Using a modified SF-36 Health Survey, they found the LAD patients scored higher in vitality on the SF-36 and also reported significant differences in matters of dress, use of bathing suits, hugging, comfort with nudity, and sex drive compared with patients undergoing mastectomy. Other dimensions of QOL showed no significant differences. Their results support that of other researchers who have found that body image is more positive in women with breast-conserving surgery and/or after reconstruction compared to mastectomy alone (Mock, 1993; Nissen et al., 2001; Pusic, 1999).

Social Well-being

Breast cancer has a great influence on family relationships and QOL. According to Northouse (1994), the effects of breast cancer on family relationships can be viewed from the developmental perspective of the family life cycle. Based on this perspective, increased family demands are associated with the care of young children. Family demands peak during school age and adolescence, then decline later in the family life cycle. Family strain is highest during early stages of the family life cycle. When the demands of illness are superimposed on the usual demands of family life, particularly a diagnosis of breast cancer, the demands on family life are heightened because families must not only cope with day-to-day care of young children, and emerging careers, but they must also cope with a life-threatening diagnosis and the effects of treatment. Some families continue to do well despite the major stressors, while others report maximum disruption of family life. Northouse, Templin, and Mood (2001) found that factors that mediate the perception of QOL include concurrent family stressors, patient and family fear of recurrence, family hardiness, employment status, and increased social support.

QOL Effects on the Marital Relationship. A few studies investigating the effects of breast cancer on the spouse demonstrate that diagnosis and treatment have a stressful impact (Northouse, 1989; Wilson, 1991). Spouses report psychosomatic problems such as eating disorders, sleep disturbances, and distress levels comparable with their wives. In a series of interviews with spouses of breast cancer patients, Samms (1999) found husbands' concerns related to their wives' breast cancer changed over time and their misunderstandings about their own personal emotions hindered their ability to provide support to their wives. These results confirmed the earlier findings of Northouse (1989), where spouses reported that one of the most difficult experiences they encountered was to help their spouses deal with the emotional impact of the illness. Husbands reported feelings of inadequacy and disclosed that they were unprepared for their wives' emotional distress. In a follow-up study, Northouse, Templin, Mood, and Oberst (1998) found couples facing breast cancer reported greater decreases in their marital and family functioning, more uncertain appraisals, and more adjustment problems associated with the illness when compared to couples with a benign diagnosis. There was also a correlation between the levels of adjustment reported by women with breast cancer and their husbands over time. Couples who reported high distress or a high number of role problems at diagnosis were likely to remain highly distressed at 60 days and 1 year. These findings underscore the importance of assisting couples, not just patients, to manage the adjustment difficulties associated with breast cancer.

Impact of Breast Cancer on Children. Children's response to maternal breast cancer is largely associated with developmental age. Issel, Erseck, and Lewis (1990) found that younger children worry about the safety of the family and the ability to stay together while older school-aged children worry about disruption in the family and the added household chores they must undertake as a result of the illness. Adolescents struggled with their desire for independence and the increased family burden. In a qualitative study, Zahlis (2001) interviewed 16 children from 11–18 years old who had been between 8 and 12 years of age when their mothers were diagnosed with early-stage breast cancer. The interviews were audiotaped, transcribed, and coded into categories of distinct worries about their mothers' breast cancer. The children voiced nine categories of worry during the interviews: (1) worrying that the mother was going to die; (2) feeling confused; (3) worrying that something bad would happen; (4) worrying about the family and others; (5) worrying when the mother did not look good; (6) worrying that their mothers would change; (7) wondering if the family would have to cut back financially; (8) worrying about talking to others; and (9) wondering if they would get cancer. The data further revealed that the children attempted to make sense of their mothers' illness for themselves and imagined how it might affect their own lives in the future.

Spiritual Well-being

Both positive and negative aspects of spiritual well-being have been identified as influences on QOL in breast cancer survivors. Uncertainty over the future was found to have a negative effect on QOL, while hope for the future, transcendence, living in the moment, and appreciation of daily living had a positve effect (Dow et al., 1996).

These unanticipated positive outcomes have spurred many breast cancer survivors to publish their experiences with breast cancer, support and educate others experiencing the disease, and initiate efforts to change health care policy (Leigh, 1992).

QOL Tools Used in Research and Breast Cancer

Several QOL instruments were designed for use specifically in breast cancer research (Cella et al., 1993; Dow et al., 1996; Fraser et al., 1993; Schag & Heinrich, 1990; Sprangers et al., 1993). These measures contain varying domains of multidimensionality and have been used to evaluate treatment and disease side effects on physical, psychological, social, and spiritual well-being. Selected breast cancer-specific QOL tools are listed and described on Table 11-1.

It is important to examine each of the QOL tools for use in research since they may emphasize different aspects of QOL. For example, the Cancer Rehabilitation Evaluation System (CARES) includes a component of assessment for identifying high-risk individuals requiring psychosocial intervention (Schag & Heinrich, 1990). The QOL instrument developed by Ferrell, Dow, and Grant (1995) captures perceived changes in spiritual well-being such as transcendence, hopefulness, and uncertainty over the future. Sprangers and colleagues (1993) use a modular approach to QOL assessment in cancer clinical trials based on the European Organisation for Research and Treatment of Cancer (EORTC) Study Group. The module incorporates a "core" instrument (QLQ-C30) that covers a range of QOL issues along with a site-specific module for breast cancer that is used to assess aspects of QOL of particular importance to specific populations. Fraser and associates (1993) used the "Qualitator," a daily diary card used to measure QOL for patients with advanced breast cancer undergoing chemotherapy. Based on results with 31 patients, the authors found that the Qualitator provided accurate prognostic data about subsequent treatment response and was easy to administer.

Interventions to Improve Quality of Life in Breast Cancer

Interventions to maintain and improve QOL are increasingly reported in the literature. The following discussion focuses on patient education and support, exercise intervention, and coping skills management.

Table 11-1.   **Breast Cancer Specific QOL Instruments**

Instrument Name	Specifications
QOL: Breast Cancer Version Ferrell, Dow, & Grant (1995).	41-item rating scale 4 subscales: Physical (8 items) Psychological (18 items) Social (8 items) Spiritual (7 items) Items rated on a scale of 0 to 10 Cronbach's alpha of entire scale (r = 0.93) Test-retest reliability = 0.89
FACT-B: Function Assessment of Cancer Treatment (Breast) Cella et al. (1993).	33-item ordinal measure 5 subscales: Physical Social/Family Emotional Relationship with Doctor Functional well-being Items rated on scale of 0 to 4 Cronbach's alpha of entire scale (r = 0.89) Test-retest reliability = 0.92
CARES: Cancer Rehabilitation Evaluation System Schag & Heinrich (1990).	139 potential problems experienced by patients Items rated on scale of 0 (no problems) to 4 (severe) 5 summary scales: physical, psychosocial, marital, medical interaction, and sexual Test-retest ≥ 0.82 Alpha coefficients from 0.82–0.94

Patient Education and Support Groups

The oldest known patient education program for breast cancer is the "Reach for Recovery" program, an American Cancer Society (ACS) sponsored group that was started in 1969. Despite its widespread and nearly universal appeal, there are few reports in the literature that evaluate the QOL outcomes of this program. One study of telephone interviews with 652 women found that most found it helpful (Rogers, Bauman, & Metzger, 1985). However, there was no significant difference in the emotional state of women who participated in Reach for Recovery versus those who did not. A similar result was obtained by Ashbury and colleagues (1998) who found that Reach for Recovery patients were generally satisfied with the program, had significantly higher functional social support, and reported having significantly better relationships with their physicians. However, they did not find any significant differences between the program participants and nonparticipants on other QOL dimensions such as emotional, psychological, social, and family well-being.

Exercise Intervention

Exercise intervention programs have also been reported to be helpful in rehabilitation by maintaining physical functioning and decreasing emotional stress (Segal et al., 2001; Mock et al., 1994; Mock et al., 1997). Segal and associates (2001) evaluated the effects of a structured exercise program, and a self-directed exercise program versus usual care in Stages I and II breast cancer patients (n = 123). They found that physical functioning, as measured by the physical functioning subscale of the SF-36, improved by 5.7 and 2.2 points in the self-directed and supervised exercise groups, respectively, while decreasing by 4.1 points in the usual care group. When patients receiving chemotherapy were removed from the analysis they also found an increase in aerobic capacity and weight loss in the structured exercise group. This report supported the findings of an earlier study that breast cancer survivors can improve their physical functioning through the use of a self-directed walking exercise program (Mock et al., 1997). Mock and colleagues did, however, report a lower level of distress among exercise participants, while no improvement in QOL scores (FACT-G and FACT-B) was found in the study by Segal (2001).

Coping Skills Management

Coping skills management programs focused primarily on behavioral interventions for physical symptoms experienced with cancer and its treatment. Ganz and colleagues (2000), in a study of an educational program for managing menopausal symptoms, found that women taking part in a comprehensive menopausal assessment intervention program experienced a significant improvement in their menopausal symptoms and sexual functioning, as measured by the CARES sexual functioning scale. However, the treatment group did not report an increased sense of vitality, nor were there any measurable improvements in general QOL.

In a randomized trial of 246 newly diagnosed breast cancer patients under 50, Gustafson and colleagues (2001) assessed the impact of a computer-based support system on social support, participation in health care, ability to acquire and deal with information, confidence in doctors, and psychosocial QOL. They used a randomized control design with pre- and post-test measures of QOL using the FACT-B. They found that the computer-based system significantly improved the patients' confidence in attaining information and interacting with the health care system, especially among underserved populations. There were, however, no significant changes in the QOL measures among participants.

It is difficult to understand how programs that are consistently evaluated as helpful by patients show no improvement in the patients' measured QOL. In their study of metastatic breast cancer patients, receiving group therapy Edmonds, Lockwood, and Cunningham (1999) also noted little long-term improvement in QOL or mood among their subjects as measured by the Profile of Mood States (POMS) and Functional Living Index of Cancer (FLIC). However, the therapists reported profound changes in patient status, indicating long-term changes may elude measurement by standard tools. Other possibilities to explain the results are that women who undergo therapy or attend support groups are more conscious of their QOL changes and physical symptoms and therefore are more likely to report them in questionnaires. Further studies in this area are indicated to evaluate the sensitivity and reliability of existing tools as well as the effectiveness of education and support groups on QOL.

Issues for Future QOL Research in Breast Cancer

Several other areas for future QOL research in breast cancer are indicated. The first focuses on age differences among groups. Research has identified that breast cancer in younger women deserves special research attention (Gustafson et al., 2001; Ganz et al., 2000; Schover, 1994). Younger women are a high-risk group for psychological distress, which may relate to interference with developmental goals during the reproductive years. Second, the QOL needs of women with metastatic disease as well as the effectiveness of interventions to meet the requirements of this potentially needy population must be evaluated. Third, further work with evaluating positive aspects to surviving and living with breast cancer is needed. These positive aspects (perceived social support, transcendence, and hope) can be used as catalysts for mapping out future QOL interventions. Fourth, further studies need to be conducted on including patients in the treatment decision-making process and whether this increases their sense of control, meaning in life, and maintenance of hope.

Finally, the many survivorship groups dedicated to breast cancer have a host of information available through their networks that can be useful in designing innovative interventions, including Internet support.

The QOL in women with breast cancer continues to be a vast and fruitful area of study. A concerted effort among clinicians, researchers, educators, administrators, and survivors is needed to work toward a common goal of improving QOL in breast cancer.

REFERENCES

American Cancer Society. (2001). *Breast cancer facts and figures 2001–2002*. Atlanta: Author.

American Cancer Society. (2002). *Cancer facts and figures 2002*. Atlanta: Author.

Andrykowski, M. A., Curran, S. L., & Lighner, R. (1998). Off-treatment fatigue in breast cancer survivors: A controlled comparison. *Journal of Behavioral Medicine*, 21, 1–18.

Ashbury, F., Cameron, C., Mercer, S., Fitch, M., & Nielsen, E. (1998). One on one peer support and quality of life for breast cancer patients. *Patient Education and Counseling, 35*, 89–100.

Averette, H., Mirhashemi, R., & Moffat, F. (1999). Pregnancy after breast carcinoma: The ultimate medical challenge. *Cancer, 85*, 2301–2304.

Bachmann, G. (1994). Nonhormonal management of menopausal symptoms. *Journal of the National Cancer Institute*, Monograph 16, 161–168.

Bower, J. E., Ganz, P. A., Desmond, K. A., Rowland, J. H., Meyerowitz, B. E., & Belin, T. R. (2000). Fatigue in breast cancer survivors: Occurrence, correlates, and impact on quality of life. *Journal of Clinical Oncology, 18*(4), 743–753.

Broekel, J. A., Jacobsen, P. B., Horton, J., Balducci, L., & Lyman, G. H. (1998). Characteristics and correlates of fatigue after adjuvant chemotherapy for breast cancer. *Journal of Clinical Oncology, 16*, 1689–1696.

Buzdar, A. U., Jones, S, E., Vogel, C. L., Wolter, J., Plourde, P., & Webster, A. (1997). A phase III trial comparing anastrozole (1 and 10 milligrams), a potent and selective aromatase inhibitor, with megestrol acetate in postmenopausal women with advanced breast carcinoma. *Cancer, 79*(4), 730–739.

Buzdar, A. U., Smith, R., Vogel, C., Bonomi, P., Keller, A. M., Favis, G., Mulagha, M., & Cooper, J. (1996). Fadrozole HCL (CGS-16949A) versus megestrol acetate treatment of postmenopausal patients with metastatic breast carcinoma: Results of two randomized double blind controlled multiinstitutional trials. *Cancer, 77*(12), 2503–2513.

Carpenter, J. S., & Andrykowski, M. A. (1999). Menopausal symptoms in breast cancer survivors. *Oncology Nursing Forum, 26*(8) 1311–1317.

Carter, B. (1997). Women' experiences of lymphedema. *Oncology Nursing Forum, 24* (5), 875–882.

Cella, D. F., Tulsky, D. S., Gray, G., Sarafian, B., Linn, E., Bonomi, A., Silberman, M., Yellen, S., Vinocur, P., & Brannon, J. (1993). The functional assessment of cancer therapy scale: Development and validation of the general measure. *Journal of Clinical Oncology, 11*, 570–579.

Cobleigh, M. (2000). Managing menopausal problems. In *Diseases of the Breast* (2nd ed., pp. 1041–1050). J. R. Harris, M. Lippman, M. Morrow, & C. K. Osborne (Eds.). Philadelphia: Lippincott Williams & Wilkins.

Cobleigh, M., Berris, B. F., Bush, T., Davidson, N. E., Robert, N. J., Sparano, J. A., Tormey, D. C., & Wood, W. C. (1994). Estrogen replacement therapy in breast cancer survivors. A time for change. Breast cancer committee cooperative oncology group. *JAMA, 272*(7), 540–545.

Couzi, R. J., Helzlsouer, K. J., & Fetting, J. H. (1995). Prevalence of menopausal symptoms among women with a history of breast cancer and attitudes toward estrogen replacement therapy. *Journal of Clinical Oncology, 13,* 2737–2744.

Danforth, D. (1991). How subsequent pregnancy affects outcome in women with a prior breast cancer. *Oncology, 5*(11), 23–29.

Day, L., Ganz, P. A., Costanzo, J. P., Cronin, W. M., Wickerham, D. L., & Fisher, B. (1999). Health-related quality of life and tamoxifen in breast cancer prevention: A report from the National Surgical Adjuvant Breast and Bowel Project P-1 Study. *Journal of Clinical Oncology, 17*(9), 2659–2669.

Donegan, W. (1977). Pregnancy and breast cancer. *Obstetrics and Gynecology, 50,* 244–251.

Dorval, M., Maunsell, E., Deschenes, L., and Brisson, J. (1998). Type of mastectomy and quality of life for long term breast carcinoma survivors. *Cancer, 83*(10), 2130–2138.

Dow, K. H. (1994). Having children after breast cancer. *Cancer Practice, 2,* 407–413.

Dow, K. H., Ferrell, B., Leigh, S., Ly, J., & Gulasekaram, P. (1996). An evaluation of the quality of life among long-term survivors of breast cancer. *Breast Cancer Research and Treatment, 39,* 261–263.

Dow, K. H., Ferrell, B., Leigh, S., & Melancon, C. (1997). The cancer survivor as co-investigator: The benefits of collaborative research with advocacy groups. *Cancer Practice, 5,* 255–257.

Dow, K. H., Harris, J., & Roy, C. (1994). Pregnancy after breast conserving surgery and radiation therapy. *Journal of the National Cancer Institute, Monograph 16,* 131–137.

Edmonds, C., Lockwood, G., & Cunningham, A. (1999). Psychological response to long term group therapy: A randomized trial with metastatic breast cancer patients. *Psychooncology, 8,* 74–91.

Ferrell, B. R., Dow, K., & Grant, M. (1995). Measurement of the quality of life in cancer survivors. *Quality of Life Research, 4,* 523–531.

Ferrell, B., Grant, M., Funk, B., Otis-Green, S., & Garcia, N. (1998). Quality of life in breast cancer survivors as identified by focus groups. *Psychooncology, 6,* 13–23.

Ferrell, B., Grant, M., Funk, B., Otis-Green, S., & Garcia, N. (1997). Quality of Life in breast cancer survivors: Implications for developing support services. *Oncology Nursing Forum, 25*(5), 887–895.

Fraser, S., Ramirez, A., Ebbs, S., Fallowfield, L., Dobbs, H., Richards, M., Bates, T., & Baum, M. (1993). A daily diary for quality of life measurement in advanced breast cancer trials. *British Journal of Cancer, 67*, 341–346.

Ganz, P. (1997). Sexual functioning after breast cancer: A conceptual framework for future studies. *Annals of Oncology, 2*, 105–107.

Ganz, P., Greendale, G., Peterson, L., Zibecchi, L., Kahn, B., & Belin, T. (2000). Managing menopausal sumptoms in breast cancer survivors: Results of a randomized controlled trial. *Journal of the National Cancer Institute, 92*(13), 1054–1064.

Ganz, P. A., Rowkind, J. H., Desmond, K., Meyerowitz, B. G., & Wyatt, G. E. (1998). Life after breast cancer: Understanding women's health-related issues and sexual functioning. *Clin Oncol 16*(2), 501–514.

Gustafson, D., Hawkins, R., Pingree, S., McTavish, B. Arora, N., Mendenhall, J., Cella, D., Serlin, R., Apantaku, F., Stewart, J., & Salner, A. (2001). Effect of computer support on younger women with breast cancer. *Journal of General Internal Medicine, 16*(7), 435–446.

Harrington, S. (1937). Carcinoma of the breast: Results of surgical treatment when the carcinoma occurred in the course of pregnancy or lactation and when the pregnancy occurred subsequent to operation. *Annals of Surgery, 106*, 690–700.

Issel, L., Ersek, M., & Lewis, F. (1990). How children cope with mother's breast cancer. *Oncology Nursing Forum, 17*, 5–12.

Jemal, A., Thomas, A., Murray, T., & Thun, M. (2002) Cancer Statistics 2002. *CA: Cancer Journal for Clinicians, 52*, 23–47.

King, C. R., Haberman, M., Berry, D., Bush, N., Butler, L., Dow, K. H, Ferrell, B., Grant, M., Gue, D., Hinds, P., Kreuer, J., Padilla, G., & Underwood, S. (1997). Quality of life and the cancer experience: The state of the knowledge. *Oncology Nursing Forum, 24*(1), 27–41.

Koyama, H., Wada, T., & Nishiwzawa, Y. (1977). Cyclophosphamide-induced ovarian failure and its therapeutic significance in patients with breast cancer. *Cancer, 39*, 1403–1409.

Kroman, N., Wohlfahrt, J., Anderson, K., Mouridsen, H., Westergaard, T., & Melbye, M. (1998). Parity, age at first childbirth and the prognosis of primary breast cancer. *British Journal of Cancer, 78*(11), 1529–1533.

Leigh, S. (1992). Myths, monsters, and magic: Personal perspectives and professional challenges of survival. *Oncology Nursing Froum, 19*, 1475–1480.

Loprinzi, C., Kugler, J., Sloan, J., Malliard, J. A., LaVasseur, B. I., Bartin, D. L., Novotny, P. J., Dakhil, S. R., Rodger, K., Rummans, T. A., & Christensen, B. J.

(2000). Vanlafaxine in management of hot flashes in survivors of breast cancer: A randomised controlled trial. *Lancet, 356,* 2059–2063.

Mock, V. (1993). Body image in women treated for breast cancer. *Nursing Research, 42,* 153–157.

Mock, V., Barton Burke, M., Creaton, E., Winningham, M., McKenney-Tedder, S., Powel Schwager, L., & Liebman, M. (1994). A nursing rehabilitation program for women receiving adjuvant chemotherapy for breast cancer. *Oncology Nursing Forum, 16,* 899–908.

Mock, V., Dow, K., Meares, C., Grimm, P., Dienemann, J., Haisfield-Wolfe, M. E., Quitasol, W., Mitchell, S., Chakravarthy, A., & Gage, I. (1997). Effects of exercise on fatigue, physical functioning, and emotional distress during radiation therapy for breast cancer. *Oncology Nursing Forum, 24*(6), 991–1000.

Moschen, R., Kemmler, G., Schweigkofler, H., Holzner, B., Dunser, M., Richter, R., Fleischhacker, W. W., & Sperner-Unterweger, B. (2001). Use of alternative/complementary therapy in breast cancer patients—a psychological perspective. *Support Care Cancer, 9*(4), 267–274.

Moore, H. (2000). Fertility and the impact of systemic therapy on hormonal status following treatment for breast cancer. *Current Oncology Reports, 2,* 587–593.

National Institutes of Health. (2000). *Adjuvant Therapy for Breast Cancer.* NIH Consensus Statement 2000. November 1–3, 17(4), 1–35.

Nissen, M., Swenson, K., Ritz, L., Farrell, J., Sladek, M., & Lally, R.(2001). Quality of life after breast carcinoma surgery: A comparison of three surgical procedures. *Cancer, 91*(7), 1238–1246.

Northouse, L. (1989). The impact of breast cancer on patients and husbands. *Cancer Nursing, 12,* 276–284.

Northouse, L. (1994). Breast cancer in younger women: Effects on interpersonal and family relations. *Journal of the National Cancer Institute, Monograph 16,* 183–190.

Northouse, L., Templin, T., & Mood, D. (2001). Couples' adjustment to breast disease during the first year following diagnosis. *Journal of Behavioral Medicine, 24*(2), 115–136.

Northouse L., Templin, T., Mood, D., & Oberst, M. (1998). Couples' adjustment to breast cancer and benign breast disease: A longitudinal analysis. *Psychooncology, 7*(1), 37–48.

Passik, S., & McDonald, M. V. (1998). Psychosocial aspects of upper extremity lymphedema in women treated for breast carcinoma. *Cancer supplement, 83*(12), 2817–2820.

Petrek, J., Pressman, P., & Smith, R. (2000). Lymphedema: Current issues in research and management. *Cancer Journal for Clinicians, 50,* 292–307.

Pusic, A., Thompson, T., Kerrigan, C. Sargeant, R., Chang, B., Kelsouer, K., and Manson, P. (1999). Surgical options for the early-stage breast cancer: Factors associated with patient choice and postoperative quality of life. *Plastic Reconstructive Surgery, 104*(5), 1325–1333.

Reichman, B. S., & Green, K. B. (1994). Breast cancer in young women: Effects of chemotherapy on ovarian function, fertility, and birth defects. *Journal of the National Cancer Institute, Monograph 16*, 125–130.

Rogers, T., Bauman, L., & Metzger, L. (1985). An assessment of the Reach to Recovery program. *Cancer Journal for Clinicians, 36*, 116–124.

Samms, M. C. (1999). The husband's untold account of his wife's breast cancer: A chronologic analysis. *Oncology Nursing Forum 26*(8), 1351–1358.

Sankila, R., Heinavaara, S., & Hakulinen, T. (1994). Survival of breast cancer patients after subsequent term pregnancy: "healthy mother effect." *American Journal of Obstetrics and Gynecology, 170*(3), 818–823.

Schag, C., & Heinrich, R. (1990). Development of a comprehensive quality of life measurement tool: CARES. *Oncology, 4*(5), 135–138.

Schover, L. (1994). Sexuality and body image in younger women with breast cancer. *National Cancer Institute, Monograph 16*, 177–182.

Schwartz, A. L. (1999). Fatigue mediates the effects of exercise on quality of life. *Qual Life Res, 8*(6), 529–538.

Segal, R., Evans, W., Johnson, D., Smith, J., Colletta, S., Gayton, J., Woodard, S., Wells, G., & Reid, R. (2001). Structured exercise improves physical functioning in women with stages I and II breast cancer: Results of a randomized controlled trial. *Journal Clinical Oncology, 19*(3), 657–665.

Shapiro, C., & Recht, A. (1994). Late effects of adjuvant therapy for breast cancer. *Journal of the National Cancer Institute, Monograph 16*, 101–112.

Sprangers, M., Cull, A., Bjordal, K., Groenvold, M., & Aaronson, N. (1993). The EORTC. Approach to quality of life assessment: Guidelines for developing questionnaire modules. *Quality of Life Research, 2*, 287–295.

Stein, K. D., Jacobsen, P. B., Hann, D. M., Greenberg, H., & Lyman, G. (2000). Impact of hot flashes on quality of life among postmenopausal women being treated for breast cancer. *Journal of Pain and Symptom Management 19*(6) 436–445.

Sutton, R., Buzdar, A., & Hortobagyi, G. (1990). Pregnancy and offspring after adjuvant chemotherapy in breast cancer patients. *Cancer, 65*, 847–850.

Swain, S., Santen, R., Burger, H., & Pritchard, K. (1999). Treatment of estrogen deficiency symptoms in women surviving breast cancer. Part 4: Urogenital atrophy, vasomotor instability, sleep disorders, and related symptoms. *Oncology, 13*, 551–575.

Theriault, R., & Vassilopoulou-Sellin, R. (1994). Estrogen-replacement therapy in younger women with breast cancer. *Journal of the National Cancer Institute, Monograph 16*, 149–152.

Valagussa, P., DeCandis, D., & Antonelli, G. (1996). Reproductive potential after adjuvant chemotherapy for breast cancer. *Recent Results in Cancer Research, 140,* 277–283.

Velentgas, P., Daling, J., & Malone, K. (1999). Pregnancy after breast carcinoma: Outcomes and influence on mortality. *Cancer, 85,* 2424–2432, 2301–2305.

Von Schoultz, E., Johansson, J., Wilking, N., & Rutquist (1995). Influence of prior and subsequent pregnancy on breast cancer prognosis. *Journal of Clinical Oncology, 13,* 430–434.

Wapnir, I., Cody, R., & Greco, R. (1999). Subtle differences in quality of life after breast cancer surgery. *Annals of Surgical Oncology, 6(4),* 359–366.

Wang, X., Cosby, L., Harris, M., & Liu, T. (1999). Major concerns and needs of breast cancer patients. *Cancer Nursing, 22(2),* 157–163.

Wilson, H. (1991). Living with a wife undergoing chemotherapy. *Image: Journal of Nursing Scholarship, 23,* 78–84.

Wilson, K., Dowling, A., Abdolell, M., & Tannock, I. (2000). Perception of quality of life by patients, partners and treating physicians. *Quality of Life Research, 9,* 1041–1052.

Yellen, S., & Cella, D. (1995). Something to live for: Social well-being, parenthood status, and decision-making in oncology. *Journal of Clinical Oncology, 13,* 1255–1264.

Zahlis, E. H. 2001. The child's worries about the mother's breast cancer: Sources of distress in school-age children. *Oncology Nursing Forum 28(6),* 1019–1025.

Chapter

12

Clinical Implications of
Quality of Life

CYNTHIA R. KING

Quality of life for oncology patients and QOL research are relevant to oncology nursing clinical practice. One of the primary goals of any type of nursing care is to assess human response to illness. Nurses know that human responses to illness, and specifically cancer, are influenced not only by the disease, but also by psychological influences, social influences (e.g., interpersonal, family, and cultural), and spiritual issues. These four areas of influence are similar to the four domains of QOL displayed in the City of Hope Medical Center Conceptual Model of Quality of Life (Figure 12-1). Thus, there is a tie between the concept of QOL and oncology nursing goals across the illness trajectory. But how do oncology nurses in clinical practice directly tie the concept of QOL to, and apply QOL research in, clinical practice?

First imagine that a newly diagnosed cancer patient is like a novice dancer and an experienced nurse is the dance instructor. As the patient develops a relationship with the nurse, they start dancing. The dance may be a duet (a nurse and a patient together), a company of dancers (nurse and patient along with family, caregivers, or other health care professionals), or a solo dance (patient dances and the nurse, family, and others support from the sidelines). This dance is not only about the movements, but also about attitude, motivation, and physical, psychological, social, and spiritual influences (Figure 12-2). For cancer patients this is analogous to living with a positive attitude and not about concentrating on dying (King, 2001).

Nurses' Perceptions of Quality of Life

Nurses play an integral role in the care of all oncology patients. Unfortunately, nurses in clinical practice cannot assume they know how patients and families feel about their quality of life while living with cancer or undergoing treatment. Several studies

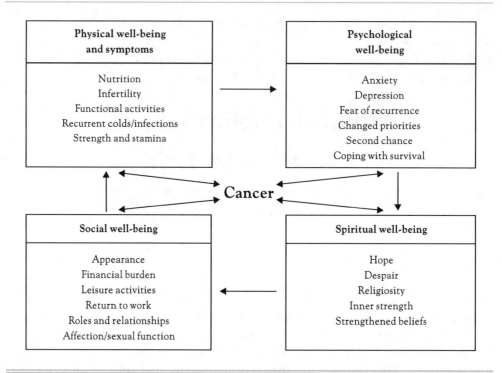

Figure 12-1. **Quality of life model for cancer survivors.**

Source: Adapted with permission from Ferrell, Grant et al., at City of Hope Medical Center.

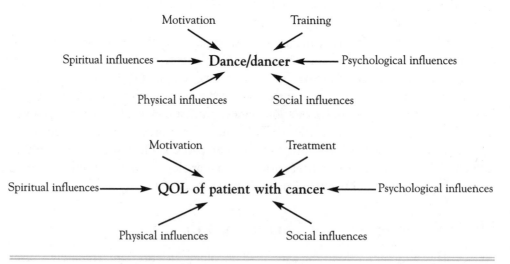

Figure 12-2. **Similarity of dance and quality of life.**

Permission granted from ONS. King, C. R. *Dance of Life* (2001).

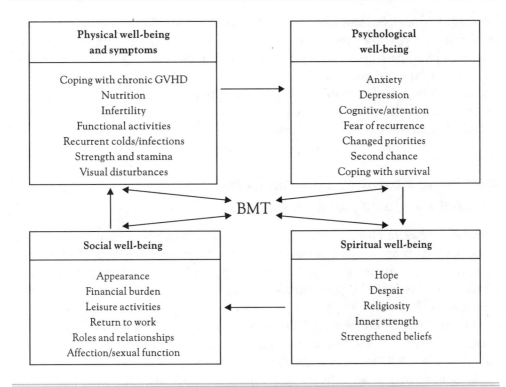

Figure 12-3. Quality of life model for bone marrow transplant survivors.
Source: Adapted with permission from Ferrell, Grant et al., at City of Hope Medical Center.

have been performed to assess nurses' perceptions of quality of life. In one study, King, Ferrell, Grant, and Sakurai (1995) explored nurses' perceptions of the impact of bone marrow transplantation on the QOL of survivors. The study was conducted using the City of Hope Medical Center Conceptual Model of QOL (Figure 12-3). The nurses' responses to a QOL questionnaire were compared with the responses of the BMT survivors. Significant differences were found between the nurses' and patients' perceptions of the impact of BMT on QOL. Even though nurses could describe both positive and negative consequences of BMT, they perceived patients to have a poorer QOL than that actually reported by patients.

Other nursing studies have reported similar discrepancies in perceptions of the patient's QOL between the patient, nurse, and physician (Aaronson, 1986; Carr & Higginson, 2001; Cochran & Ganong, 1989; Dow, Ferrell, Haberman, & Eaton, 1999; Farrell, 1991; Ferrell & Dow, 1996; Johnston, 1982; Larson, 1984; Larson, 1986; Mayer, 1987; Schipper & Levitt, 1985; von Essen & Sjoden, 1991; Wilson,

Dowling, Abdollel, & Tannock, 2000; von Essen & Sjoden, 1991). Additionally, 86% of health care practitioners equate treatment efficacy with extension of survival, whereas 45% of patients view treatment efficacy as preserving QOL, 29% view it as extension of expected life, and 13% perceive it as delaying disease progression (Crawford et al., 1997). Unfortunately, these misperceptions can result in lack of appropriate comprehensive care for patients, provision of care that is not required by patients, or lack of attention to issues other than physical ones.

Barriers to Providing Nursing Care Focused on Quality of Life Issues

Although nurses in clinical practice are in an ideal position to support the importance of QOL as an outcome measure of cancer treatment, numerous obstacles prevent nurses from assessing QOL and providing support to this important concept. Lindley and Hirsch (1994) performed a study to assess oncology nurses' attitudes, perceptions, and knowledge of QOL in patients with cancer. An exploratory survey was conducted at the 1990 Oncology Nursing Society Congress. Six hundred twenty-one nurses completed two questionnaires regarding the impact of treatment on QOL, the importance of QOL assessment, barriers to measuring QOL, and knowledge about QOL measurement issues. The authors concluded that nurses do value QOL as an outcome measure, but lack knowledge regarding its measurability, especially related to reliable tools and time to assess QOL in clinical practice. Specifically, 68 percent of the respondents indicated that a lack of time was a barrier to measuring QOL in clinical practice, while 63 percent responded that a lack of valid tools for measuring patient QOL was a barrier. Other obstacles cited were (a) lack of physician and patient time, (b) patient unwillingness to complete questionnaires, (c) health care professionals' unwillingness to administer questionnaires, (d) nurses not liking research, and (e) health care professionals believing it is an invasion of patient's privacy to measure QOL.

It would appear from this study that nurses have difficulty overcoming barriers to its use. Despite the fact that QOL can best be assessed by the patient, and that many reliable and valid self-administered questionnaires for patients exist, nurses perceived the amount of time health care professionals would need to administer QOL tools as a major obstacle.

In 1995, the Oncology Nursing Society held a State-of-the-Knowledge conference concerning QOL issues for patients with cancer, their families, and health care providers. A recommendation from this conference was to evaluate the applicability of available information about QOL to nurses in clinical practice (King et al., 1997).

This recommendation combined with the knowledge that there are barriers to assessing and measuring QOL led to recent research by King, Hinds, Dow, Schum, and Lee (2002). This qualitative research by King and associates explored patients' QOL as defined by nurses and examined the knowledge needed to apply QOL outcomes in clinical practice. Focus group discussions were held with adult and pediatric oncology nurses in three states in the United States. Participants were provided a copy and asked to read the article "Quality of life and the cancer experience: The state-of-the-knowledge" (King et al., 1997) prior to the discussion. Forty-seven unique themes were reported in response to three key questions used to facilitate discussions. The three questions included: (1) QOL—could you say what the term means to you in terms of your practice; (2) what helps you to use QOL information in your own nursing practice on any day; and (3) was there any particular content in the article that you found helpful about QOL. The six most frequently reported themes were: (a) Using the patient's standard; (b) Nursing strategies; (c) Differences decrease QOL care; (d) Maintenance of social interest; (e) Insightful relations with patient; and (f) Nurse-patient communication.

The theme "using the patient's standard" represents nurses' beliefs that the best measure of QOL is what the patient believes it to be and this can vary based on the situation. This was the most frequently reported code in response to question 1. "Nursing strategies" recognizes that nurses can implement certain tactics and procedures to increase a patient's QOL. This was the second most common theme in response to question 1, but also was a common theme in response to questions 2 and 3. The theme "differences decrease QOL care" recognizes that cultural, economic, and behavioral differences may cause barriers for nurses attempting to assess or improve QOL for patients. "Maintenance of social interest," "insightful relations with patient," and "nurse-patient communication" were common themes in response to question 3. In the theme of "maintenance of social interest" nurses recognized the importance of patients remaining involved in life events as part of QOL. "Insightful relations with patient" and "nurse-patient communication" both deal with the importance of the nurse-patient relationship to improve QOL. From this research and key themes it was apparent that clinically based oncology nurses did not find research-based information relevant to their clinical practice for assessment of QOL or interventions to positively affect QOL (King et al., 2002).

From this research King and colleagues (2002) developed a conceptual model of the nurses' relationship-based perception of patients' QOL (Figure 12-4 and Table 12-1). This model demonstrates that an oncology nurse's QOL assessment is mostly based on a strong nurse-patient relationship.

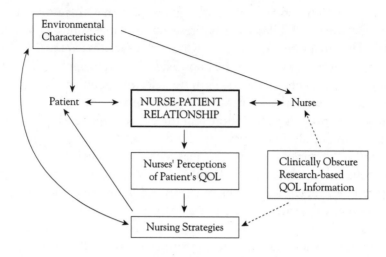

Figure 12-4. **Nurses' relationship-based perception of patient's quality of life.**
Legend: A solid line means a strong influence for clinical nurses, while a dashed line means the
researched-based QOL information is not helpful for clinical purposes so it is infrequently used.
Adapted from King, Hinds, Dow, Schum, & Lee (2002). Used with permission from ONS Press.

Patients' and Nurses' Perceptions of Quality of Life

Despite the research demonstrating that nurses cannot assume they understand how
patients view their QOL and potential barriers to providing nursing care focused on
QOL, recently nurses have learned that information gained from patients regarding
QOL issues throughout the cancer trajectory may be useful in clinical practice. For
instance, information gained from cancer patients regarding QOL issues at diagnosis
may be used by nurses to provide newly diagnosed patients with realistic expectations
of the impact of cancer and therapies on QOL. From this knowledge nurses and
patients can work together to train other patients and provide support and encouragement through the cancer journey (King, 2001).

One way to obtain this knowledge is through patients' stories. Nurses can gather
stories from patients individually or in groups to help them understand patients'
perspectives of QOL. Hinds and King (Hinds & King, 1998; King, 2001) have found
several key characteristics throughout numerous patients' stories regarding QOL.
These include: (a) a profound sense of vulnerability; (b) inability to avoid frightening aspects of cancer and treatment; (c) changes in priorities in life; (d) a desire to
make life better for others; (e) a need to be respected by other individuals; (f) a need

Table 12-1. **Model Concepts and Their Definitions**

Concept	Definition
Nurse–Patient Relationship	Nurses rely on establishing strong rapport with patients and their family members, being physically present, being technically competent to complete quality of life assessments, and to adjust their own behavior, mood, and pace of providing treatment-related information.
Nurses' Perceptions of Patients' Quality of Life	Nurses' recognize that their most valid measure of an individual's quality of life is what that individual believes it to be, and that this belief could differ from what others (including health care professionals and family members) believe it to be, and that this belief could vary by situation.
Nursing Strategies	Actions initiated by nurses and directed toward improving the patient's physical condition, functional abilities, and social interests, and implemented in consideration of the patient's values, preferences, definition of normalcy, and need for hope.
Clinically Obscure Research-based QOL Information	Nurses' belief that the lack of (a) a single or clear definition of quality of life, (b) clinical guidelines to assess a patient's quality of life, and (c) population-specific strategies to influence quality of life all contribute to their conclusion that the findings from studies on quality of life are not useful to them and contribute to the low likelihood of their using the findings in their practice.
Environmental Characteristics	Nurses describe how rules and procedures and the general atmosphere of a health care setting as well as coworkers' views can affect a patient's quality of life and the nurses' abilities to influence patient's quality of life.

Adapted from King, Hinds, Dow, Schum, & Lee (2002). Used with permission from ONS Press.

for loving connections with other individuals; (g) learning to deal with alienation from the "norms" of society; (h) greater appreciation of daily life and activities; and (i) a need to be taken seriously. Listening to patients' stories and finding common experiences such as vulnerability and changes in priorities can be helpful for nurses to share with patients as they start and continue their "dance of life" with cancer.

Patients' Perceptions of What Nurses Can Do to Improve Quality of Life

Although nurses perceive numerous barriers to assessing and supporting the concept of QOL, patients have reported specific interventions that nurses and physicians can utilize to improve QOL for patients. In 1992 Ferrell and colleagues surveyed bone marrow transplant (BMT) survivors concerning the meaning of QOL. One of the questions asked was, "What could physicians or nurses do to improve QOL?" Six themes were identified from the 119 responses. The first theme was for health care providers to *Be Accessible*. Specifically, survivors wanted physicians and nurses to be available to respond to questions and problems. The second theme focused on survival and was identified as *Discover a Cure*. The third theme, *Provide Support Groups* to benefit patients and their families, is a recurrent theme for BMT survivors as well as all cancer survivors. The fourth theme involved a need to *Reinforce Current Education*. Survivors and families continue to need both support and information/education posttreatment. Specifically, survivors want information concerning long-term effects and symptoms. *Provide Additional Coping Strategies* was the fifth theme. Survivors and families suggested support groups as well as individual counseling to enhance coping. Lastly, respondents suggested that providers *Increase Patient Participation in Decision Making*. Survivors wanted to continue to make informed decisions. Having cancer, undergoing treatment, and surviving cancer are considered "out of control" situations. Survivors felt that having information to make informed decisions helped them to maintain control in an "out of control" situation. This study validated the need for nurses to be involved throughout the many stages of cancer and to be concerned about QOL issues for patients and families (Table 12-2). It is important for nurses to understand QOL changes over time in relationship to individual patients and how they respond to cancer.

How Can Clinical Nurses Affect Quality of Life for Patients with Cancer?

Knowing that controversies regarding the definition and measurement of QOL prevail, how can clinical nurses positively affect QOL for patients with cancer? The first step is for clinical nurses to increase their knowledge and skills regarding QOL issues (Table 12-2). Few, if any, QOL courses for nurses exist, but nurses can attend presentations, seminars, or workshops on QOL. Books, articles, and the Internet can be helpful resources for clinical nurses. Networking with colleagues in nursing organizations such as the National Oncology Nursing Society can provide valuable information on how other clinical nurses have assessed QOL and developed interventions to positively affect QOL. Because nurses are present throughout the cancer journey, they develop a relationship or partnership with the patient and family and seek to help them cope with living with cancer. As nurses continue to help cancer patients with problems such as fatigue, pain, nausea and vomiting, organ toxicities, sexual dysfunction, and suffering, they are ultimately working to improve each patient's QOL (King, 2001).

As Grant and Dean point out in Chapter 1, some factors of QOL may not be amenable to nursing intervention (e.g., diagnosis, family illness history, predisposing characteristics, and medical treatment). Yet, other factors are amenable to nursing interventions (e.g., the environment, information provided to patients and families, and symptom management). Additional recommendations for clinical practice are presented in Table 12-2.

Table 12-2. Tips for Positively Affecting QOL for Patients with Cancer

Increase knowledge and skills related to QOL:
    Attend presentations, seminars, workshops.
    Read articles, books.
    Use the Internet.
    Network with colleagues.
    Start a journal club.

Assess QOL, specifically, how patients perceive their illness, treatment, and recovery.

Understand that QOL is evaluated subjectively by the patient.

Help patients and families identify what makes their QOL better or worse.

Be accessible to patients and families.

Be sensitive to individual situations.

Provide support groups for patients and families.

Provide information/education for patients/families.
    Concentrate on concrete objective information.
    Provide information on symptoms and symptom management.

Be aware of potential long-term effects of treatment and the impact on QOL.

Encourage patients to participate in activities that improve QOL.

Address the negative effects of cancer treatments on QOL.

Help patients learn new coping techniques
    Guided imagery
    Progressive muscle relaxation
    Meditation

Nurses in clinical practice can use what has been learned from QOL research, patient stories, and their relationship with patients to: (a) use established tools to assess the QOL of patients throughout the cancer experience; (b) understand that QOL is evaluated subjectively; (c) evaluate symptoms within a framework of QOL and developing interventions for symptom management; (d) help patients and families determine what makes QOL better or worse; (e) provide education and support groups to patients and families; and (f) address the negative impact of cancer treatments on QOL (King et al., 1997).

In Chapter 15, "Fatigue and Quality of Life: A Question of Balance," Burke describes fatigue as a clinical symptom requiring intervention. In discussing fatigue as a symptom that significantly affects QOL, Burke offers practical interventions to reduce fatigue and improve QOL. She also provides examples of teaching tools to conserve energy. Eilers and King (Chapter 13) stress the importance of appropriate symptom management and providing appropriate information and education to transplant patients and their families in their chapter "Quality of Life Issues Related to Marrow Transplantation." In Chapter 9, "Quality of Life and Symptoms," Ferrell and Grant describe how clinically managing symptoms is an important QOL concern across settings of cancer care (acute, home care, outpatient). In Chapter 11, Kuhn and Hassey Dow highlight the importance of patient education, exercise interventions, coping skills in behavioral and cognitive management, and support groups in improving QOL in patients with breast cancer.

CONCLUSION

Even though nurses and other health care professionals cannot know exactly what any specific patient experiences on the cancer journey, the nurses are still instructors or leaders along the journey. Nurses have an important role with cancer patients and their families because they have more direct and prolonged contact with them. This places nurses in an optimal position to assess and positively affect the quality of life of oncology patients. Nurses need to learn from each patient what physical, psychological, social, and spiritual aspects increase or decrease his or her QOL. As advocates, educators, and leaders of the dance, nurses can use their relationship-based perceptions of patients' QOL to help patients understand their strengths, needs, and important physical, psychological, social, and spiritual aspects of QOL during the journey. It is also essential that clinicians develop knowledge and skills in order to be a significant force in affecting the QOL of patients with cancer. Currently, nursing curricula stress the physical and social skills (e.g., communication and counseling). Little, if any, content is provided regarding QOL issues for patients and families. The knowledge and skills of oncology nurses, and nurses in general, are critical to advancing QOL as an accepted treatment outcome.

REFERENCES

Aaronson, N. K. (1986). Methodological issues in psychosocial oncology with special reference to clinical trials. In V. Ventafridda, F. S. A. M. van Dam, R. Yancik, & M. Tamburini (Eds.), *Assessment of Quality of Life and Cancer Treatment* (pp. 29–41). Amsterdam: Excerpta Medica.

Carr, A. J., & Higginson, I. J. (2001). Are quality of life measures patient centered? *British Medical Journal, 322,* 1357–1360.

Cochran, J., & Ganong, L. H. (1989). A comparison of nurses' and patients' perceptions of intensive care unit stressors. *Journal of Advances in Nursing, 14,* 1038–1043.

Crawford, E. D., Benneti, C. L., Stone, N. N., Knight, S. J., De Anton, E., Sharp, L. Granick, M. B., & Porterfield, H. A. (1997). Comparison of perspectives on prostate cancer. Analysis of survey data. *Urology, 50,* 366–372.

Dow, K. H., Ferrell, B. R., Haberman, M. R., & Eaton, L. (1999). The meaning of quality of life in cancer survivorship. *Oncology Nursing Forum, 26,* 519–528.

Farrell, G. A. (1991). How accurately do nurses perceive patients' needs? A comparison of general and psychiatric settings. *Journal of Advances in Nursing, 16,* 1062–1070.

Ferrell, B. R., & Dow, K. H. (1996). Portraits of cancer survivorship: A glimpse through the lens of survivors' eyes. *Cancer Practice, 4,* 76–80.

Ferrell, B., Grant, M., Schmidt, G. M., Rhiner, M., Whitehead, C., Fonbuena, P., & Forman, S. J. (1992a). The meaning of quality of life for bone marrow transplant survivors. Part 1: The impact of bone marrow transplant on quality of life. *Cancer Nursing, 15* (3), 153–160.

Ferrell, B., Grant, M., Schmidt, G. M., Rhiner, M., Whitehead, C., Fonbuena, P., & Forman, S. J. (1992b). The meaning of quality of life for bone marrow transplant survivors. Part 2: Improving quality of life for bone marrow transplant survivors. *Cancer Nursing, 15* (4), 247–253.

Johnston, M. (1982). Recognition of patients' worries by nurses and other patients. *British Journal of Clinical Psychology, 21,* 255–261.

King, C. R. (2001). The Dance of life. *Clinical Journal of Oncology Nursing, 5*(1).

King, C. R., Ferrell, B. R., Grant, M., & Sakurai, C. (1995). Nurses' perceptions of the meaning of quality of life for bone marrow transplant survivors. *Cancer Nursing, 18,* 118–129.

King, C. R., Haberman, M., Berry, D. L., Bush, N., Butler, L., Dow, K. H., Ferrell, B., Grant, M., Gue, D., Hinds, P., Kreuer, J., Padilla, G., & Underwood, S. (1997). Quality of life and the cancer experience: The state-of-the-knowledge. *Oncology Nursing Forum, 24*(1), 27–41.

King, C. R., Hinds, P., Dow, K.H., Schum, L., & Lee, C. (2002). The nurse's relationship-based perceptions of patient quality of life. *Oncology Nursing Forum, 29*(10), 1409. (on-line only)

Larson, P. J. (1984). Important nurse caring behaviors perceived by patients with cancer. *Oncology Nursing Forum, 11,* 46–50.

Larson, P. J. (1986). Cancer nurses' perceptions of caring. *Cancer Nursing, 9,* 86–91.

Lindley, C. M., & Hirsch, J. D. (1994). Oncology nurses' attitudes, perceptions, and knowledge of quality-of-life assessment in patients with cancer. *Oncology Nursing Forum, 21*(1), 103–110.

Mayer, D. K. (1987). Oncology nurses' versus cancer patients' perceptions of nurse caring behaviors: A replication study. *Oncology Nursing Forum, 14,* 48–52.

Schipper, H., & Levitt, M. (1985). Measuring quality of life: Risks and benefits. *Cancer Treatment, 69,* 1115–1123.

von Essen, L., & Sjoden, P. O. (1991). Patient and staff perceptions of caring. *Journal of Advances in Nursing, 16,* 1363–1374.

Wilson, K. A., Dowling, A. J., Abdolell, M., & Tannock, I. F. (2000). Perception of quality of life by patients, partners and treating physicians. *Quality of Life Research, 9,* 1041–1052.

13

Quality of Life
Issues Related to
Marrow Transplantation

JUNE G. EILERS • CYNTHIA R. KING

Although bone marrow transplants (BMT) were first attempted in 1891 and then again in the late 1950s and early 1960s, there is limited information available regarding quality of life (QOL) of the first recipients. In the 1950s and 1960s numerous difficulties were encountered, and, thus, there was limited success with few long-term survivors. This degree of difficulty was due in part to inadequate tissue typing, the lack of adequate supportive care during aplasia, and the side effects of the high doses of cytotoxic therapy (Wingard, 1991). As knowledge increased and support therapies such as blood products and antibiotics became available, results improved. The greatest advances have occurred since the early 1980s, with increased understanding regarding marrow typing, improved approaches for aplasia management, and the utilization of critical care support therapies.

Because of the multiple potential problems with transplant, much of the initial effort focused primarily on survival of the acute phases and extending the length of this survival. Thus, limited data exist regarding QOL for the early transplant recipients. As the survival rates from the acute phase of transplant improved and posttransplant cure rates increased (Pavletic & Armitage, 1996), practitioners have broadened their concern from merely length of survival to QOL. Response to the ever-upward spiraling cost of health care in our society also fueled examination of quality of life outcomes in light of the cost of the procedure. This chapter will address QOL in BMT and issues related to the examination of QOL in this arena.

Transplantation as a Treatment

Bone marrow transplantation (BMT) is the term that traditionally has been used to describe the treatment modality used to replace malfunctioning marrow in a person whose marrow is diseased or deficient due to such conditions as leukemia, aplastic anemia, and immune deficiencies. This form of treatment is also used to replace or "rescue" the marrow destroyed by high doses of cytotoxic treatment in individuals with cancers such as lymphoma, breast cancer, and germ cell tumors that have not responded adequately to traditional doses of therapy. In these situations, the goal of the cytotoxic treatment is to destroy all of the cancer cells. Due to their high mitotic index, the cells in the marrow (e.g., white blood cells, red blood cells, and platelets) are also destroyed. Thus, the marrow must be recovered, or "rescued," to overcome the otherwise lethal state of the cytotoxic-induced aplasia.

The bone marrow typically has been the primary source of the cells used for the replacement or rescue of the marrow. These cells, called pluripotent stem cells, have the potential to produce the early forms of red blood cells, white blood cells, and platelets. With additional laboratory study, hematopoietic stem cells capable of reconstituting the marrow were also identified in the peripheral circulation (Juttner et al., 1988; Kessinger, Armitage, Landmark, Smith, & Weisenburger, 1986; Reiffers et al., 1986) and umbilical cord blood (Gluckman et al., 1989). As these sources of stem cells became more widely used, different terminology for marrow transplant evolved. *Hematopoietic stem cell transplant* (HSCT) is the term that encompasses the marrow, peripheral circulation, and umbilical cord blood as sources of the stem cells for use in transplantation (Pavletic & Armitage, 1996). The transplant itself merely involves the infusion of the pluripotent stem cells. This process is very similar to a blood transfusion.

Transplant brings together many of the treatment-related advances that have developed over the years into a modality that offers hope to individuals with otherwise life-threatening conditions (Thomas, 1994). Discovery of the role of stem cells in the production of the cells in the marrow provided the groundwork for rescue of the marrow. Human leukocyte antigen (HLA) typing allowed the identification of potential donors for individuals whose marrow was malfunctioning (Beatty et al., 1985). Advances regarding dose-response curves for chemotherapy agents led to administration of higher doses of drug for optimal cell kill in transplant. The ability to administer pluripotent stem cells intravenously for marrow engraftment and repopulation of the marrow decreased the concern regarding marrow aplasia seen with high doses of chemotherapy. New and improved antimicrobial agents and better management of aplasia-related infections have also been crucial to improved survival during transplant (Wingard, 1991).

An understanding of the approaches for providing major organ support, such as dialysis and mechanical ventilation, has been essential to supporting patients through transplantation. The administration of pharmaceuticals, including diuretics, volume expanders, and pressors, has added to the success of supportive care during the crises that occur with transplant. Blood product harvesting for administration to individuals with low blood counts has provided additional support until the marrow recovers adequate production. In addition to this use of blood products, growth factors have been used to enhance peripheral stem cell collection and hematopoietic recovery, thus shortening the duration of aplasia. Nutritional support to facilitate normal cell recovery from the cytotoxic treatments and recovery of the immune system has improved the overall success. Careful orchestration of each of these components of the whole process is critical to the success of HSCT.

Frequently, transplant can be performed without major complications, especially in the autologous arena, in which clients with limited disease receive their own marrow. This has contributed greatly to the increased interest in HSCT, to the skyrocketing increase in the number of transplants performed, and to the increased number of transplant programs in the 1990s (Horowitz, 1995). Multiple programs now perform small numbers of transplants using a variety of protocols. This has led to improved access for individuals requiring transplant; however, it has impacted the ability to track the success of this modality and to follow the HSCT recipients. What then is the best way to measure success in transplantation, and what place does QOL have in that measurement?

As discussed in other chapters, QOL has evolved as a significant theme in the health care literature over the last several decades. This increased interest in QOL has also been experienced in the transplant setting. Several aspects of HSCT combine to provide the basis for the perceived importance of QOL in transplant.

Transplantation as a Unique Experience

Awareness of the unique aspects of transplantation facilitates an enhanced understanding of QOL for this population. Candidates for HSCT are most generally individuals with life-threatening conditions. They have been informed they will likely die secondary to the disease process unless a more aggressive treatment strategy is used. Therefore, these potential recipients must come to terms with the issue of possible death. The immediacy of the life-threatening phase of the disease varies for each individual and depends on such factors as age and diagnosis. HSCT is a more aggressive treatment strategy that offers these individuals an alternative. It is not, however, without significant risk. Candidates are informed of the potential complications of the procedure. These include the risk of premature death secondary to complications seen with the toxicity of the high dose antineoplastic therapy. HSCT patients and their families must face the paradox that the treatment offering them hope against fairly certain death may actually result in premature death. They must be willing to acknowledge and accept the significance of the risk of death from the disease in order to be willing to face the risk of life-threatening complications. It is the hope of a new lease on life that enables them to face this risk (Eilers, 1991). And, with the excellent support therapies available, some recipients have few major problems and actually do very well. The impact of this paradox on QOL will be addressed in more detail later in the chapter.

Potential HSCT recipients have a wide variety of diseases and are in different stages of the disease process (Pavletic & Armitage, 1996). Additionally, they have had varying amounts and types of treatments and experience with symptoms and complications prior to HSCT. Therefore, no two recipients enter the world of HSCT at the same point in terms of disease trajectory; symptom, complication, and treatment history; and risk for complications.

Depending on the underlying disease process and patient age, different types of transplants are used. They are identified based on the donor of the pluripotent stem cells for the rescue of the marrow (Table 13-1). Allogeneic transplants utilize stem cells from an HLA-matched donor. Initially used primarily for patients with leukemia, these transplants were the mainstay of the modality of transplant for the first several decades. Over time, the principle of marrow rescue with hematopoietic stem cells was applied in autologous transplants for other malignancies. These transplants use the individual's own stem cells for collection, storage, and later reinfusion posttreatment. Syngeneic transplants, which are much fewer in number, involve the use of marrow (stem cells) from an identical twin. Since the donor and recipient are HLA identical, syngeneic transplants are very similar to autologous transplants.

Although the different types of transplants use the same principle of marrow rescue, allogeneic transplants differ significantly from autologous and syngeneic transplants. The major difference is related to the potential complication of graft-

Table 13-1. **Types of Hematopoietic Stem Cell Transplants**

Type of Transplant	Source of Cells
Autologous	Patient
Syngeneic	Identical twin
Allogeneic	Donor
Related	Dnor is HLA-matched relative
Unrelated	Donor is HLA-matched nonrelative
Mismatched	Dnor is not complete HLA match

versus-host disease (GVHD) in allogeneic transplant. This process involves the graft or new hematopoietic system actually rejecting its host (the recipient). Due to this risk, allogeneic recipients require additional immune suppression, increasing the risk for infections throughout the period of suppression. In addition to the difference between allogeneic transplants and autologous and syngeneic transplants, there is a potential difference within the grouping of allogeneic transplant based on donor match. Unrelated and mismatched transplants, used when an HLA matched sibling is not available, have an increased risk of complications related to GVHD.

Not only do the types of transplants differ, the cytotoxic protocols used have varied toxicities and therefore have potentially different effects on the HSCT recipients and their families. Some patients have relatively simple, uncomplicated courses with minimal side effects. Others experience multiple life-threatening complications and latent effects (King, 1995).

HSCT is a very costly procedure. The need for multiple support therapies and the necessary high level of critical care support contribute to the costs involved in transplant. Although practitioners have attempted to provide transplant at a lower cost with a movement to the outpatient setting, costs remain a significant factor. Pharmaceuticals alone comprise a significant portion of the costs.

Due to the cost involved and the potential level of toxicity, both in the acute phase and long term, QOL is especially important to consider in HSCT. Mast (1995) identified that historically a major goal of QOL research has been to justify expensive and often toxic treatment regimens in terms of patients' psychosocial, function, and pathophysiologic responses to treatment. Awareness of QOL posttransplant is vital for pretransplant counseling, informed consent, and evaluating outcomes after different types of conditioning therapy. Moreover, this awareness can assist care providers in limiting problems by providing appropriate rehabilitative support and counseling regarding long-term expectations. Knowing that HSCT is a costly, life-threatening procedure with a lasting impact on QOL, health care providers are frequently challenged with the question: Is HSCT worth the risk and cost? This chapter addresses issues related to determining the QOL outcomes of HSCT.

Information regarding the QOL of HSCT recipients is essential to answer this question. As the results in transplantation improve and increasing numbers of HSCT recipients survive, there is an expanding pool of potential subjects for QOL studies. As the recipients live longer after HSCT, not only is there an expanded time period for potential study of QOL, but also more knowledge is gained regarding longer-term complications that may not have developed in the shorter-term survivors of the past.

The changes over time in HSCT that have led to improved results and wider application of the treatment modality also affect the generalizability of QOL findings from survivors of the early transplants. As supportive therapies have advanced and treatment results have improved, HSCT has been utilized in a broader spectrum of diagnoses. With the advances in technology and knowledge, transplant teams have learned how to respond to clinical situations when they occur to decrease the morbidity and mortality related to treatment. Components of transplant that may have contributed to the impact on the recipient in the past may no longer be state of the art.

Measuring QOL in HSCT requires an awareness of the heterogeneity of the population being studied and differences in the procedures currently being used as compared to those of the past. Not only is there heterogeneity in the types of transplant (autologous versus allogeneic, related versus unrelated, and matched versus mismatched), but there are also differences in terms of the level of wellness of the individual at the time of transplant, the level of aggressiveness of the underlying disease, and the age of the HSCT recipient. Furthermore, different treatment protocols have different toxicities. Thus, it becomes difficult to compare outcomes across the entire spectrum of HSCT.

Theoretical Approach to QOL

The volume of literature in the area of transplantation has increased dramatically over the last several decades. Evidence of this increase is found in the development of a journal devoted to bone marrow transplantation. However, investigators have made very limited progress in terms of systematic, theory-driven analysis of QOL related to HSCT. Numerous articles on HSCT address physical complications that may be seen with transplantation and topics related to marrow engraftment (Buchsel, 1986; Buchsel & Kelleher, 1989; Eilers, Berger, & Petersen, 1988; Ersek, 1992; Ezzone et al., 1993; Ford & Eisenberg, 1990; Ford & Ballard, 1988; Franco & Gould, 1994; Haberman, 1988; Hutchison & King, 1983; Klemm, 1985; McConn, 1987; McGuire et al., 1993; Nims & Strom, 1988; Parker & Cohen, 1983; Shaffer & Wilson, 1993; Wujcik, Ballard, & Camp-Sorrell, 1994). Clinical articles have discussed the process of HSCT and the care requirements. Psychological and emotional factors during and after treatment have been addressed in a number of earlier studies (Andrykowski, Henslee, & Barnett, 1989; Hengeveld, Houtman, & Zwaan, 1988; Wolcott, Wellisch, Fawzy, & Landsverk, 1986a, 1986b), but they focused primarily on the allogeneic transplant recipient and donor. Furthermore, the use of a theoretical approach to studies in this area has been limited. Prior to the late 1990s, only a limited number of the studies of QOL in BMT identified the conceptual or theoretical framework for the study (Andrykowski, Greiner et al., 1995; Baker et al., 1994; Belec, 1992; Bush, Haberman, Donaldson, & Sullivan, 1995; Ferrell et al., 1992a, 1992b; Grant et al., 1992; Haberman, Bush, Young, & Sullivan, 1993; Molassiotis, Boughton, Burgoyne, & van den Akker, 1995; Nespoli et al., 1995; Schmidt et al., 1993). More recently researchers have started to refer to the multidimensional nature of QOL. Interestingly, nursing research is more likely to address the theoretical approach used in QOL research.

There does appear to be agreement that QOL is dependent on the client's perception. Nevertheless, due to ambiguity regarding its meaning (Ferrans, 1990; King et al., 1997; Mast, 1995), consensus has not been reached regarding conceptual or operational definitions for QOL (Cella & Tulsky, 1990; King et al., 1997; Mast, 1995). In fact prior to the late 1990s some studies have not even offered a definition of QOL before attempting to measure it (Andrykowksi, Greiner et al., 1995; Belec, 1992; Bush et al., 1995; Gaston-Johansson & Foxall, 1996; Grant, Ferrell et al., 1992; Haberman et al., 1993; Nespoli et al., 1995; Schmidt et al., 1993). One definition that has been used by several researchers presents QOL as the degree of satisfaction with present life circumstances as perceived by the individual (Belec, 1992; Gaston-Johansson & Foxall, 1996).

Just as there is a lack of a consistent definition for QOL, there is a lack of agreement regarding the dimensions or domains of QOL studied by various researchers (King et al., 1997). Some examine only physical aspects of transplant, while others include social, economic, and spiritual components. The spiritual component is most likely to be present in studies including narrative questioning or building on the City of Hope model for QOL (Figure 13-1). The varied and atheoretical approaches to the study of QOL have limited the ability to build theory and to establish sound tools for measuring QOL in the HSCT population.

Ferrell and colleagues developed a model to examine the impact of BMT on QOL (Ferrell et al., 1992a). This model was based on previous research and surveys of long-term BMT survivors. The conceptual model includes the four domains of physical well-being and symptoms, psychological well-being, social well-being, and spiritual well-being (see Figure 13-1). QOL is depicted as a series of interrelationships between the domains. This model was used in a sequential article (Ferrell et al., 1992b) to discuss the results of a survey of long-term survivors. It has subsequently been used by other investigators. Byar and colleagues, Saleh and Brockopp, and Whedon and associates used the model in a QOL study of long-term survivors of autologous transplant (Byar, Eilers, & Vose, 1999; Saleh & Brockopp, 2001; Whedon, Stearns, & Mills, 1995); Dow and Ferrell (1994) used it to compare the meanings of changes in QOL for HSCT, breast cancer, and thyroid cancer patients; and King, Ferrell, Grant, and Sakurai (1995) used it in a study of nurses' perceptions of QOL in transplant. Further research is needed to determine the applicability of this model to groups beyond those included in the studies to date.

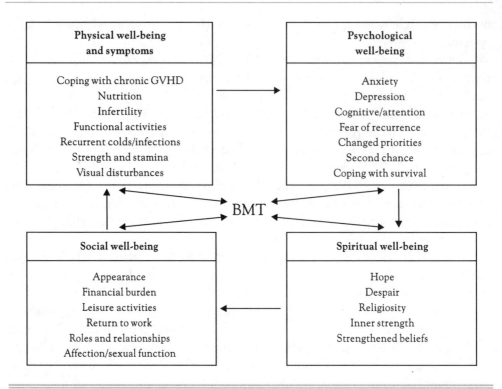

Figure 13-1. **Quality of life model for bone marrow transplant survivors.**
Source: Adapted with permission from Ferrell, Grant et al., at City of Hope Medical Center.

QOL in HSCT Research

Most early QOL-related studies of transplant patients examined psychological aspects from the case study or anecdotal approach (Brown & Kelly, 1976; Gardner, August, & Githens, 1977; Patenaude, Szymanski, & Rappeport, 1979; Pfefferbaum, Lindamood, & Wiley, 1977; Popkin, Moldow, Hall, Branda, & Yarchoan, 1977; Wolcott, Fawzy, & Wellisch, 1987; Wolcott, Wellisch, Fawzy, & Landsverk, 1986a; Wolcott, Wellisch, Fawzy, & Landsverk, 1986b). As the number of HSCT recipients increased and survival rates improved, interest in QOL for these individuals has also increased. Advances in research knowledge and the availability of larger samples has facilitated research in the area.

A number of reviews of studies regarding QOL in HSCT have been presented in the literature, with some overlap across the reviews. In 1994 Whedon and Ferrell reviewed reports of post-HSCT QOL studies to examine the findings regarding QOL beyond the first year posttransplant. Their review included the numbers of subjects, their ages, the types of transplant, the time post-HSCT, the measures used in the studies, and the major findings. King (1995) presented a review of the physical, psychological, social, and spiritual residual effects of transplant remaining after one year, with particular emphasis on the incidence of the physical effects. Decker's (1995) review of a select group of transplant studies highlighted particular psychosocial concerns of transplant recipients before, during, and after HSCT; perceived QOL after transplant; and the impact of family, friends, and caregivers on the hospitalization and recovery phases of HSCT. The most extensive review of studies and abstracts assessing QOL and psychosocial issues in adults with cancer who had been treated with HSCT was completed by Hjermstad and Kaasa (1995). Their review of 48 QOL studies included (a) type of transplant and number of subjects, (b) use of comparison group, (c) study design, (d) times of measurement, (e) methods of assessment (tools), (f) inclusion of performance status, and (g) conclusions. In terms of overall results (although specific symptoms and problems have emerged from the findings of the studies reviewed), generally the participating subjects in each of the reviews reported fairly good QOL. A later review by Neitzert and colleagues (1998) focused on residual difficulties in transplant survivors including: (a) fatigue and general functioning/psychological distress; (b) sexual functioning; and (c) endocrine functioning. Once again the reviewers noted that although there are residual difficulties, survivorship is often associated with high global QOL. A later review by Neitzert and colleagues (1998) focused on residual difficulties in transplant survivors including: (a) fatigue and general functioning/psychological distress; (b) sexual functioning; and (c) endocrine functioning. Once again the reviewers noted that, although there are residual difficulties, survivorship is often associated with high global QOL.

As an overview, with the exception of one chart review study for endocrine function, sample size in the studies reviewed ranged from 6 to 238, with allogeneic being the most common type of transplant. The majority of the subjects were adults. Most of the studies were cross-sectional or retrospective, with the time post-HSCT ranging from 3 months to over 12 years. Only a limited number of studies included data from the time of admission or pretransplant. Few of the longitudinal studies followed subjects for greater than one year posttransplant. The studies used chart data, mailed questionnaires, phone interviews, and personal interviews. Comparison groups were used infrequently. The instruments used varied greatly. Although progress has been made in the study of QOL in HSCT, significant gaps and weaknesses remain. These will be discussed later.

A number of studies of QOL in HSCT not included in the reviews and published since 1995 have added to the knowledge base by addressing some area of weakness. Characteristics of these studies that will be reviewed include study design (longitudinal versus cross-sectional), instruments, the use of narrative/interview data, inclusion criteria based on type of transplant and cancer diagnosis, use of a nontransplant comparison group, neuro/cognitive changes, and QOL in pediatric transplant survivors.

Although the majority of the studies continue to be cross-sectional, a number of longitudinal studies have been reported. Andrykowski, Bruehl, Brady, and Henslee-Downey (1995) reported data from prior to and 12 to 16 months after transplant. McQuellon and colleagues (1996) reported data from prior to and 103 to 502 days posttransplant while Meyers and associates (1994) had longitudinal data from four time points, pretransplant, two weeks, discharge, and eight months after transplant. McQuellon and colleagues (1998) also had data at four time points over the first year; pretransplant, discharge, 100 days, and at one year. Molassiotis, van den Akker, Milligan, and Goldman (1997) reported data from three time points, pretransplant, three to four weeks later, and at one to two years.

Only the study by Broers and colleagues, reported in two articles (Broers, Hengeveld, Kaptein, LeCessie, van de Loo, & de Vries, 1998; Broers, Kaptein, Le-Cessie, Fibbe, & Hengeveld 2000) covered a longer period of time, with data from pretransplant to three years. Pretransplant data only were reported by Baker, Marcellus, Zabora, Polland, and Jordrey (1997). Gaston-Johansson and Foxall (1996) and Ahles, Tope, Furstenberg, Hann, and Mills (1996) reported pretransplant and acute phase data in their reports. The longitudinal study by Andrykowski and associates (1997) involved survivors at least 12 months (mean 43.5 months) posttransplant and again 18 months later.

Cross-sectional studies have examined subjects at a variety of time points posttransplant. Kopp and colleagues (1998) grouped their data to compare subjects less than 1-year posttransplant with subjects more than one year posttransplant. In another article, Kopp and associates (2000) reported on the same group of subjects. Five studies included individuals from as early as one month posttransplant with those many years posttransplant with clustering for the expected differences in QOL during the initial year posttransplant as compared to beyond the first year. Hann and associates (1997) conducted follow-up at 3.5–62.5 months posttransplant; Heinonen, Volin, Uutela, Zevon, Barrick, and Ruutu (2001) at 4–171 months posttransplant; Molassiotis and colleagues (1996) at 6–122 months; McQuellon and associates (1998) at 6–156 months; Sutherland and colleagues (1997) at 1–253 months; and Parsons, Barlow, Levy, Supran, and Kaplan (1999) conducted follow-up on children less than 6 months and greater than 12 months posttransplant.

Three QOL studies focused on the time after the first year posttransplant. This is when subjects could be expected to be more stable. Saleh and Brockopp (2001) evaluated subjects 12–210 months posttransplant; Schimmer and colleagues (2001) evaluated subjects at 2.8 to 4.6 years posttransplant; and Zittoun and associates (1997) assessed subjects less than one year posttransplant. Fromm, Andrykowski, and Hunt (1996) compared subjects from greater than one year to four years posttransplant with those five to ten years posttransplant.

Data collection involved numerous self-report instruments (presented in more detail in Table 13-2). The use of narrative/interview data to enhance findings is seen

Table 13-2. **Instruments Used in Quality of Life Studies of Hematopoietic Stem Cell Transplant Recipients**

Instrument	Studies Using Instrument
A Brief Measure of Social Support (SSQ6)	Heinonen, Volin, Uutela, Zevon, Barrick, & Ruutu, 2001
Achenbach Behavior Check List (ABCL)	Lesko, Ostroff, Mumma, Mashberg, & Holland, 1992; Phipps, Brenner, Heslop, Krance, Jayawardene, & Mulhern, 1995
Affect Balance Scale (ABS)	Schimmer, Elliott, Abbey, Raiz, Keating, Beanlands, McCay, Messner, Lipton, & Devins, 2001
Atkinson Life Happiness Rating	Schimmer, Elliott, Abbey, Raiz, Keating, Beanlands, McCay, Messner, Lipton, & Devins, 2001
Beck Depression Inventory (BDI)	Ahles, Tope, Furstenberg, Hann, & Mills, 1996; Gaston-Johansson & Foxall, 1996; Gaston-Johansson, Franco, & Zimmerman, 1992; Hengeveld, Houtman, & Zwaan, 1988; Rodrigue, Boggs, Weiner, & Behen, 1993; Schimmer, Elliott, Abbey, Raiz, Keating, Beanlands, McCay, Messner, Lipton, & Devins, 2001; Syrjala, Chapko, Vitaliano, Cummings, & Sullivan, 1993
Beery Development Test of Visual Motor Integration (VMI)	Phipps, Brenner, Heslop, Krance, Jayawardene, & Mulher, 1995
Bradburn Positive and Negative Affect Scale (BPNAS)	Andrykowski, Bruehl, Brady, & Henslee-Downey, 1995; Baker, Curbow, & Wingard, 1991; Bush, Haberman, Donaldson, & Sullivan, 1995
Brief Symptom Inventory (BSI)	Lesko, Ostroff, Mumma, Mashberg, & Holland, 1992; Mumma, Mashberg, & Lesko, 1992; Syrjala, Chapko, Vitaliano, Cummings, & Sullivan, 1993
Busnelli Anxiety Scale	Nespoli, Verri, Locatelli, Bertuggia, Taibi, & Burgio, 1995
Cantril Self-Anchoring Ladder of Life Scale (CSAL)	Baker, Curbow, & Wingard, 1991; Bush, Haberman, Donaldson, & Sullivan, 1995; Curbow, Somerfield, Baker, Wingard, & Legro, 1993; Wingard, Curbow, Baker, Zabora, & Piantadosi, 1992; Saleh & Brockopp, 2001

continues

Table 13-2. **continued**

Instrument	Studies Using Instrument
Center for Epidemiologic Studies—Depression Scale (CES-D)	Baker, Marcellus, Zabora, Polland, & Jordrey, 1997; McQuellon, Craven, Russell, Hoffman, Cruz, Perry, & Hunt, 1996; McQuellon, Russell, Rambo, Craven, Radford, Perry, Cruz, & Hurd, 1998; Schimmer, Elliott, Abbey, Raiz, Keating, Beanlands, McCay, Messner, Lipton, & Devins, 2001
Children's Depression Scale	Nespoli, Verri, Locatelli, Bertuggia, Taibi, & Burgio, 1995
City of Hope Quality of Life-BMT QOL-BMT-Survivors Tool	Grant, Ferrell, Schmidt, Fonbuena, Niland, & Forman, 1992; Saleh & Brockopp, 2001; Whedon, Stearns, & Mills, 1995
Composite International Diagnostic Interview	Jenkins, Liningtton, & Whittaker, 1991; Jenkins, Lester, Alexander, & Whittaker, 1994; Murphy, Jenkins, & Whittaker, 1996
Coping Strategy Questionnaire (CSQ)	Gaston-Johansson, Franco, & Zimmerman, 1992
Death Anxiety Questionnaire (DAQ)	Mumma, Mashberg, & Lesko, 1992
Demands of BMT Recovery Inventory	Bush, Haberman, Donaldson, & Sullivan, 1995
Dementia Rating Scale (DRS)	Meyers, Weitzner, Byrne, Valentine, Champlin, & Przepiorka, 1994
Derogatix Sexual Functioning Scale (DSF)	Lesko, Ostroff, Mumma, Mashberg, & Holland, 1992; Mumma, Mashberg, & Lesko, 1992
DSM III	Lesko, Ostroff, Mumma, Mashberg, & Holland, 1992
ECOG Performance Status Rating Scale (PSR)	Hann, Jacobsen, Martin, Kronish, Azzarello, & Fields, 1997; McQuellon, Russell, Rambo, Craven, Radford, Perry, Cruz, & Hurd, 1998

continues

Table 13-2. **continued**

Instrument	Studies Using Instrument
European Organization for Treatment and Research of Cancer QOL Questionnaire (EORTC QLQ0Q30)	Bush, Haberman, Donaldson, & Sullivan, 1995; Kopp, Schweigkofler, Holzner, Nachbaur, Niedwewieser, Fleischhacker, & Sperner-Unterweger, 1998; Kopp, Schweigkofler, Holzner, Nachbaur, Niedwewieser, Fleischhacker, Kemmler & Sperner-Unterweger 2000; Zittoun, Suciu, Watson, Solbu, Muus, Mandelli, Stryckmans, Peetermans, Thaler, Resegotti, Dardenne, & Willemze, 1997
Eysenck Personality Questionnaire (EPQ)	Jenkins, Liningtton, & Whittaker, 1991
FACES Life Satisfaction	Wingard Curbow, Baker, Zabora, & Piantadosi, 1992
Family APGAR	Baker, Wingard, Curbow, Zabora, Jodrey, Fogarty, & Legro, 1994; Baker, Marcellus, Zabora, Polland, & Jordrey, 1997
Functional Assessment of Cancer Therapy—Bone Marrow Transplant (FACT-BMT)	Heinonen, Volin, Uutela, Zevon, Barrick, & Ruutu, 2001; Kopp, Schweigkofler, Holzner, Nachbaur, Niedwewieser, Fleischhacker & Sperner-Unterweger, 1998; Kopp, Schweigkofler, Holzner, Nachbaur, Niedwewieser, Fleischhacker, Kemmler, & Sperner-Unterweger, 2000; McQuellon, Craven, Russell, Hoffman, Cruz, Perry, & Hunt, 1996; McQuellon, Russell, Rambo, Craven, Radford, Perry, Cruz, & Hurd, 1998; Saleh & Brockopp, 2001
Functional Limitations Battery (FLB)	Broers, Hengeveld, Kaptein, LeCessie, van de Loo, & de Vries, 1998; Broers, Kaptein, LeCessie, Fibbe, & Hengeveld, 2000
Functional Living Index Cancer (FLIC)	Andrykowski, Altmaier, Barnett, Otis, Gingrich, & Henslee-Downey, 1990; Andrykowski, Bruehl, Brady, & Henslee-Downey, 1995; Andrykowski, Henslee, & Barnett, 1989; Andrykowski, Henslee, & Farrall, 1989; Andrykowski, Carpenter, Greiner, Altmaier, Burish, Antin, Gingrich, Cordova, & Henslee-Downey, 1997; Broers, Hengeveld, Kaptein, LeCessie, van de Loo, & de Vries, 1998

continues

Table 13-2. **continued**

Instrument	Study Using Instrument
General Health Questionnaire (GHQ)	Broers, Hengeveld, Kaptein, LeCessie, van de Loo, & de Vries, 1998; Fromm, Andrykowski, & Hunt, 1996; Prieto, Saez, Carreras, Atala, Sierra, Rovira, Batlle, Blanch, Escobar, Vieta, Gomez, Rozman, & Cierera, 1996
Health Locus of Control	Broers, Hengeveld, Kaptein, LeCessie, van de Loo, & de Vries, 1998
Health Perceptions Questionnaire	Bush, Haberman, Donaldson, & Sullivan, 1995
Hospital Anxiety and Depression Scale (HADS)	Bush, Haberman, Donaldson, & Sullivan, 1995; Jenkins, Liningtton, & Whittaker, 1991; Jenkins, Lester, Alexander, & Whittaker, 1994; Leigh, Wilson, Burns, & Clark, 1995; Molassiotis, Boughton, Burgoyne, & van den Akker, 1995; Molassiotis, van den Akker, Milligan, Goldman, Boughton, Holmes, & Thomas, 1996
Illness Intrusiveness Rating Scale	Schimmer, Elliott, Abbey, Raiz, Keating, Beanlands, McCay, Messner, Lipton, & Devins, 2001
Impact of Event Scale (IES)	Lesko, Ostroff, Mumma, Mashberg, & Holland, 1992; Mumma, Mashberg, & Lesko, 1992
Internal-External Locus of Control Scale	Kopp, Schweigkofler, Holzner, Nachbaur, Niedwewieser, Fleischhacker, & Sperner-Unterweger, 1998
Jalowiec Coping Scale	Molassiotis, van den Akker, Milligan, & Goldman, 1997
Leukemia-BMT module	Zittoun, Suciu, Watson, Solbu, Muus, Mandelli, Stryckmans, Peetermans, Thaler, Resegotti, Dardenne, & Willemze, 1997
Life Questionnaire Test	Baker, Marcellus, Zabora, Polland, & Jordrey, 1997; Curbow, Somerfield, Baker, Wingard, & Legro, 1993

continues

Table 13-2. **continued**

Instrument	Study Using Instrument
Mastery Scale	Baker, Marcellus, Zabora, Polland, & Jordrey, 1997
Medical Coping Modes Questionnaire (MCMQ)	Litwins, Rodrigue, & Weiner, 1994; Rodrigue, Boggs, Weiner, & Behen, 1993
Medical Outcomes Study— Short Form-36 (MOS SF-36)	Hann, Jacobsen, Martin, Kronish, Azzarello, & Fields, 1997; Heinonen, Volin, Uutela, Zevon, Barrick, & Ruutu, 2001; McQuellon, Craven, Russell, Hoffman, Cruz, Perry, & Hunt, 1996; McQuellon, Russell, Rambo, Craven, Radford, Perry, Cruz, & Hurd, 1998; Sutherland, Fyles, Adams, Hao, Lipton, Minden, Meharchand, Atkins, Tejpar, & Messner, 1997
Memorial Symptom Assessment Scale (MSAS)	Hann, Jacobsen, Martin, Kronish, Azzarello, & Fields, 1997
Mental Attitude to Cancer Scale	Jenkins, Lester, Alexander, & Whittaker, 1994; Murphy, Jenkins, & Whittaker, 1996
Mental Health Inventory (MHI)	Lesko, Ostroff, Mumma, Mashberg, & Holland, 1992
Multidimensional Health Locus of Control (MHLC)	Gaston-Johansson, Franco, & Zimmerman, 1992
Minnesota Multiphasic Personality Inventory (MMPI)	Rodrigue, Boggs, Weiner, & Behen, 1993
Neuropsychologic Battery [Trail Making Test B, Visual Retention Tests (VRT), Controlled Oral Work Association (COWA), Temporal Oral Orientation all from the Benton Iowa Screening Battery for Mental Decline]	Ahles, Tope, Furstenberg, Hann, & Mills, 1996
Norbeck Social Support Questionnaire	Kopp, Schweigkofler, Holzner, Nachbaur, Niedwewieser, Fleischhacker, & Sperner-Unterweger, 1998; Molassiotis, van den Akker, Milligan, Goldman, Boughton, Holmes, & Thomas, 1996
Nottingham Health Profile	Prieto, Saez, Carreras, Atala, Sierra, Rovira, Batlle, Blanch, Escobar, Vieta, Gomez, Rozman, & Cierera, 1996

continues

Table 13-2. **continued**

Instrument	Study Using Instrument
Offer Self-Image Questionnaire	Nespoli, Verri, Locatelli, Bertuggia, Taibi, & Burgio, 1995
Pain-o-Meter (PoM)	Gaston-Johansson, Franco, & Zimmerman, 1992
Perceived Health Questionnaire (PHQ)	Andrykowski, Altmaier, Barnett, Otis, Gingrich, & Henslee-Downey, 1990; Andrykowski, Greiner, Altmaier, Burish, Antin, Gingrich, McGarigle, & Henslee-Downey, 1995
Perceived Quality of Life Questionnaire (PQOL)	Andrykowski, Greiner, Altmaier, Burish, Antin, Gingrich, McGarigle, & Henslee-Downey, 1995
Personality Research Form	Neuser, 1988
Piers-Harris Self Concept, Play Performance Scale for Children	Phipps, Brenner, Heslop, Krance, Jayawardene, & Mulhern, 1995
Pittsburgh Sleep Quality Index	Andrykowski, Carpenter, Greiner, Altmaier, Burish, Antin, Gingrich, Cordova, & Henslee-Downey, 1997
Play Performance Scale for Children	Phipps, Brenner, Heslop, Krance, Jayawardene, & Mulhern, 1995
Positive and Negative Affect Scale (PNAS)	Andrykowski, Brady, Greiner, Altmaier, Burish, Antin, Gingrich, McGarigle, & Henslee-Downey, 1995; Fromm, Andrykowski, & Hunt, 1996
Present State Examination (PSE)	Leigh, Wilson, Burns, & Clark, 1995
Princess Margaret Hospital—Symptom Experience Report	Schimmer, Elliott, Abbey, Raiz, Keating, Beanlands, McCay, Messner, Lipton, & Devins, 2001

continues

Table 13-2. **continued**

Instrument	Study Using Instrument
Profile of Mood State (POMS)	Andrykowski, Altmaier, Barnett, Burish, Gingrich, & Henslee-Downey, 1990; Andrykowski, Altmaier, Barnett, Otis, Gingrich, & Henslee-Downey, 1990; Andrykowski, Brady, Greiner, Altmaier, Burish, Antin, Gingrich, McGarigle, & Henslee-Downey, 1995; Andrykowski, Bruehl, Brady, & Henslee-Downey, 1995; Andrykowski, Carpenter, Greiner, Altmaier, Burish, Antin, Gingrich, Cordova, & Henslee-Downey, 1997; Andrykowski, Greiner, Altmaier, Burish, Antin, Gingrich, McGarigle, & Henslee-Downey, 1995; Andrykowski, Henslee, & Barnett, 1989; Andrykowski, Henslee, & Farrall, 1989; Baker, Curbow, & Wingard, 1991; Baker, Wingard, Curbow, Zabora, Jodrey, Fogarty, & Legro, 1994; Baker, Marcellus, Zabora, Polland, & Jordrey, 1997; Bush, Haberman, Donaldson, & Sullivan, 1995; Curbow, Somerfield, Baker, Wingard, & Legro, 1993; Fromm, Andrykowski, & Hunt, 1996; Heinonen, Volin, Uutela, Zevon, Barrick, & Ruutu, 2001; Jenkins, Lester, Alexander, & Whittaker, 1994; Molassiotis, van den Akker, Milligan, Goldman, Boughton, Holmes, & Thomas, 1996, Molassiotis, van den Akker, Milligan, Goldman, & Boughton, 1996; Molassiotis, van den Akker, Milligan, & Goldman, 1997; McQuellon, Craven, Russell, Hoffman, Cruz, Perry, & Hunt, 1996; McQuellon, Russell, Rambo, Craven, Radford, Perry, Cruz, & Hurd, 1998; Saleh & Brockopp, 2001
Psychiatric Diagnostic Interview (PDI)	Ahles, Tope, Furstenberg, Hann, & Mills, 1996
Psychosexual Functioning Questionnaire	Molassiotis, van den Akker, Milligan, Goldman, Boughton, Holmes, & Thomas, 1996
Psychosocial Adjustment to Illness Scale (PAIS)	Andrykowski, Altmaier, Barnett, Burish, Gingrich, & Henslee-Downey, 1990; Andrykowski, Altmaier, Barnett, Otis, Gingrich, & Henslee-Downey, 1990; Andrykowski, Brady, Greiner, Altmaier, Burish, Antin, Gingrich, McGarigle, & Henslee-Downey, 1995; Andrykowski, Bruehl, Brady, & Henslee-Downey, 1995; Fromm, Andrykowski, & Hunt 1996; Jenkins, Liningtton, & Whittaker, 1991; Molassiotis, Boughton, Burgoyne, & van den Akker, 1995; Molassiotis, van den Akker, Milligan, Goldman, Boughton, Holmes, & Thomas, 1996; Mumma, Mashberg, & Lesko, 1992; Saleh & Brockopp, 2001 *continues*

Table 13-2. **continued**

Instrument	Study Using Instrument
Pryer Personality Assessment Scale	Leigh, Wilson, Burns, & Clark, 1995
Quality of Life Index (QLI)	Gaston-Johansson & Foxall, 1996
Recovery of Function Scale (ROF)	Andrykowski, Brady, Greiner, Altmaier, Burish, Antin, Gingrich, McGarigle, & Henslee-Downey, 1995
Relational Support Scale	Baker, Wingard, Curbow, Zabora, Jodrey, Fogarty, & Legro, 1994; Baker, Marcellus, Zabora, Polland, & Jordrey, 1997
Rey Auditory-Verbal Learning Task	Phipps, Brenner, Heslop, Krance, Jayawardene, & Mulhern, 1995
Rosenberg Self-Esteem Scale (RSE)	Andrykowski, Brady, Greiner, Altmaier, Burish, Antin, Gingrich, McGarigle, & Henslee-Downey, 1995; Baker, Wingard, Curbow, Zabora, Jodrey, Fogarty, & Legro, 1994; Broers, Hengeveld, Kaptein, LeCessie, van de Loo, & de Vries, 1998; Fromm, Andrykowski, & Hunt, 1996; Molassiotis, van den Akker, Milligan, Goldman, Boughton, Holmes, & Thomas, 1996
Rotterdam Symptom Checklist	Molassiotis, van den Akker, Milligan, Goldman, Boughton, Holmes, & Thomas, 1996
Satisfaction with Life Domains Scale	Baker, Curbow, & Wingard, 1991; Baker, Wingard, Curbow, Zabora, Jodrey, Fogarty, & Legro, 1994; Schimmer, Elliott, Abbey, Raiz, Keating, Beanlands, McCay, Messner, Lipton, & Devins, 2001; Wingard, Curbow, Baker, Zabora, & Piantadosi, 1992
Self Report Karnofsky Performance Scale	Baker, Marcellus, Zabora, Polland, & Jordrey, 1997

continues

Table 13-2. **continued**

Instrument	Study Using Instrument
Sickness Impact Profile (SIP)	Andrykowski, Altmaier, Barnett, Burish, Gingrich, & Henslee-Downey, 1990; Andrykowski, Altmaier, Barnett, Otis, Gingrich, & Henslee-Downey, 1990; Andrykowski, Bruehl, Brady, & Henslee-Downey, 1995; Andrykowski, Henslee, & Barnett, 1989; Fromm, Andrykowski, & Hunt, 1996; Litwins, Rodrigue, & Weiner, 1994; Syrjala, Chapko, Vitaliano, Cummings, & Sullivan, 1993
Simmons Scale	Wolcott, Wellisch, Fawzy, & Landsverk, 1986b
Sleep, Energy, and Appetite Scale (SEAS)	Altmaier, Barnett, Otis, Gingrich, & Henslee-Downey, 1990; Andrykowski, Bruehl, Brady, & Henslee-Downey, 1995
Sleep Experience Report (SER)	Andrykowski, Carpenter, Greiner, Altmaier, Burish, Antin, Gingrich, Cordova, & Henslee-Downey, 1997
Social Adjustment Scale (SAS)	Leigh, Wilson, Burns, & Clark, 1995; Lesko, Ostroff, Mumma, Mashberg, & Holland, 1992; Wolcott, Willisch, Fawzy, & Landsverk, 1986b
Spielberger State-Trait Anxiety Inventory	Ahles, Tope, Furstenberg, Hann, & Mills, 1996; Gaston-Johansson, Franco, & Zimmerman, 1992; Gaston-Johansson & Foxall, 1996; Rodrigue, Boggs, Weiner, & Behen, 1993; Kopp, Schweigkofler, Holzner, Nachbaur, Niedwewieser, Fleischhacker, & Sperner-Unterweger, 1998
Symbol Digits Modality Test (SDMT)	Phipps, Brenner, Heslop, Krance, Jayawardene, & Mulhern, 1995
Symptom Check-List 90-R (SCL-90-R)	Broers, Hengeveld, Kaptein, LeCessie, van de Loo, & de Vries, 1998
Symptom Distress Scale (SDS)	Molassiotis, van den Akker, Milligan, Goldman, Boughton, Holmes, & Thomas, 1996; Molassiotis, van den Akker, Milligan, & Goldman, 1997
Symptom Experience Report (SER)	Andrykowski, Altmaier, Barnett, Otis, Gingrich, & Henslee-Downey, 1990; Andrykowski, Bruehl, Brady, & Henslee-Downey, 1995; Andrykowski, Brady, Greiner, Altmaier, Burish, Antin, Gingrich, McGarigle, & Henslee-Downey, 1995

continues

Table 13-2. **continued**

Instrument	Study Using Instrument
State-Trait Anger Expression Inventory (STAXI)	Rodrigue, Boggs, Weiner, & Behen, 1993
Weschler Intelligence	Phipps, Brenner, Heslop, Krance, Jayawardene, & Mulhern, 1995
Wide Range Achievement Test (WRAT-R)	Phipps, Brenner, Heslop, Krance, Jayawardene, & Mulhern, 1995
Zung Depression Inventory	Kopp, Schweigkofler, Holzner, Nachbaur, Niedwewieser, Fleischhacker, & Sperner-Unterweger, 1998

in a number of studies reported during this time (Fromm, Andrykowski, & Hunt, 1996; Molassiotis and Morris, 1998; McQuellon and colleagues, 1998).

As autologous transplants became more prevalent in the late 1980s and 1990s, autologous subjects also became more common in QOL research studies. Most QOL studies included both autologous and allogeneic subjects. In some studies, the number of autologous and allegoric subjects were similar (Andrykowski et al., 1997; Baker et al., 1997; Broers et al., 1998; Broers et al., 2000; Fromm, Andrykowski, & Hunt, 1996; Meyers et al., 1994; Zittoun et al., 1997). Allogeneic subjects were more common in the following studies: (a) Heinonen, Volin, Uutela, Zevon, Barrick, & Ruutu (2001) with 108 allogeneic and 1 syngeneic subjects; (b) Kopp and associates (1998) with 16 autologous and 40 allogeneic subjects; (c) Kopp and colleagues (2000) with the same group as their 1998 study; (d) Molassiotis, van den Akker, Milligan, and Goldman (1997) with 10 autologous and 21 allogeneic subjects; and (e) Prieto and colleagues (1996) with 43 autologous and 70 allogeneic subjects. In contrast autologous subjects outnumbered allogeneic subjects in studies by Molassiotis and colleagues (1996) with 53 autologous and 38 allogeneic subjects; McQuellon and associates (1998) with 70 autologous and 16 allogeneic subjects; and Saleh and Brockopp (2001) with 32 autologous and 7 allogeneic patients. Subjects were restricted to autologous transplant in the studies conducted by Gaston-Johansson and Foxall (1996), Whedon, Stearns, and Mills (1995), Ahles, Tope, Furstenberg, Hann, and Mills (1996), McQuellon and colleagues (1996), and Schimmer and associates

(2001). In contrast the study reported by Sutherland and colleagues (1997) evaluated 231 allogeneic (5% syngeneic) subjects and the study performed by Molassiotis and Morris (1998) reported results from 28 unrelated allogeneic transplant recipients.

With the exception of the study by McQuellon and associates (1996) that focused on breast cancer transplant subjects, the diagnosis of the subjects within the studies varied greatly. The most common diagnoses included lymphoma (Hodgkins and non-Hodgkin's), leukemia, breast cancer, multiple myeloma, aplastic anemia, and myelodysplastic syndrome.

Use of a comparison group was only reported in four studies. These included Prieto and colleagues' (1996) study comparing transplant with bone cancer and *normal* individuals; Hann and associates' (1997) study comparing autologous transplants with noncancer; Molassiotis and associates' (1996) study comparing autologous and allogeneic transplant recipients with a maintenance chemotherapy group; and Zittoun and colleagues' (1997) study comparing autologous and allogeneic recipients with a chemotherapy group.

As oncology/hematology teams are acknowledging and reporting neuro/cognitive changes with high doses of antineoplastic therapy, awareness of and concern for the neuro/cognitive changes with transplantation is beginning to surface in QOL studies (Ahles, Tope, Furstenberg, Hann, & Mills, 1996; and Meyers et al., 1994). Pediatric QOL studies continue to be few in number. Studies by Kanabar and colleagues (1995), Nespoli and colleagues (1995), and Phipps and colleagues (1995) focused on QOL in pediatric recipients of transplants. Felder-Puig and associates (1999) focused on pediatric allogeneic transplant survivors 15–27 years old who were from 2 to 13 years (mean 7 years) posttransplant. Three research groups included teenagers in their studies with adult subjects. These studies were reported by Prieto and colleagues (1996) including individuals 15–54 years old, Jenkins, Lester, Alexander, and Whittaker (1994) including 15–56-year-old individuals, and Sutherland and associates (1997) including 16–56-year-old individuals. Parsons, Barlow, Levy, Supran, and Kaplan (1999) compared childrens' scores with parents and also with physician disease severity ratings. In general the respondents (and their parents) reported limited problems. Difficulties included neuropsychological disturbances; declines in social competence, self-esteem, and general emotional well-being; and anxiety regarding recurrence.

Measurement of QOL in HSCT

In spite of the growing interest in QOL and the awareness of its importance, ambiguity prevails regarding measurement of the concept (Ferrans, 1990; King et al., 1997). Various tools and global life satisfaction questions have been used to assess QOL in HSCT. Table 13-2 provides a listing of tools that have been used. In addition, studies frequently included specific, researcher-developed questions and instruments. At times studies have included only questions pertaining to specific physical aspects of QOL, such as pain, and have made global reference to QOL. In such instances it is important to acknowledge that only one domain of the multidimensional concept has been partially addressed. Although this dimension is a component of QOL, one must be cautious regarding generalization to global QOL. As will be noted by examination of Table 13-2, many of the tools listed do not focus on the multidimensional aspects of QOL. In fact, some of those listed are not truly QOL measures and are regarded as insufficient measures of health-related QOL (Osoba, 1994).

Measurement of global QOL is another area for attention. The ability of single items to measure this multidimensional concept is worth questioning. If the level of function in the different domains is not similar, subjects may have difficulty identifying an overall rating. When the level of function varies, the question may be answered based on the influence of a particular domain in subjects' lives.

The combination of disease-specific scales and global aspects of QOL, such as life satisfaction, is seen as an effort to address specific health situation concerns and the global aspects perceived as important by many of the individuals being evaluated (Mast, 1995). Although it is important for QOL tools to address disease- and treatment-specific areas of concern, the development and use of unique tools impact the ability to compare across groups. In contrast, however, some of the tools currently available do not specifically address areas pertaining to HSCT survivors in terms of long-term effects of the transplant. Examination of cognitive changes is one example of an area of concern (Ahles, Tope, Furstenberg, Hann, & Mills, 1996; Meyers et al., 1994). Two studies (Kemmler et al., 1999; King, Dobson, & Harnett, 1996) are noteworthy for their comparison of QOL instruments.

Another area of concern is the development of tools by a specific discipline. If QOL is truly dependent on the perception or interpretation of the individual, is there a need for discipline-specific tools? Should interventions to improve QOL be discipline or subject specific?

Measurement of QOL in pediatric subjects is also an area of concern (Parsons, Barlow, Levy, Sappran, & Kaplan, 1999). Instruments used in most QOL studies to date have been developed and tested on adults. Numerous questions regarding the best approach to measure QOL in children need to be addressed as there are increasing numbers of long-term survivors of pediatric HSCT. In addition to the heterogeneity issues related to type of transplant, disease process, and treatment discussed previously, because of the normal developmental changes that occur in the pediatric patient, age at the time of transplant, and at the time of study, must also be taken into account. Pediatric research has primarily focused on physiologic and psychologic effects of HSCT, rather than attempting to address the concept of QOL from the perspective of the recipient in this population.

Mast (1995) encourages researchers to address the appropriateness of the match of the QOL instrument(s) and definitions of QOL in proposed studies. The list of questions she identified to be addressed in the process of instrument selection include those shown in Table 13-3.

Qualitative studies such as those by Haberman and colleagues (1993) and Molassiotis and Morris (1998) have been helpful to tap HSCT recipients' dynamic, highly individual, and often very positive QOL experiences. The use of narrative questions, such as those in the City of Hope Quality of Life in Bone Marrow Transplant Survivors (see Appendix 2) has also produced rich data (Byar, Eilers, & Vose, 1999). Due to the current state of QOL instrument development and the ever-changing status of HSCT treatment protocols, the triangulation of quantitative data and descriptive qualitative data should be given strong consideration in order to adequately describe and measure this multidimensional concept (Eilers, Byar, & Nuss, 2000).

Future Research

The majority of QOL research in HSCT to date has been retrospective, cross-sectional studies of relatively small numbers of adults who have had transplants. There is a need for baseline pretransplant data to determine if the QOL changes noted are secondary to the HSCT conditioning regimen, the effects of the disease, treatments received prior to transplant, or unknown factors. Longitudinal studies that follow subjects over time will contribute to the knowledge base regarding the normal

---

Table 13-3. **Questions Used to Select an Instrument**

1. Which measures reflect your conceptual definition of QOL?

2. What degree of detail in QOL measurement is useful and practical, yet consistent with your conceptual definition?

3. Which of the operational definitions of QOL can you justify theoretically to suit the purpose and aims of measurement?

4. Are indicators of QOL in the instruments derived from actual patient responses rather than professional opinion?

5. Do the measures address areas of specific and overall QOL concern for your patients that are influenced by your nursing interventions?

6. Is a cancer-specific, disease-specific, or general-illness-specific QOL measure most useful?

Source: Adapted from Mast, 1995, p. 963. Used with permission.

recovery pattern and provide information regarding the point at which the effects noted become long-term effects as compared to merely a delay in recovery. Rehabilitation efforts also need to be addressed. For instance, did transplant survivors who had less physical, psychological, social, and spiritual problems receive more rehabilitation, have fewer side effects, or did they have better coping skills? The majority of studies have examined QOL in adults, which is important, yet in terms of long-term effects, the potential impact of HSCT on the surviving child should not be overlooked. Assessment of the real impact of HSCT on long-term physical and psychosocial functioning has been hampered by the paucity of prospective research that starts with pre-HSCT data and follows subjects for an extended period posttransplant.

There is a need for theory-driven, longitudinal, prospective studies that follow larger numbers of subjects over a longer period of time, using consistent, valid, and reliable instruments. Due to the heterogeneity of HSCT recipients, large samples are essential to allow broader generalization of findings. This would help to overcome the problems seen when individuals a few months to many years psottransplant are studied as one group. Although the group of choice is difficult to identify, the use of comparison groups would add strength to the findings of such studies. There is also a need for studies that include pediatric subjects and studies that look at the impact on the QOL of families involved in HSCT.

Clinicians and researchers must address questions regarding research methods and design in a joint effort to expand our body of knowledge regarding the impact of HSCT on QOL. Although consensus exists regarding the need for baseline data, the best time for obtaining those data is less clear. Due to the heterogeneity of potential HSCT candidates, perhaps baseline data may demonstrate a large variation in QOL pre-HSCT. The intent of the measures should be to determine not only the impact of the disease and previous treatment on QOL, but also recent changes in QOL secondary to the disease or treatment. For example, has the individual been in a fairly stable, declining, or improving state? Perhaps rather than QOL measures during the acute phase of HSCT, it would be more important to have consistent and accurate assessment of the morbidity associated with transplant, and relate it to changes in QOL from pre- to post-HSCT.

The exclusion from research of individuals with active recurrent disease also has significant implications. While it is important to protect vulnerable subjects, exclusion of these individuals only tells us the QOL of the individuals for whom HSCT successfully irradicated their disease. What about those who continue to struggle with disease? Does HSCT affect the end-stage disease experience for these individuals? Some of this information could be obtained from the medical records, but investigators must identify approaches for sensitively obtaining additional information in this area. The difficulty that persists is determining the alteration, if any, in the expected disease trajectory caused by HSCT. For example, how would the person have died if

HSCT had not been attempted? Such information is essential to assist individuals considered at high risk for death from their initial disease to make an informed decision regarding consenting for transplant or considering another treatment option. How do HSCT recipients whose disease has relapsed feel about their QOL? Does transplant alter symptomatology as the recipients die? What about the recipients who die—can we do a better job of palliative care for these individuals?

When to study QOL is also an issue to consider. Studies have frequently set one-year post-HSCT as the criterion for inclusion in research samples. Although the rationale for this approach can be justified based on waiting for stabilization and avoiding unnecessary subject burden during recovery, it has resulted in a gap in our knowledge base. We do not have a clear picture of QOL during the recovery phase posttransplant, and thus do not know the trajectory of the recovery process.

The period from 100 days to one year is marked by many physical effects and frequent checkups. It is more accurately viewed as a continuation of acute posttreatment recovery (Whedon & Ferrell, 1994). During this time the patient's status may be very labile in all QOL domains. Rehabilitation needs during this time period need to be articulated. Beyond the first year many latent physical effects resolve. Yet, some continue as chronic health problems. Existence during the first year is characterized as a tightrope walk or roller coaster because the individual is moving cautiously forward through each month of survival beyond the state of having chronic cancer and very slowly reaching toward an identity of cure. Shouldn't health care providers be concerned regarding the impact this has on QOL during the first year posttransplant? This is especially important since this is also the time when HSCT recipients may die with recurrent disease.

Studies to date have focused on the time beyond one year and as far out as 20-plus years as posttransplant, without breakdowns for different lengths of time. Is it appropriate to combine recipients from such a large range of time? What about the many changes in treatment protocols over that time? If longitudinal studies were used more extensively, then the question of when to study might change to: at what intervals should the survivors be followed? Some studies have offered data regarding a ceiling effect after one year (Whedon, Stearns, & Mills, 1995). Others refer to this stabilization after three years (Broers et al., 1998; Broers, Kaptein, LeCessie, Fibbe, & Hengeveld, 2000).

Researchers must look not only at when the transplant was performed, but also at the type of transplant and type of preparatory regimen to determine if generalization can be made to other types of HSCT. Perhaps some of the findings apply only to autologous, related allogeneic, or unrelated allogeneic transplants. At times the findings may apply only to certain preparatory regimens especially with the rapidity of changes in HSCT.

Who Should Provide the Information Regarding QOL?

In addition to HSCT recipients, other sources of information could increase our understanding of QOL. The intent of approaching each source must be clearly understood in order to facilitate appropriate utilization of the information collected. With the exception of when the HSCT recipient cannot respond, as in the situation with young children, the intent would be to use these groups not as proxies, but as supplemental sources of information. This is based on the assumption that QOL must be determined by the individual experience. Epstein and colleagues (1989) discussed the use of proxies to evaluate QOL. Their findings indicated that family members who were more involved with the subject were more likely to be able to evaluate QOL. However, when the care burden increased, QOL was usually evaluated as lower.

Family members can provide information regarding the assessment of the HSCT recipient's experience and the effect of the transplant on the QOL of the recipient's family. This is especially important to consider when HSCT recipients must travel great distances to tertiary treatment centers and when treatment for GVHD necessitates extended stays in the locality of the transplant center. As with other types of family research, one must address who the best family member is to ask and how to handle the family data (e.g., as one unit with the HSCT recipient or as individuals). Responses will depend on multiple factors including the relationship with the recipient, direct involvement with care, physical proximity to the transplant center, additional family and work responsibilities, the nature of the transplant course, and the outcome of the transplant. Family members interviewed at the time of the recipient's admission for transplant have frequently discussed the sense of "preparing for the worst and hoping for the best." This paradox keeps them in a state of uncertainty (Eilers, 1991, 1992). Another factor that should be considered is the residual effect on family survivors when the HSCT recipient dies.

Health care professionals can provide information regarding their perception of the effects of the transplant on an individual and provide assessment of the recipient's pre- and posttransplant status. It is important for professional health care providers' perceptions of HSCT QOL to be accurate, as their perceptions will influence the teaching, care, and counseling provided to recipients and family members. King, Ferrell, Grant, and Sakurai (1995) reported that nurses' perceptions of QOL for HSCT recipients were generally poorer than those reported by the recipients themselves. Although physicians have been involved in the study of QOL in HSCT, no data exist to date regarding physicians' perceptions of HSCT-related QOL.

Concerns Related to Assessing QOL in HSCT

A number of underlying concerns must be considered when assessing QOL in HSCT recipients. Some survivors report an unexpectedly high QOL (Whedon & Ferrell, 1994). It may be that survivors do not want to appear ungrateful to care providers, or they may be so consumed with "being alive" that they may not be able to recognize or accurately describe their QOL issues. What is the best approach to explore this issue?

Does the experience of a life-threatening condition such as cancer alter an individual's outlook on life, and thus, influence assessment of issues related to QOL? Just as paraplegics after critical accidents have adjusted to disability and identify their QOL higher than may be expected by others, do individuals with cancer experience a similar change in their assessment of priorities? Does dealing with a life-threatening illness alter one's concept of QOL? Are survivors just happy to be alive and not as concerned regarding alterations from *normal*? At the same time, if QOL assessment is to be provided by HSCT recipients, how can we question if their views have been altered by the experience of having a life-threatening condition? Perhaps we need to take into account that just as HSCT recipients tend to evaluate satisfaction with care higher due to a sense of indebtedness (Ferrell et al., 1992b), they may tend to be more accepting of residual effects of HSCT that may be seen as less desirable by others.

Challenges Related to QOL

One challenge is to evaluate the adjustment to limitations experienced by HSCT recipients. Such an effort would not be in an attempt to alter the adjustment, but rather to provide rehabilitation to decrease limitations and to facilitate coping in individuals with residual effects of transplant.

How do the following influence the quantitative measurement of the philosophically abstract and contextually dependent concept of QOL: (a) the paradox of risking death to live; (b) the meaning of the experience; and (c) the second opportunity for life? Symptoms and problems experienced by HSCT recipients in adaptation might be mediated by the individual's perspective on his or her situation (Altmaier, Gingrich, & Fyfe, 1991).

Another factor that is difficult to assess is the impact of what was expected by the individuals prior to HSCT. If the current level of function or outcome is much less than expected, does that influence assessment of the current situation and QOL? Likewise, if the expectation of HSCT was merely to buy time, are those individuals more accepting of residual effects? Also, how do expectations influence or alter the recipient's and the family's reception and understanding during informed consent process, and thus, their evaluation of posttransplant QOL.

Whedon and colleagues (1995) questioned whether some aspects of QOL are traitlike and prone to more stability while others are statelike and predisposed to instability. Are the traitlike aspects related to underlying diagnosis and history, or experience? Are these aspects that are traitlike similar across individuals or are these aspects traitlike for some and statelike for others? When examining changes in QOL over time posttransplant, how should one interpret improvements in some domains and worsening in others?

Since treatment protocols are ever-changing in transplant, there will be a potentially ever-changing spectrum of residual effects. Frequently, the long-term effect is not really known before protocols are altered to improve short-term results. Thus, researchers must address the unique challenge of attempting to account for differences in treatment protocols and the morbidity during the acute phase of transplant.

There has been a gradual evolution in the study of the concept of QOL in HSCT. But, as health care providers have improved the quality of research, changes in protocols and improved supportive treatment may have actually altered the potential impact of the complications previously identified. New medications may potentially increase or decrease the effect on QOL.

It may not always be easy to identify relationships between alterations from disease and HSCT as causative factors. When HSCT recipients are dealing with progressive disease and/or nonresponse to the transplant therapy, how can we ascertain if the impact on QOL is secondary to the underlying disease process or secondary to the treatment administered as part of the transplant? The importance of some changes or residual effects, such as alterations in fertility, will probably be different for the 22-year-old as compared to the 56-year-old HSCT recipient. Other residual effects such as fatigue and pain may function as confounding variables that actually affect assessment of QOL. Are these symptoms or effects that should be more appropriately managed, or irreversible residual effects? If the latter, how can professionals provide the necessary counseling to patients and families? In addition, some effects may actually be related to underlying disease or treatment prior to HSCT, such as sterility caused by disease or previous treatment.

Use of a Comparison Group

Although it would be helpful to compare HSCT survivors with another group, identification of the appropriate comparison group remains unclear, especially if attempting to identify an equivalent group. Chemotherapy patients have been used in comparison studies (Altmaier et al., 1991; Litwins et al., 1994; Molassiotis et al., 1996; Zittoun et al., 1997). Felder-Puig and associates (1999) compare three groups of pediatric transplant survivors, individuals with bone cancer, and normal individuals. Andrykowski and colleagues (Andrykowski, Altmaier, Barnett, Otis, Gingrich, & Henslee-Downey, 1990) used renal transplant recipients as a comparison and proposed that the solid organ transplant recipients, patients treated for other life-threatening conditions, and even the general population could serve as comparisons for HSCT recipients. Wolcott and associates (1986b) compared HSCT recipients with donors in a study of psychological adjustment. When generic instruments are included subjects are compared to population norms (Hann et al., 1997).

Implications for Nursing Practice

Nursing implications will be discussed in terms of application to nurses working with potential transplant candidates, nurses directly involved in transplant, and those caring for individuals posttransplant. The implications will be addressed for the same three time periods in terms of transplantation—pretransplant, during the acute phase, and posttransplant, with discussion of immediate and long-term posttransplant. Accurate information regarding QOL posttransplant is essential for nurses providing care to recipients and family members in this arena. As discussed in the study by King (1995), nurses' knowledge regarding QOL does have the potential to impact the care delivered. This knowledge or lack of it can influence both the information shared with potential recipients and families and the direct care delivered. Obtaining this information and remaining current regarding the implications for practice is not always an easy task.

Since HSCT encompasses a broad spectrum of recipients both in terms of diagnoses and treatment protocols, QOL outcomes for one segment of individuals may or may not be applicable to others. Thus, it is important for nurses to know the outcomes related to like scenarios. Due to the time required for adequate documentation regarding long-term effects and the rapidity with which transplant protocols change, this information frequently is not readily available. Therefore, it is often the role of staff working with potential transplant recipients and family members to facilitate information gathering and interpretation of the applicability of the findings. This is especially important in light of the fact that since potential recipients often are dealing with a life-threatening diagnosis, they may have an intense need to hear only stories with positive outcomes. In other situations, they may have difficulty sorting through information shared by former recipients and family members. At times such information may not be applicable to a given situation and may require some interpretation by knowledgeable professionals.

The process of adequately informing potential recipients and family members regarding transplant is a transdisciplinary responsibility that occurs in both formal and informal settings. Nurses caring for individuals receiving traditional treatment for high-risk diseases may find themselves being approached with statements such as, "The doctor mentioned that we might have to consider other options in the future, such as transplant. What do you think?" "Have you ever taken care of anyone who has had a transplant? Is it really as bad as it sounds?" Verbal and nonverbal responses in such situations have the potential to influence the individual's decisions regarding treatment choices. It is important that all nurses caring for potential HSCT recipients have adequate knowledge to be able to respond appropriately and know how to refer the individuals for additional information. All of the information shared with potential HSCT recipients and family members prior to the consent signing must be accurate and up-to-date in order to allow them to make the appropriate decision regarding treatment for their unique situation. Nurses not directly involved in transplant and therefore not in possession of current knowledge need to be aware of available resources to provide the potential recipient and family with the necessary information. Lack of sufficient data regarding the QOL of HSCT recipients over time interferes with this process.

Nurses caring for individuals scheduled for HSCT preparatory regimens must ensure that the individuals have an understanding of transplant and have had an opportunity to get their questions answered clearly. The nurse attempting this affirmation process must proceed with astute caution and be aware of findings indicating that the recipient may have been informed of probable death secondary to disease if more aggressive treatment isn't used. The positive attitude often displayed may be a manifestation of "hoping for the best" in light of having been "prepared for the worst" (Eilers, 1991, 1992). Once the transplant process has been initiated, recipients and family members must be supported in the decision they made. Nurses must exercise caution to avoid a sense of concern regarding the appropriateness of the decision for transplant.

Although there is limited outcomes data in HSCT to link specific nursing interventions with decreased posttransplant morbidity, astute nursing care is regarded as important. During HSCT, adequate symptom management, especially in terms of nausea, vomiting, and pain control, can decrease the discomfort associated with the acute phase of the treatment. Prevention of complications will decrease the likelihood of long-term effects related to major organ failure. Family members require support during this phase to decrease the negative impact of HSCT on them. Often family members can benefit from additional educational sessions regarding the process, side effects, and care expectations. Teaching regarding what to expect, an explanation of changes, and a discussion of the cause of certain signs and symptoms can provide information and decrease the stress for many families. Support groups can also decrease the sense of isolation and aloneness that family members may experience. Maintaining a whole-person focus will decrease the psychosocial and spiritual distress often experienced by recipients and family members.

Professionals teaching and providing support groups during the acute phase of HSCT must be aware of expected outcomes, so that the information can be accurately shared as questions arise. This awareness includes knowing that we should not generalize from one aspect of one domain identified in a given study to the impact on the multidimensional concept of QOL in general related to transplant.

After the acute phase of transplant, recipients and family members require reinforcement of earlier teaching regarding what to expect as they anxiously seek a return to *normal*. Therefore, it is important for staff to have adequate information regarding usual patterns of recovery. Awareness of these patterns can also guide decisions to initiate appropriate rehabilitative measures to expedite optimal recovery.

For some individuals there may be a need to facilitate the process Mishel and Murdaugh (1987) referred to as "redesigning the dream." HSCT recipients and family members may have approached transplant in anticipation of full recovery and find themselves dealing with a new array of problems, especially in the case of allogeneic recipients experiencing persistent difficulties with GVHD. These individuals may require support as the concept of an evolving or new normal becomes a reality for them.

HSCT recipients have identified "finding a cure" as an important thing for staff to do related to QOL (Ferrell et al., 1992a, 1992b). Professionals must work together to facilitate study in this area and collect the essential data regarding QOL post-HSCT. Participating in multidisciplinary studies will also increase the awareness of activities in various disciplines. Multidisciplinary collaborative approaches can also help to identify the preferred approach for working together in the most cost-effective manner to achieve the desired outcome in terms of survival and optimum QOL.

CONCLUSION

Many advances have been made in the field of hematopoietic stem cell transplantation since the first transplant in 1891. As overall survival rates have improved, there has been increased concern with QOL issues for transplant survivors. HSCT is a costly, life-threatening procedure with long-term effects on QOL. Even though interest in QOL has increased significantly, there have been limited systematic, theory-driven analyses of QOL related to HSCT. Few studies identify the conceptual or theoretical framework used, and some studies have failed to define QOL before measuring this concept. Furthermore, studies have frequently measured only one domain of QOL, and few of the tools used to measure QOL in transplant survivors have specifically addressed issues related to transplant. There is a need now for theory-driven, longitudinal prospective studies from patients' perspectives using reliable and valid tools. Clinicians need information regarding QOL in order to provide accurate information and education to potential patients and families and to improve the care delivered. Nurses caring for patients scheduled for HSCT are responsible for assuring that patients and families understand the transplant process and QOL issues. Additionally, information gathered through research about symptoms experienced and psychological, social, and spiritual problems will help nurses to improve symptom management and provide support for patients and families.

REFERENCES

Ahles, T., Tope, D., Furstenberg, C., Hann, D., & Mills, L. (1996). Psychologic and neurologic impact of autologous bone marrow transplantation. *Journal of Clinical Oncology, 14*(5), 1457–1462.

Altmaier, E. M., Gingrich, R. D., & Fyfe, M. A. (1991). Two year adjustment of bone marrow transplant survivors. *Bone Marrow Transplantation, 7*(4), 311–316.

Andrykowski, M. A., Altmaier, E. M., Barnett, R. L., Burish, T. B., Gingrich, R., & Henslee-Downey, P. J. (1990). Cognitive dysfunction in adult survivors of allogeneic marrow transplantation: Relationship to dose of total body irradiation. *Bone Marrow Transplantation, 6,* 269–276.

Andrykowski, M. A., Altmaier, E. M., Barnett, R. L., Otis, M. L., Gingrich, R., & Henslee-Downey, P. J. (1990). The quality of life in adult survivors of allogeneic bone marrow transplantation. Correlates and comparison with matched renal transplant recipients. *Transplantation, 50*(3), 399–406.

Andrykowski, M. A., Brady, M. J., Greiner, C. B., Altmaier, E. M., Burish, T. G., Antin, J. H., Gingrich, R., McGarigle, C., & Henslee-Downey, P. J. (1995). "Returning to normal" following bone marrow transplantation: Outcomes, expectations and informed consent. *Bone Marrow Transplantation, 15*(4), 573–581.

Andrykowski, M. A., Bruehl, S., Brady, M. J., & Henslee-Downey, P. J. (1995). Physical and psychosocial status of adults one year after bone marrow transplantation: A prospective study. *Bone Marrow Transplantation, 15,* 837–844.

Andrykowski, M. A., Carpenter, J. S., Greiner, C. B., Altmaier, E. M., Burish, T. G., Antin, J. H., Gingrich, R., Cordova, M. J., & Henslee-Downey, P. J. (1997). Energy level and sleep quality following bone marrow transplantation. *Bone Marrow Transplantation, 20,* 669–679.

Andrykowski, M. A., Greiner, C. B., Altmaier, E. M., Burish, T. G., Antin, J. H., Gingrich, R., McGarigle, C., & Henslee-Downey, P. J. (1995). Quality of life following bone marrow transplantation: Findings from a multicentre study. *British Journal of Cancer, 71,* 1322–1329.

Andrykowski, M. A., Henslee, P. J., & Barnett, R. L. (1989). Longitudinal assessment of psychosocial functioning of adult survivors of allogeneic bone marrow transplantation. *Bone Marrow Transplantation, 4,* 505–509.

Andrykowski, M. A., Henslee, P. J., & Farrall, M. G. (1989). Physical and psycho-social functioning of adult survivors of allogeneic bone marrow transplantation. *Bone Marrow Transplantation* 4(1), 75–81.

Badell, I., Igual, L., Gomez, P., Bureo, E., Ortega, J. J., Cubells, J., Muñoz, A., Martinez, A., Madero, L., Vergeguer, A., Torres, A., Richard, C., Olivè, T., Danile, M., & Bayé, R. (1998). Quality of life in young adults having received a BMT during childhood: a BETMON study. *Bone Marrow Transplantation,* 21:Suppl 2, S68–S71.

Baker, R., Curbow, B., & Wingard, J. R. (1991). Role retention and quality of life of bone marrow transplant survivors. *Social Science in Medicine,* 32(6), 697–704.

Baker, F., Marcellus, D., Zabora, J., Polland, A., & Jodrey, D. (1997). Psychological distress among adult patients being evaluated for bone marrow transplantation. *Psychosomatics,* 38(1), 10–19.

Baker, F., Wingard, J. R., Curbow, B., Zabora, J., Jodrey, D., Fogarty, L., & Legro, M. (1994). Quality of life of bone marrow transplant long-term survivors. *Bone Marrow Transplantation,* 13, 589–596.

Beatty, P. G., Clift, R. A., Mickelson, E. M., Nisperos, B. B., Flournoy, N., Martin, P. J., Sanders, J. E., Stewart, P., Buckner, C. D., Storb, R., & Hansen, J. A. (1985). Marrow transplantation from related donors other than HLA-identical siblings, *New England Journal of Medicine,* 313(13), 765–771.

Belec, R. H. (1992). Quality of life: Perceptions of long-term survivors of bone marrow transplantation. *Oncology Nursing Forum,* 19(1), 31–37.

Broers, S., Hengeveld, M. W., Kaptein, A. A., LeCessie, S., van de Loo, F., & de Vries, T. (1998). Are pretransplant psychological variables related to survival after bone marrow transplantation? A prospective study of 123 consecutive patients. *Journal of Psychosomatic Research,* 45(4), 341–351.

Broers, S., Kaptein, A.A., LeCessie, S., Fibbe, W., & Hengeveld, M. W. (2000). Psychological functioning and quality of life following bone marrow transplantation: a 3-year follow-up study. *Journal of Psychosomatic Research,* 48(1), 11–21.

Brown, H. N., & Kelly, M. J. (1976). Stages of bone marrow transplantation: A psychiatric perspective. *Psychosomatic Medicine,* 38(6), 439–446.

Buchsel, P. C. (1986). Long-term complications of allogeneic bone marrow transplantation: Nursing implications. Oncology Nursing Forum, 13(6), 61–70.

Buchsel, P. C., & Kelleher, J. (1989). Bone marrow transplantation. *Nursing Clinics of North America,* 24(4), 907–938.

Bush, N. E., Haberman, M., Donaldson, G., & Sullivan, K. M. (1995). Quality of life of 125 adults surviving 6–18 years after bone marrow transplantation. *Social Science and Medicine,* 40, 479–490.

Byar, K., Eilers, J., & Vose, J. (1999). Quality of life of individuals at least five years or more post-autologous blood and marrow stem cell transplant. *Oncology Nursing Forum, 26*(2), 387, Abstract #132A.

Cella, D. F., & Tulsky, D. S. (1990). Measuring quality of life today: Methodological aspects. *Oncology, 4*(5), 29–38.

Chao, N. J., Tierney, D. K., Bloom, J. R., Long, G. D., Barr, T. A., & Stallbaum, B. A. (1992). Dynamic assessment of quality of life after autologous bone marrow transplantation. *Blood, 80*(3), 825–830.

Colon, E. A., Callies, A. L., Popkin, M. K., & McGlave, P. B. (1991). Depressed mood and other variables related to bone marrow transplantation survival in acute leukemia. *Psychosomatics, 32*, 420–425.

Curbow, B., Somerfield, M. R., Baker, F., Wingard, J. R., & Legro, M. W. (1993). Personal changes, dispositional optimism, and psychological adjustment to bone marrow transplantation. *Journal of Behavioral Medicine, 16*(5), 423–443.

Decker, W. A. (1995). Psychosocial considerations for bone marrow transplant recipients. *Critical Care Nursing Quarterly, 17*(4), 67–73.

Dow, K. H., & Ferrell, B. R. (1994). Long-term cancer survival: A quality of life model. *Quality of Life—A Nursing Challenge, 3*(4), 81–86.

Eilers, J. (1991). *Family member perception of bone marrow transplant: A qualitative pilot study.* Unpublished research pilot study, University of Nebraska Medical Center, Omaha, NE.

Eilers, J. (1992). *Uncertainty in family members of bone marrow transplant patients.* Unpublished research study, University of Nebraska Medical Center, Omaha, NE.

Eilers, J., Berger, A. M., & Petersen, M. C. (1988). Development, testing and application of the Oral Assessment Guide. *Oncology Nursing Forum, 15*(3), 325–330.

Eilers, J., Byar, K., and Nuss, S. (2000). The lived experience of autologous blood and marrow stem cell transplant survivors. *Oncology Nursing Forum, 27*(2), 352, Abstract #202.

Epstein, A. M., Hall, J. A., Tognetti, J., Son, L. H., & Conant, L. (1989). Using proxies to evaluate quality of life. *Medical Care, 27*(3) (Suppl.), 591–598.

Ersek, M. (1992). The process of maintaining hope in adults undergoing bone marrow transplantation for leukemia. *Oncology Nursing Forum, 19*(6), 883–889.

Ezzone, S., Jolly, D., Replogle, K., Kapoor, N., & Tutschka, P. T. (1993). Survey of oral hygiene regimens among bone marrow transplant centers. *Oncology Nursing Forum, 20*(9), 1375–1381.

Felder-Puig, R., Peters, C., Matthes-Martin, S., Lamche, M., Felsberger, C., Gadner, H., & Topf, R. (1999). Psychosocial adjustment of pediatric patients after allogeneic stem cell transplantation. *Bone Marrow Transplantation, 24*, 75–80.

Ferrans, C. E. (1990). Quality of life: Conceptual issues. *Seminars in Oncology Nursing, 6*, 248–254.

Ferrell, B., Grant, M., Schmidt, G. M., Whitehead, C., Fonbuena, P., & Forman, S. J. (1992a). The meaning of quality of life for bone marrow transplant survivors. Part 1: The impact of bone marrow transplant on quality of life. *Cancer Nursing, 15*(3), 153–160.

Ferrell, B., Grant, M., Schmidt, G. M., Whitehead, C., Fonbuena, P., & Forman, S. J. (1992b). The meaning of quality of life for bone marrow transplant survivors. Part 2: Improving quality of life for bone marrow transplant survivors. *Cancer Nursing, 15*(4), 247–253.

Ford, R., & Ballard, B. (1988). Acute complications after bone marrow transplantation. *Seminars in Oncology Nursing, 4*(1), 15–24.

Ford, R., & Eisenberg, S. (1990). Bone marrow transplant: Recent advances and nursing implications. *Nursing Clinics of North America, 25*(2), 405–422.

Franco, T., & Gould, D. (1994). Allogeneic bone marrow transplantation. *Seminars in Oncology Nursing, 10*(1), 3–11.

Fromm, K., Andrykowski, M. A., & Hunt, J. (1996). Positive and negative psychosocial sequelae of bone marrow transplantation: Implications for quality of life assessment. *Journal of Behavioral Medicine, 19*(3), 221–240.

Gardner, G. G., August, C. S., & Githens, J. (1977). Psychological issues in bone marrow transplantation. *Pediatrics, 60*(4), 625–631.

Gaston-Johansson, F., & Foxall, F. (1996). Psychological correlates of quality of life across the autologous bone marrow transplant experience. *Cancer Nursing, 19*(3), 170–176.

Gaston-Johansson, F., Franco, T., & Zimmerman, L. (1992). Pain and psychological distress in patients undergoing autologous bone marrow transplantation, *Oncology Nursing Forum, 19*(1), 41–48.

Gluckman, E., Broxmeyer, H. E., Auerbach, A. D., Friedman, H. S., Douglas, G. W., Gevergie, A., Esperou, H., Thierry, D., Socie, G., Lehn, P., Cooper, S., English, D., Kurtzberg, J., Bard, J., & Boyse, E. A. (1989). Hematopoietic reconstitution in a patient with Fanconi's anemia by means of umbilical cord blood from an HLA-identical sibling. *New England Journal of Medicine, 321*, 1174–1178.

Grant, F., Ferrell, B., Schmidt, G. M., Fonbuena, P., Niland, J. C., Forman, S. J. (1992). Measurement of quality of life in bone marrow transplantation survivors. *Quality of Life Research*, 375–384.

Haberman, M. R. (1988). Psychosocial aspects of bone marrow transplantation. *Seminars in Oncology Nursing, 4*, 55–59.

Haberman, M., Bush, N., Young, K., & Sullivan, K. M. (1993). Quality of life of adult long-term survivors of bone marrow transplantation: A qualitative analysis of narrative data. *Oncology Nursing Forum, 20*(10), 1545–1553.

Hann, D. M., Jacobsen, P. B., Martin, S. C., Kronish, L. E., Azzarello, L. M., & Fields, K. K. (1997). Quality of life following bone marrow transplantation for breast cancer: A comparative study. *Bone Marrow Transplantation, 19*, 257–264.

Heinonen, H., Volin, L., Uutela, A., Zevon, M., Barrick C., & Ruutu, T. (2001). Gender-associated differences in the quality of life after allogeneic BMT. *Bone Marrow Transplantation, 28*, 503–509.

Hengeveld, M. W., Houtman, R. B., & Zwaan, F. E. (1988). Psychological aspects of bone marrow transplantation: A retrospective study of 17 long-term survivors. *Bone Marrow Transplantation, 3*, 69–75.

Hjermstad, M. J., & Kaasa, S. (1995). Quality of life in adult cancer patients treated with bone marrow transplantation—a review of the literature. *European Journal of Cancer, 31A*(2), 163–173.

Holzner, B., Kemmler, G., Sperner-Unterweger, B., Kopp, M., Dünser, M., Margreiter, R., Marchitz, I., Nachbaur, D., Fleischhacker, W. W., & Greil, R. (2001). Quality of life measurement in oncology—a matter of the assessment instrument? *European Journal of Cancer, 37*, 2349–2356.

Horowitz, M. M. (1995). New IBMTR/ABMTR slides summarize current use and outcome of allogeneic and autologous transplants. IBMTR News Letter 2, 1–8.

Hutchison, M. I., & King, A. (1983). A nursing perspective on bone marrow transplantation. *Nursing Clinics of North America, 18*(3), 511–520.

Jenkins, P. L., Liningtton, A., & Whittaker, J. A. (1991). A retrospective study of psychosocial morbidity in bone marrow transplant recipients. *Psychosomatics, 32*(1), 65–71.

Juttner, C. A., To, L. B., Ho, J. Q. K., Bardy, P. G., Dyson, P. G., Haylock, D. N., & Kimber, R. J. (1988). Early lympho-hemopoietic recovery after autografting using peripheral blood stem cells in acute non-lymphoblastic leukemia. *Transplantation Proceedings, XX*(1), 40–43.

Kanabar, D. J., Attard-Montalto, S., Saha, M., Kingston, J. E., Malpas, J. E., & Eden, O. B. (1995). Quality of life in survivors of childhood cancer after megatherapy with autologous bone marrow rescue. *Pediatric Hematology and Oncology, 12*, 29–36.

Kessinger, A., Armitage, J. O., Landmark, J. D., Smith, D. M., & Weisenburger, D. D. (1986). Autologous peripheral hematopoietic stem cell transplantation restores hematopoietic function following marrow ablative therapy. *Blood, 71*(3), 723–727.

King, C. R. (1995). Latent effects and quality of life one year after marrow and stem cell transplantation. *Quality of Life—A Nursing Challenge, 4*(2), 40–45.

King, C. R., Ferrell, B. R., Grant, M., & Sakurai, C. (1995). Nurses' perceptions of the meaning of quality of life for bone marrow transplant survivors. *Cancer Nursing, 18*(2), 118–129.

King, C. R., Haberman, M., Berry, D. L., Bush, N., Butler, L., Dow, K. H., Ferrell, B., Grant, M., Gue, D., Hinds, P., Kreuer, J., Padilla, G., & Underwood, S. (1997). Quality of life and the cancer experience: The state-of-the-knowledge. *Oncology Nursing Forum, 24*(1), 27–41.

Klemm, P. (1985). Cyclosporin A: Use in preventing graft-versus-host disease. *Oncology Nursing Forum, 12*(5), 25–32.

Kopp, M., Schweigkofler, H., Holzner, B., Nachbaur, D., Niedwewieser, D., Fleischhacker, W. W., Kemmler, G., & Sperner-Unterweger, B. (2000). EORTC QLQ-C30 and FACT-BMT for the measurement of quality of life in bone marrow transplant recipients: A comparison. *Eurpoean Journal of Haematology, 65,* 97–103.

Kopp, M., Schweigkofler, H., Holzner, B., Nachbaur, D., Niedwewieser, D., Fleischhacker, W. W., & Sperner-Unterweger, B. (1998). Time after bone marrow transplantation as an important variable for quality of life: Results of a - cross-sectional investigation using two different instruments for quality-of-life assessment. *Annals of Hematology, 77*(1–2), 27–32.

Leigh, S., Wilson, K. C. M., Burns, R., & Clark, R. E. (1995). Psychosocial morbidity in bone marrow transplant recipients: A prospective study. *Bone Marrow Transplantation, 16*(5), 635–640.

Lesko, L. M., Ostroff, J. S., Mumma, G. H., Mashberg, D. E., & Holland, J. C. (1992). Long-term psychological adjustment of acute leukemia survivors: Impact of bone marrow transplantation versus conventional chemotherapy. *Psychosomatic Med, 54,* 30–47.

Litwins, N. M., Rodrigue, J. R., & Weiner, R. S. (1994). Quality of life in adult recipients of bone marrow transplantation. *Psychological Reports, 75,* 323–328.

Mast, M. E. (1995). Definition and measurement of quality of life in oncology nursing research: Review and theoretical implications. *Oncology Nursing Forum, 22*(6), 957–964.

McConn, R. (1987). Skin changes following bone marrow transplantation. *Cancer Nursing, 10*(2), 82–84.

McGuire, D. B., Altomonte, V., Peterson, D. E., Wingard, J. R., Jones, R. J., & Grochow, L. B. (1993). Patterns of mucositis and pain in patients receiving preparative chemotherapy and bone marrow transplantation. *Oncology Nursing Forum, 20*(10), 1493–1502.

McQuellon, R. P., Craven, B., Russell, G. B., Hoffman, S., Cruz, J. M., Perry, J. J., & Hurd, D. D. (1996). Quality of life in breast cancer patients before and after autologous bone marrow transplantation. *Bone Marrow Transplantation, 18,* 579–584.

McQuellon, R. P., Russell, G. B., Cella, D. F., Craven, B. L., Brady, M., Bonomi, A., & Hurd, D. D. (1997). Quality of life measurement in bone marrow transplantation: Development of the Functional Assessment of Cancer Therapy-Bone Marrow Transplant (FACT-BMT) scale. *Bone Marrow Transplant, 19,* 357–368.

McQuellon, R. P., Russell, G. B., Rambo, T. D., Craven, B. L., Radford, J., Perry, J. J., Cruz, J., & Hurd, D. D. (1998). Quality of life and psychological distress of bone marrow transplant recipients: The "time trajectory" to recovery over the first year. *Bone Marrow Transplantation, 21,* 477–486.

Meyers, C., Weitzner, M., Byrne, K., Vlentine, A., Champlin, R. E., & Przepiorka, D. (1994). Evaluation of the neurobehavioral functioning of patients before, during, and after bone marrow transplantation. *Journal of Clinical Oncology, 12*(4), 820–826.

Mishel, M. H., & Murdaugh, C. (1987). Family adjustment to heart transplantation: Redesigning the dream. *Nursing Research, 36*(6), 332–338.

Molassiotis, A., Boughton, B. J., Burgoyne, T., & van den Akker, O. B. A. (1995). Comparison of the overall quality of life in 50 long-term survivors of autologous and allogeneic bone marrow transplantation. *Journal of Advanced Nursing, 22,* 509–516.

Molassiotis, A., & Morris, P. J. (1998). The meaning of quality of life and the effects of unrelated donor bone marrow transplants for chronic myeloid leukemia in adult long-term survivors. *Cancer Nursing, 21*(3), 205–211.

Molassiotis, A., van den Akker, O. B. A., Milligan, D. W., Goldman, J. M., & Boughton, B. J. (1996). Psychological adaptation and symptom distress in bone marrow transplant recipients. *Psycho-Oncology, 5,* 9–22.

Molassiotis, A., van den Akker, O. B. A., Milligan, D. W., Goldman, J. M., Boughton, B. J., Holmes, J. A., & Thomas, S. (1996). Quality of life in long-term survivors of marrow transplantation: Comparison with a matched group receiving maintenance chemotherapy. *Bone Marrow Transplantation, 17*(2), 249–258.

Molassiotis, A., van den Akker, O. B. A., Milligan, D. W., & Goldman, J. M. (1997). Symptom distress, coping style and biological variables as predictors of survival after bone marrow transplantation. *Journal of Psychosomatic Research 42*(3), 275–285.

Mumma, G. H., Mashberg, D., & Lesko L. M. (1992). Long-term psychosexual adjustment of acute leukemia survivors: Impact of marrow transplantation versus conventional chemotherapy. *General Hospital Psychiatry, 14,* 43–55.

Murphy, K. C., Jenkins, P. L., & Whittaker, J. A. (1996). Psychosocial morbidity and survival in adult bone marrow transplant recipients—a follow-up study. *Bone Marrow Transplantation, 18,* 199–201.

Neitzert, C. S., Ritvo, P., Dancey, J., Weiser, K., Murray, C., & Avery, J. (1998). The psychosocial impact of bone marrow transplantation: a review of the literature. *Bone Marrow Transplantation, 22,* 409–422.

Nespoli, L., Verri, A. P., Locatelli, F., Bertuggia, L., Taibi, R. M., & Burgio, G. R. (1995). The impact of pediatric bone marrow transplantation on quality of life. *Quality of Life Research, 4*, 233–240.

Neuser, J. (1988). Personality and survival time after bone marrow transplantation. *Journal of Psychosomatic Research, 32*(4/5), 451–455.

Nims, J., & Strom, S. (1988). Late complications of bone marrow transplant recipients: Nursing care issues. *Seminars in Oncology Nursing, 4*(1), 47–54.

Osoba, D. (1994). Lessons learned from measuring health-related quality of life in oncology. *Journal of Clinical Oncology, 12*(3), 608–616.

Parker, N., & Cohen, T. (1983). Acute graft-versus-host disease in allogeneic marrow transplantation. A nursing perspective. *Nursing Clinics of North America, 18*(3), 569–577.

Parsons, S. K., Barlow, S. E., Levy, S. L., Supran, S. E., & Kaplan, S. H. (1999). Health-related quality of life in pediatric bone marrow transplant survivors: According to whom? *International Journal of Cancer, Supplement, 12*, 46–51.

Patenaude, A. F., Szymanski, L., & Rappeport, J. (1979). Psychological costs of bone marrow transplantation in children. *American Journal of Orthopsychiatry, 49*(3), 409–422.

Pavletic, Z. S., & Armitage, J. O. (1996). Bone marrow transplantation for cancer—An update. *The Oncologist, 1*, 159–168.

Pfefferbaum, B., Lindamood, M., & Wiley, W. F. (1978). Stages in pediatric bone marrow transplantation. *Pediatrics, 61*(4), 625–628.

Phipps, S., Brenner, M., Heslop, H., Krance, R., Jayawardene, D., & Mulhern, R. (1995). Psychological effects of bone marrow transplantation on children and adolescents: Preliminary report of a longitudinal study. *Bone Marrow Transplantation, 15*, 829–835.

Popkin, M. K., Moldow, C. F., Hall, R. C. W., Branda, R. F., & Yarchoan, R. (1977). Psychiatric aspects of allogeneic bone marrow transplantation for aplastic anemia. *Diseases of the Nervous System, 38*(11), 925–927.

Prieto, J. M., Saez, R., Carreras, E., Atala, J., Sierra, J., Rovira, M., Batlle, M., Blanch, J., Escobar, R., Vieta, E., Gomez, E., Rozman, C., & Cierera, E. (1996). *Bone Marrow Transplantation, 17*, 1133–1142.

Reiffers, J., Bernard, P., David, B., Bezon, G., Sarrat, A., Marit, G., Moulinier, J., & Broustet, A. (1986). Successful autologous transplantation with peripheral blood hematopoietic cells in a patient with acute leukemia. *Experimental Hematology, 14*, 312–315.

Rodrigue, J. R., Boggs, S. R., Weiner, R. S., & Behen, J. M. (1993). Mood, coping style, and personality functioning among adult bone marrow transplant candidates. *Psychosomatics, 34*(2), 159–165.

Saleh, U. S., & Brockopp, D. V. (2001). Quality of life one year following bone marrow transplantation: Psychometric evaluation of the quality of life in bone marrow transplant survivors tool. *Oncology Nursing Forum, 28*(9), 1457–1464.

Schimmer, A. D., Elliott, M. E., Abbey, S. E., Raiz, L. Keating, A., Beanlands, H. J., McCay, E., Messner, H. A., Lipton, J. H., & Devins, G. M. (2001). Illness intrusiveness among survivors of autologous blood and marrow transplantation. *Cancer, 92*(12), 3147–3154.

Schmidt, G. M., Niland, J. C., Forman, S. J., Fonbuena, P. P., Dagis, A. C., Grant, M. M., Ferrell, B. R., Barr, T. A., Stallbaum, B. A., Chao, N. J., & Blume, K. G. (1993). Extended follow-up in 212 long-term allogeneic bone marrow transplant survivors. Issues of quality of life. *Transplantation, 55*(3), 551–557.

Shaffer, S., & Wilson, J. N. (1993). Bone marrow transplantation: Critical care implications. *Critical Care Nursing, Clinics of North America, 5*(3), 531–542.

Sutherland, H. J., Fyles, G. M., Adams, G., Hao, Y., Lipton, J. H., Minden, M. D., Meharchand, J. M., Atkins, H., Tejpar, I., & Messner, H. A. (1997). Quality of life following bone marrow transplantation: A comparison of patient reports with population norms. *Bone Marrow Transplantation, 19*, 1129–1136.

Syrjala, K. L., Chapko, M. K., Vitaliano, P. P., Cummings, C., & Sullivan, K. M. (1993). Recovery after allogeneic marrow transplantation: Prospective study of predictors of long-term physical and psychosocial functioning. *Bone Marrow Transplantation, 11*, 319–327.

Thomas, E. D. (1994). Nobel lecture, December 8, 1990. Bone marrow transplantation—Past, present and future. *Scand Journal Immunol, 39*, 339–345.

Vose, J. M., Kennedy, B. C., Bierman, P. J., Kessinger, A., & Armitage, J. O. (1992). Long-term sequelae of autologous bone marrow or peripheral stem cell transplantation for lymphoid malignancies. *Cancer, 69*, 784–789.

Whedon, M., & Ferrell, B. R. (1994). Quality of life in adult bone marrow transplant patients: Beyond the first year. *Seminars in Oncology Nursing, 10*(1), 42–57.

Whedon, M., Stearns, D., & Mills, L. E. (1995). Quality of life of long-term adult survivors of autologous bone marrow transplantation. *Oncology Nursing Forum, 22*(10), 1527–1537.

Wingard, J. R. (1991). Historical perspectives and future directions. In M. B. Whedon (Ed.), *Bone marrow transplantation principles, practice, and nursing insights* (pp. 3–19). Boston: Jones and Bartlett.

Wingard, J. R., Curbow, B., Baker, F., & Piantadosi, S. (1991). Health, functional status, and employment of adult survivors of bone marrow transplantation. *Annals of Internal Medicine, 114*(2), 113–118.

Wingard, J. R., Curbow, B., Baker, R., Zabora, J., & Piantadosi, S. (1992). Sexual satisfaction in survivors of bone marrow transplantation. *Bone Marrow Transplantation, 9*, 185–190.

Wolcott, D. L., Fawzy, F. I., & Wellisch, D. K. (1987). Psychiatric aspects of bone marrow transplantation: A review and current issues. *Psychiatric Medicine, 4,* 299–317.

Wolcott, D. L., Wellisch, D. K., Fawzy, F. I., & Landsverk, J. (1986a). Adaptation of adult bone marrow transplant recipient long-term survivors. *Transplantation, 41*(4), 478–484.

Wolcott, D. L., Wellisch, D. K., Fawzy, F. I., & Landsverk, J. (1986b). Psychological adjustment of adult bone marrow transplant donors whose recipient survives. *Transplantation, 4,* 484–488.

Wujcik, D., Ballard, B., Camp-Sorrell, D. (1994). Selected complications of allogeneic bone marrow transplantation. *Seminars in Oncology Nursing, 10*(1), 28–41.

Zittoun, R., Suciu, S., Watson, M. Solbu, G., Muss, P., Mandelli, F., Stryckmans, P., Peetermans, M., Thaler, J., Resegotti, L., Dardenne, M., & Willemze, R. (1997). Quality of life in patients with acute myelogenous leukemia in prolonged first complete remission after bone marrow transplantation (allogeneic or autologous) or chemotherapy: A cross-sectional study of the EORTC-Gimenma AML 8A trial. *Bone Marrow Transplantation, 20*(4), 307–315.

Chapter

14

A European Perspective on
Quality of Life
of Stem Cell Transplantation Patients

MONICA C. FLIEDNER

Nursing aspects of quality of life (QOL) of patients who underwent a bone marrow transplantation (BMT) or peripheral blood cell transplantation (PBCT) has been assessed for many years. There are several organizations that investigate aspects of QOL. The most important organization in Europe, the European Group for Blood and Marrow Transplantation (EBMT), is primarily examining all medical and nursing aspects of the stem cell transplanted (SCT) patient. In 1975, a group of ten physicians from Switzerland, France, and the Netherlands started discussing medical and scientific aspects of BMT annually. Two years later, scientists from Germany, Italy, and Great Britain joined this growing organization. These countries were followed by all other European countries in the following years. In 1985, the first EBMT nurses' conference was organized by nurses to improve networking nurses involved in bone marrow (and later blood cell) transplantations. Since then the conference has been organized on an annual basis and the number of attendees has grown from 20 to more than 400 per conference. The conference is organized and held at the same time as the EBMT conference for the physicians and scientists. Since the beginning the physicians and nurses have worked closely together, resulting in a combined session for the two groups since 1995. The medical side of the EBMT has many different working parties such as acute leukemia, solid tumors, aplastic anemia, and infection. The Late Effect and Infection Working parties may be of special interest to nurses and collaborators.

The purpose of this chapter is to provide an overview of the many studies and experiences concerning the QOL of the SCT patient, which were presented at the EBMT Nurses Conferences between 1985 and 2001. This overview will facilitate international communication among nurses working on units where blood or marrow transplantations are performed. Geographical differences between participating countries in SCT (Goldman 1993; Gratwohl, Hermans, Goldman, & Gahrton, 1993) will be considered in the overview.

It is important for the patient to realize the impact that transplantation may have on his or her later life. Therefore, nurses need to define patients at risk and areas where special attention is necessary to promote, enhance, and support the quality of the patients' lives. Some of the goals of nursing, therefore, are to promote the strength of the patients to optimize their abilities and to improve their QOL. Consideration of QOL should play an important role each time the nursing and medical staff, together with the patient and his or her family, discuss the continuity of treatment (Fliedner, 1992). However, how can nurses improve the QOL of patients after a transplantation if the concept is unclear and if the goal is still ambiguous? The caring medical staff should realize that nurses, doctors, and the patient perceive the quality of the patient's life differently. To measure and evaluate the QOL of the patient there should be an agreed-upon definition. In other chapters of this book definitions are discussed; therefore, it will not be the purpose of this chapter to completely accomplish the task of defining QOL but rather to give an overview of different aspects on which nurses, working with the transplant patients, may choose to focus.

The meaning of life is altered immediately once a patient is diagnosed with cancer. When a person is evaluated for SCT, in a sense, everything that promotes life satisfaction is taken away. The independence of the person is *significantly* restricted. The individual is limited in his or her freedom to walk around and do whatever pleases him or her. The person usually has to stay close to the unit or hospital and during the aplastic phase, or the isolation period, he or she is even more restricted. The person's intimacy with loved ones can be interrupted as it takes energy for the individual to stay in contact physically and mentally. One's sense of well-being, vitality, and "health" is distorted by the treatment and it takes quite a long time for the patient to feel healthy again. The struggle to survive the disease and its treatment can overshadow the concern for QOL for each patient. What makes the patient's life worth living and what contributes to his or her QOL are different for each patient and, if asked, each patient would give a different answer. It seems obvious that QOL is unique for every individual and it can also change over time and even during a given day. Cultural, spiritual, ethical, and religious values, and other life experiences influence perceptions of meaning and consequences of QOL (Zhan, 1993). Since the phrase QOL was first coined soon after World War II, it has become a significant consideration for society in general and specifically in health care. It was not until 1977 that the term QOL first received a separate heading in the *Index Medicus* (Frank-Stromborg, 1992).

An overall definition of what QOL is cannot be found in the literature. There seems as many definitions for the concept as there are people who use it. Almost all authors emphasize the subjective and individualized nature of QOL. Often, satisfaction of needs in the physical, psychological, social, activity, material, and structural domains of life are evaluated (Meeberg, 1993). Other authors look at the dimension in terms of fulfillment of life plans or emotional well-being. It is important to accept that QOL is what the person thinks and says it is at that particular moment, because it can change quickly. It is not always possible to reduce QOL to a simple measurement because it is a multifaceted phenomenon (Yang, 1990). This makes it hard to understand in a society that is more and more materialistic and in which things are only considered real when they can be measured and made visible (Yang, 1990). Happiness and a feeling of well-being will result from attending to issues that improve QOL. When individuals rate their life as high quality, they are experiencing a positive sense of self-esteem, self-concept, and pride.

Most clinical trials also include examining how QOL is affected by the treatment. Specific questions should be included when investigating the SCT population. However, it is important that the outcomes of the research not only be analyzed, but also be considered when developing a new protocol. Five major dimensions should be included in any assessment of QOL (Aaronson, 1988; Ferrell et al., 1992a, 1992b; Haberman, Bush, Young, & Sullivan, 1993; Spilker, 1990).

1. *Physical status* and functional abilities such as activity level and/or physical symptoms including infertility.

2. *Psychological status* such as life satisfaction and achievement of life goals, affect, perceived stress, self-esteem, psychological defense mechanisms, and coping.

3. *Social interactions* such as friendship and social support, family, marriage, including sexual satisfaction.

4. *Economic status* such as occupation, education, and financial status.

5. *Spiritual aspects* such as religiosity, inner strength, hope, and despair.

A stem cell transplantation has a serious impact on divergent dimensions of life. SCT influences physical well-being by the problems of infertility, coping with chronic graft-versus-host disease (GVHD), impaired nutrition, cataracts, and ongoing fatigue. Psychological well-being is influenced by anxiety, depression, and coping with survival. SCT acts on social well-being by causing a change in roles, relationships, and by burdening caregivers. Spiritual well-being is affected by altered beliefs, different values, and changes in religiosity (Ferrell et al., 1992a, 1992b).

Prior to any research involving patients and/or families or partners, one should consider that participating in tests may add another stress factor. However, most patients and family members welcome being asked how they feel and appreciate the attention given to them. It must be realized that participation in a research project evaluating the psychosocial burden of a transplantation usually does not involve any other therapeutic actions or interventions. Thus, it is important to follow up after completion of the study or develop specific intervention as needed.

EBMT Nurses Group Research

In the past 15 years, European nurses have contributed some interesting projects and studies to the research on the concept of QOL. QOL prior to, during, and after transplantation has been a topic since the beginning of the EBMT conferences. The work by nurses has developed over the years from describing personal experiences to empirical research studies. More and more systematic approaches have been used to look more closely at how QOL is affected by treatment and how nurses can play a role in promoting QOL. All of these approaches have been published in the proceedings of the EBMT nurses' conference from 1985 to 1991. Since 1992 many presentations have been published in the *EBMT Nurses Group Newsletter*, which changed its name in 1993 to *EBMT Nurses Group Journal*.

Aspects of Adult Psychosocial Care Prior to the Transplantation

Patients diagnosed with a life-threatening disease such as leukemia are confronted with important decisions that will change their lives. It is crucial that these patients are closely involved in the informed consent procedure, and that they know about their disease, their prognosis, and the problems that might arise prior, during, and after transplantation (Dillon, 1985). Usually these patients are still in the prime of their life, they might just be finishing school or starting their career, or have just married and are about to start a family. All these factors should be considered in the communication and support the patients receive throughout the entire transplantation process. Patients can show extreme anxiety prior to their SCT (Keogh, O'Riordan, McCann, & McNamara, 1995). The anxiety usually diminishes after the first steps are taken for the transplantation, when patients reach a "point of no return" and have to go through with the transplantation procedure.

By providing adequate information beforehand (Larsen et al., 1989) caregivers can anticipate and mitigate difficulties during admission for transplantation or after discharge. Although there is always a discussion about the extent to which patients and families should be told about the risk factors (Morgan, 1991), patients and families must be told what they can expect in easily understandable terms. In many countries it is mandatory by law to inform patients undergoing an intensive treatment about the risk factors and short- and long-term side effects. Such disclosure will facilitate two-way communication with the patient. In addition to verbal information, folders, videos, and illustrated booklets have been developed to provide additional information and help the patient visualize the procedure (Boyd, 1994; Defendini, Midon, & Perrot, 1994; Haupt & Keller, 1989; Kersteman & van de Loo, 1991; Keskimäki & Tammisto, 1994; Larsen, Strenstrup, Lerche, & Olsen, 1989; Saudubray, Tellaa, Feral, Moarau, & André, 1989). Authors agree that this written or audiovisual information should not be substituted for conversation between the physician, the nurse, and the patient and family. The information should be carefully planned so as to not overinform patients inappropriately or make them more frightened than necessary. Many patients will share the written information with their families (Boyd, 1994) and feel they can share the burden of transplantation with others.

Patients who undergo a peripheral stem cell transplantation will need special attention in the phase of harvesting the stem cells. In the near future we also should pay specific attention to the donors who have to mobilize stem cells for harvest. The psychological pressure of the mobilization and harvesting for the patient or donor should not be underestimated. Feelings of fear, anxiety, and worry can be experienced by the patient or the donor (Charley, 1996). Initially, the written information about the procedure itself is providing the patient with information on how to prepare for the procedure (such as eating breakfast beforehand and drinking milk during the harvest). Privacy is important for these patients, as is having a close friend or relative accompany them. Since the harvest takes time, nurses can be creative in suggesting the patient listen to music or watch movies during the procedure. In using the nursing process, if a thorough assessment of risk factors and coping strategies is obtained, it can deliver important information for the team responsible for the caring for the transplant patient.

Aspects of Adult Care During the Transplantation

The care of the patient during the admission phase of the transplantation is intensive and challenging for nurses. All aspects of QOL need attention to support the patient in dealing with the situation.

Assessing the needs of the SCT patient is important as a basis for nursing care planning. One model used to provide a framework for the nursing process is the Mead Model, which is adapted from the intensive care unit of a hospital in London (Kretzer, Morgan, & Swan, 1994). The Mead Model uses a dependence or independence continuum to assess the needs of the patient. The goals are set in terms of short-term goals, achievable within 24 hours. The patient is scored for every criterion. There are five stages ranging from total independence via intervention/prevention to total dependence. The scores indicate the independence or dependence of the patient.

Physical Status

It is important to consider the experience of the patient in previous treatment phases and the patient's reaction to possible physical side effects of chemotherapy or irradiation. Physical symptoms such as nausea and vomiting, mucositis, diarrhea, and pain can tremendously affect the QOL during transplantation. Nutritional status is influenced by these symptoms, and the bacterial limitations of the type of food patients are allowed to eat can limit the energy level. Lienhart (2001) suggests several complementary therapy methods to prevent or relieve side effects of the high-dose treatment such as nausea and vomiting. Among the possibilities described are acupuncture, acupressure, aromatherapy, and several relaxation techniques. Lienhart points out that these treatments should only be applied in addition and not as substitute to conventional drugs. Another possibility to enhance coping is foot massage (Chabot & Legaré, 1997).

One strategy to overcome physical limitations and to keep in shape—although space is very limited in isolation rooms—is any kind of physiotherapy and specifically active and passive kinesiology and isometric exercises (Planzer & Baumann, 1987). Active kinesiology is used to maintain physical fitness of the patient. It is important for the patient to maintain mobility by special movements and stretching exercises. If the condition of the patient no longer allows active exercises, passive kinesiology should be applied to stimulate circulation and prevent thrombosis or other side effects of immobility (Planzer & Baumann, 1987). To prevent pneumonia and stimulate proper and deep breathing, active or passive respiration therapy can be applied (Planzer & Baumann 1987). The positioning of the patient during respiration therapy is essential.

Research is increasingly being undertaken to look at specific symptoms during the transplantation, such as mucositis, pain, and optimal care for the central venous access device of the patient. These studies might need a metaanalysis in the near future to reach a consensus on the state-of-the-art care of handling these often-distressing symptoms. More research on each symptom, including an easy-to-use and reliable measurement tool, is still required in the near future.

Psychological Status

Many patients have difficulty with the lifestyle change that occurs during the transplantation procedure. Signs of anxiety and depression have been evaluated during the different stages of the treatment (Gloriod et al., 1992). Studies show a correlation between the physical condition and signs of depression. In some cases psychiatric interventions are necessary to support the patient in coping with the situation. Many patients have a feeling of deprivation (Dillon, 1985) because when they enter the isolation period they have to leave behind small things that characterize their personality, such as their wallet, special clothes, jewelry, and other things from home. They experience helplessness and try to escape through unusual behavior (Baumgartner, 1990), such as retreat, regression, or aggression. Therefore, it is important that patients remain responsible for themselves. It is important to break through the vicious circle and support the patient in an appropriate defense mechanism.

For many patients the completion of the conditioning regimen brings feelings of relief and optimism because they passed the "point of no return" (Dillon, 1985). Many patients experience the feeling of being able to make a new start and often celebrate their transplantation day as their second birthday. Although many allogeneic transplanted patients do not worry at that time about infection or GVHD (Dillon, 1985), they must realize that a period filled with waiting for the blood counts to return and potential complications is yet to come. The first contact with the donor can be very emotional and is crucial for patients (Baumgartner, 1990) because patients often worry about the well-being of the donor after the donation.

Physical exercise is not only necessary for the prevention of side effects of the treatment due to immobility, but it also supports the motivation of the patient (Planzer & Baumann, 1987) by providing a feeling of self-confidence resulting from the ability to do something instead of having things done for him or her. Other recreational means such as games, television and video, writing letters, or listening to music are important to give patients the opportunity to occupy themselves (Amrane & Legree, 1991; Baumgartner, 1990). Some patients look for mental support from complementary therapies such as meditation and relaxation, visualization, guided imagery, and special diets (Naylor, 1987). These techniques help patients survive the isolation period, view the transplantation as a positive experience, and maintain control of the situation as much as possible. Patients can also discover something about the reality and mystery of the quality of their own lives (Yang, 1990). To give structure to the isolation period patients are advised to have a daily routine and to keep busy, which makes the time pass more quickly (Naylor, 1987). Many centers emphasize the importance of creating a personal atmosphere for each patient. This can include not only a personal approach, but also accepting personal belongings of the patient within the limitations of the protective care policy. Patients might want to bring pictures or photographs of their friends, fill the room with artificial flowers, or bring their own computers or stereos. The isolation procedure holds many possibilities, and the team should consider carefully the wishes of the patient.

Volunteers who were in the same position as the patient (similar age, similar background) but have already successfully passed therapy for a malignancy may provide mental and emotional support for patients and families during the transplant procedures (Ilves, Salovaara, Vepsalainen, & Tuomarila, 1990). However, the volunteers should not answer any medical and nursing questions. The importance of confidentiality also needs to be emphasized. Volunteers are very valuable in sharing their experience, encouraging patients and families, giving realistic practical advice for daily life, and giving information on services for cancer patients. It is important that patients also share with volunteers their experiences and feelings, which might be too painful to share with family members.

Social Interaction

Patients are admitted to the hospital as part of a family unit in which each member has a personal role (Hucklesby, 1992). The patient must understand that the social interaction during the transplant period is considerably limited. Patients may have to deal with lack of privacy. Although patients show admirable flexibility and adaptation studies indicate that having decreased contact with friends might lead to depression, demotivation, decrease of mobility, sleeping disorders, boredom, apathy, and introversion (Van Nierop, 1992; Neyens, 1987). In this situation it is important for nurses to listen not only to what is said, but also to what is not said. Silence sometimes indicates more. Transplantation places the patient in a complex situation requiring special care. Thus, nurses need to pay extra attention to all signs of social isolation. It is also very important for SCT patients to receive mail or phone calls from friends on a regular basis (Naylor, 1987). This gives them the feeling of still being in contact with friends. Patients must be able to stay in contact with the outside world through frequent visitors (on a planned and regular basis), the daily newspaper and television, or school courses (Baumgartner, 1990).

Relatives, partners, and children play an important role not only in supporting and encouraging the patient throughout the transplant procedure (Andersson, 1991; Entonen & Wiren, 1992; Hucklesby, 1992; Keskimäki et al., 1997; Wendel, van Benthem, & Fliedner, 1991), but also in helping with any physical needs. Often the presence of a relative is required by the unit to actively assist in the care of the patient (Goldberg, Segal, Armeli, Sharon, & Akerling, 1992). The patient should decide whether to have a family caregiver involved in all aspects of care and who that caregiver should be. Many relatives experience the intensive time with the patient valuable. But, the economic, social, and psychological burden for the patient's family members, relatives, or support persons should not be underestimated when considering their specific need for contact, information, and advice. Feelings of fear, anxiety, loneliness, and psychological distress among close friends or partners of the patient have been identified (Toy, 1989). Often family members or partners feel neglected by their friends, because much love and attention is given to the patient. Family or close friends should be included in patient care and may require help and special support. However, managing the situation without help from professionals can be a part of their coping strategy (Hucklesby, 1992). Wilke, Rudolph, Grande, Siegert, and Sowade (1989) gave specific attention to the interaction between family members and the nursing team. They proposed regular multidisciplinary conferences on the unit to exchange experiences with patients and family members and to gain a certain professional distance from the patient. Family caregivers have to be prepared in advance for the role and responsibility and have to be taught the required tasks. They should be supported by professional caregivers throughout the transplantation period (Goldberg et al., 1992).

A support group for relatives of patients with hematological malignancies was initiated in Sweden (Valdman & Lundqvist, 1995). It is important to counsel relatives in their support of the patient. Family members are expected to show strength and support, but they also have to cope with the fear of losing a loved one. The goal of support groups is not only to support the family members, but also to provide facts and enhance knowledge about the process patients are going through. Family members can learn coping strategies such as relaxation exercises and can be informed about other strategies that they can use at home. Changed roles within the family are discussed and ways to handle the difficulties are shared in group sessions. These sessions are not only directed toward the hospital stay, but also toward the period when the patient is back home. Members can be counseled on what changes to expect in all of their lives.

Economic Status

In addition to the patient's comfort with the social aspect of their lives it is very important for patients to go into the transplantation period with the knowledge that everything in their professional life has been taken care of. This is not only very difficult for patients who have their own company or business or farm, but also for people who have an insecure work situation. Losing work or status at work can be difficult to accept (Entonen & Wiren, 1992). Looking for an alternative such as going back to school or learning a new skill can become important. This can function also as a distraction from thinking too much about illness and its sequelae.

Spiritual Aspects

The spiritual aspect of QOL is becoming increasingly recognized around the world as an important domain of QOL and is further described in Chapter 5. Many patients experience support from their personal view of life. Each individual has different beliefs and values and it is important that one continue to live life in the restricted environment of the treatment procedure. Support can be found not only in religion, but also in free or abstract spiritual ideas such as positive thinking, appreciating life as it is, and making the best of the situation. Several centers offer consultation with a psychologist or spiritual advisor (Baumgartner, 1990). They can structure the confused thoughts of patients and support them when they do not know where these thoughts will take them.

Aspects of Care After Discharge of the Adult Transplant Patient

The first year after the transplantation is the most crucial year in terms of psychosocial and physical adaptation. It is important for the patient and his or her family to know that what they define as QOL will be different but not necessarily worse after SCT (Fliedner, 1992). The majority of patients and their families experience this period as much more difficult than they had expected due to the fact that the majority expect life after SCT to be exactly as before SCT (Wendel et al., 1991). The disappointment can result in disillusionment and decreased morale. Many QOL studies are designed to examine the period after transplantation and discuss ways to understand and help to cope with any kind of impairment or changes in their lives. Patients are influenced in their development not only by self-concept, but also by their environments.

The transition from the protective environment of the transplant unit to home is difficult for many patients. Being dependent on their family, friends, and the hospital makes it difficult for patients to rebuild their own lives again after surviving a life-threatening illness. Ongoing community support should be provided during this time. A nurse coordinator responsible for continuity of care should be in close contact with professionals in the community to meet the needs of the patient and his or her family members (Toy, 1989). Communication lines should also be established with agencies in the community, such as social services or home health agencies to provide additional care, identify potential problems, and prevent family breakdown.

Physical Status

After transplantation, some patients indicate, that they are feeling physically stronger (Baier, Schmid, Werner-Dreissler, & Schuster, 1987), or that they are in good physical condition (Fradique, Heitor, & Costa, 1994). On the other hand, more patients are usually feeling much less physically able to perform normal daily activities, such as housekeeping or shopping. Chronic symptoms of fatigue or lack of energy are experienced in patients after both autologous and allogeneic transplantation. Changes of the body image due to factors such as GVHD play an important role in the daily life of the patient, and it is important to demonstrate how health care workers are influenced by the appearance of patients when determining how well they are doing (Haupt & Fliedner, 1992). Sometimes a health care provider can see a patient a long time after he or she has been discharged and think that he or she looks very good. A conversation with that person, however, may reveal feelings of self-consciousness due to the patient's perceived change in appearance. On the other hand, some patients with severe chronic GVHD and assumed to be impaired in daily life may be well adapted. The physical changes patients must deal with include baldness, "moon-face" due to the use of corticosteroids, and changes of the oral mucosa resulting in dry saliva and changes of the tastebuds. Unexpected and prolonged alopecia or poor hair growth of patients who received busulfan/cyclophosphamide as a conditioning regimen prior to allogeneic SCT have also been reported (Inder, 1990). Another problem for patients can be weight and muscle loss (Hirsch, Claisse, Tabani, & Gluckman, 1994). These changes of body image can lead to embarrassment, insecurity, and emotional vulnerability (Toy 1989). Evans, Barret, and Horsler (1988) concluded in their study of the QOL of patients four to nine years post SCT that, despite important physical and developmental changes, the patients show considerable adaptation to their problems and are able to develop new approaches to life. One way to overcome difficulties in resuming a normal lifestyle quickly is to follow a physical and mental rehabilitation program, which is organized by nurses and physicians together with other practitioners such as physical therapists and social workers (Harris & Hyde, 1993; Molassiotis, Boughton, Burgoyne, & van den Akker, 1994). By following a comprehensive exercise program, the patient is able to readjust and regain strength, confidence, and motivation at home and at work. Other physical impairments such as cataracts can be a problem in recovering from the treatment and returning to an active life after transplantation. Patients have to know about these possible complications to be able to work on them or learn to live with them.

The sexuality of men and women can be affected by the transplantation treatment and its sequelae (Atlan, Kalayoglu-Besisik, & Sargin, 1999; Fliedner, 1993; Muir, 2000). Both men and women experience changes in their sex lives due to physical impairments such as symptoms of GVHD and vaginal dryness. The degree of these changes depends, among other factors, on the age at transplantation, the conditioning regimen, the kind of transplantation, and the severity of GVHD. Men might be impaired by a lack of interest, erectile failure, "dry ejaculation," or premature or retarded ejaculation (Baruch et al., 1991). Women can experience symptoms of early menopause due to failure of the reproductive organs producing hormones, with consequences such as bone demineralization (Inder, 1990; Toy, 1989). Women who experience ovarian failure might need estrogen replacement therapies. Often, estrogen cremes are prescribed to overcome vaginal dryness, although side effects (e.g., carcinogenic effects) should not be underestimated (Inder, 1990).

Health care professionals may still feel uncomfortable or embarrassed addressing the issue of sexuality. They may feel a certain lack of knowledge (Kelly, 1997), have limited education and experience, or have personal reservations about discussing sexual issues. Studies show that nurses feel more confident in discussing fertility issues or changes in body image (Kelly, 1997). It is important to remember to include the patient's partner in the discussion. Nurses can suggest alternative methods, such as olive oil for overcoming the impediment of vaginal dryness during intercourse. In addition, some patients and their partners might be in need of sexual counseling (Muir, 2002; Toy, 1989) to cope with long-term effects such as infertility. It is important that male patients get correct information about the possibility of sperm banking, and that female patients learn about the possibility of storing embryos (Braat, 2001). Knowing about such possibilities can mitigate a lot of tension, communication problems, and anger between a couple (Pugh & Toy, 1989). Medical staff should realize the importance of fertility and sexuality for patients with life-threatening disease, although the priority for many patients at diagnosis is simply survival. This does not take away the desire to have a family after surviving the treatment. It would be wrong to assume that patients do not need any information about fertility options just because they already have children. Medical staff should be informed constantly about the possibilities of fertilization and its risk factors to provide correct information to the patient and his or her partner. An option is to refer patients to a specialty unit for counseling and treatment of fertility problems (Slater, Bass, Boraks, Price, & Marcus, 1995).

In order to become independent from the hospital, patients and their families must be taught as soon as possible about food precautions and the prevention of potential infections as well as interventions to be used if infections develop. Technical aspects such as taking care of the Hickman catheter also must be taught (Dannie, 1988).

Psychological Status

Psychological problems can occur some time after SCT (Baier et al., 1987), because the patient anticipates being cured and expects life to be the same. Nonetheless, potential difficulties or risk factors should be assessed as early as possible. In this phase it is important to know about the behaviors patients express with regard to self-image. They might react with behaviors such as denial, compensation, or projection (van de Loo & Mentink 1987). The ability to solve problems may determine an individual's QOL, since every person has his or her own limit of accepting health impairments. By undergoing transplantation, the patient has to extend those limits with each step of the treatment (Fliedner, 1992). Feelings of insecurity and inadequacy can limit patients in their daily lives (Haupt & Fliedner, 1992). Feelings of anxiety due to the risk of an unsuccessful treatment or fearing unforeseen complications can play an important role in the psychological state of patients (Holtkamp et al., 1996). Problems related to social isolation, loss of motivation, and depression are signals of psychological changes (Harris & Hyde, 1993). On the other hand, many patients experience physical and mental fatigue and fear of relapse or additional complications such as infections, GVHD, or late graft failure after transplantation. These feelings are normal and generally go away with time and good results, but can affect patients psychologically (Baier et al., 1987; Dannie, 1988; van de Loo & Mentink, 1987). Fatigue often remains one of the common, long-lasting symptoms in cancer patients and it is often underestimated or still unrecognized (Lenssen, 2000). Van den Brand (2001) describes vividly her own feeling of fatigue even a decade after her transplantation and offers the professional suggestions for how to help. First of all, a subjective assessment of the symptoms is mandatory to be able to judge the severity of the problem and to oversee possible areas of improvement (Lenssen, 2000). One major asset is the caregiver's ability to recognize the problem. A thorough preparation of the patient including the surroundings would be supportive according to van den Brand (2001). In addition to the medical staff, the management of fatigue requires a comprehensive collaboration of different professionals such as dietician, psychologist, and physiotherapist. After all, it remains a very personal symptom requiring a customized strategy (Lenssen, 2000). Also, physical changes such as alopecia or lesions or scars from central venous catheters or other invasive procedures might affect the psychological status of the patient due to a changed body image.

Specific symptomatology differences in psychological dysfunction have been found between autologous and allogeneic transplant patients (Molassiotis et al., 1994). After autologous transplantation, patients tend to develop more symptoms of anxiety and depression. Nevertheless, most of the time they overcome the debilitating effects and are able to lead an active and meaningful life (Dannie, 1988, 1991). Keogh and associates' study (1995) of anxiety and depression in the posttransplant phase revealed the patients tend to experience more depression from isolation or dependency during the first three months after transplantation. These feelings are largely resolved by one year posttransplantation. At six months posttransplantation, the patient might show symptoms of anxiety, but they are often diminished by one year posttransplantation. Although patients may feel it is hard to go on with the changed conditions of their lives (Fradique et al., 1994) or discouraged (Hirsch et al., 1994) it is important that they maintain their hope for the future and attempt to live each day as fully as possible. Positive thinking and complementary therapies such as aromatherapy or relaxation techniques, music, or art can support patients' coping mechanisms (Boyd, 1994). Again a thorough assessment of the risk factors is recommended. This must be followed by careful counseling and good teaching to prevent additional stress factors.

Neuropsychologic aspects such as loss of memory, behavior changes, and lack of concentration may develop in patients who undergo multiple courses of high-dose chemotherapy followed by autologous PBCT (Holtkamp, 1996).

QOL can improve drastically the moment someone shows an active interest in a patient (Yang, 1990). Patients can feel good when someone they trust asks at the end of the day how they really feel and understands that something may be bothering them. Nurses often identify patients' need for attention and should have experience when asking patients or their loved ones about how things are going—they will get the whole story of past difficulties and joys, present concerns, and future expectations. Patients often expect nurses to listen to their concerns and appreciate when they do.

Social Interactions

Some patients have difficulties in their relationships due to rage and aggressive behavior after transplantation (Baier et al., 1987; Haupt & Fliedner, 1992). The relationship between partners is put under considerable pressure. The patient is expected to be the same as before transplantation, but this is usually not the case due to physical impairment or psychological stressors. It is important to resume the old pattern of life as much as possible, although many patients indicate various difficulties in their social interactions and the lack of acceptance and understanding for years after their transplantation. These difficulties are the consequence not only of physical impairment (e.g., continuing fatigue, lack of concentration, and infertility), but also of personality changes.

Friends are very important to patients after transplantation. Patients want to be accepted in society again. The circle of friends may change after SCT, because the transplantation period spreads over a long period of time in which life for other people moves forward and often in a different direction from the patient. Patients report that some friends become much closer and others move away (Baier et al., 1987). It is very important that patients and families take the time to socialize again and plan social and cultural activities. Resuming professional or school life often helps patients to feel that they have returned to a normal lifestyle (Hirsch et al., 1994).

The expectation of both partners that sexual life will be resumed shortly after discharge might lead to disappointment. Keogh and colleagues (1995) have shown that problems regarding sexual interest and activity may be present prior to the transplantation and during the first three months after transplantation. Frequently by one year post SCT, sexual interest and activity are restored. Talking about sexuality is not easy for many patients and their partners. Both patients and partners must find a way to express their feelings and satisfy their needs for love and understanding. Partners often say that they have to get to know each other again, as if it is their first time. Delayed recovery of satisfying sexual relations may be experienced (Hirsch et al.,

1994). The patient may be influenced by a fear for infection due to low white blood cell counts, a fear of bleeding due to low platelets, or painful intercourse due to vaginal dryness. The partner might be influenced by the need to spare and protect the patient. Body image and other physical impairments play an important role in the resumption of sexual activity (van de Loo & Mentink 1987). Emotional factors such as changes in self-image, mental fatigue, and fear of relapse or complications can cause feelings of unattractiveness and social isolation. Physical and emotional impairments might lead to feelings of guilt, shame, and frustration. An extended role for nurses when caring for patients with psychosexual problems after SCT may be to provide information and guidance to help them overcome minor problems. In any rehabilitation program both the patient and his or her partner should be included in order to restore interpersonal intimacy and sexual satisfaction to optimum levels. Every person has the potential for sexual rehabilitation with the help of proper support and counseling (Goren, 1990).

Patients' relationships with family members, especially the donor, might change. The donor becomes the most important person to the allogeneic transplantation recipient for a certain period of time, and this importance may increase the bond between them. Patients may feel guilty because they are obligated to the donor for the rest of his or her life (van de Loo & Mentink, 1987).

Changes in the social roles of the patient are very important to deal with: The housewife may have to change her duties and go to work or the father, who always earned a living for the family, may have to stay at home and take care of the kids. Many problems may arise and it is important to assess the situation carefully and look for potential difficulties, as well as prepare the family for possible changes and support the family in the process of change (Keogh et al., 1995). Often partners want to stop working during the transplant procedure and recovery period to be with the patient as much as possible, or they may find that their work is affected by the burden of the situation. Social life and leisure activities of the family members are affected by the transplantation because much time is spent in and around the hospital area. Having convenient access to support from the informal network (family and friends) is crucial.

Dependency is often also a problem for patients as well as their family. Individuals who never depended on others now need assistance from others to master activities of daily living, while other individuals who were always in the position of the dependent person might become even more dependent and passive, resulting in depression (van de Loo & Mentink, 1987).

A multidisciplinary approach to problems that might arise after SCT has to start prior the transplantation procedure to prevent as many problems as possible or to treat them in an early stage.

In several countries, support groups for patients undergoing an SCT have been established. In the Netherlands the ex-SCT contact group meets on a regular basis to talk about problems, exchange experiences, and support each other in establishing a normal life (De Bruyn et al., 2001; Fliedner, 1992). In Finland (Ilves, Tuomarila, & Jussila, 1988) patients who survived a successful SCT were asked to function as supportive individuals for recently diagnosed patients who would soon undergo a transplantation. They received specific training to help other patients in their preparation for the SCT. It is often helpful for patients to share experiences with someone who has survived a transplantation. Informal support group meetings have been established and supported by a nurse (Bilbrough, 1997; Jones, Burley, & Heron, 1995) who coordinates and organizes the group. Others organizations developed formal courses that last from one to two weeks, in which patients together share information, work on a subject in small groups, exercise, and rest (Salovaara et al., 1999). The goals of these groups are to promote the coping process and adjust to a new situation.

Economic Status

Many patients experience financial difficulties as a result of disruption in employment (Molassiotis et al., 1994; Toy, 1989). Many lose their jobs or cannot resume the same work after their transplantation. Countries differ in their social security systems and how much sickness benefit may be collected. It is obvious, however, that many patients lose a portion of their usual salary. Financial aid is not always sufficient (Fradique et al., 1994). Patients, therefore, need mental and organizational support to feel comfortable when getting back to work after a long period of treatment and convalescence. It is important that work colleagues accept the patient when returning to work.

Spiritual Aspects

SCT patients are in a very vulnerable situation and may look for support in spirituality. Baier and associates (1987) found that some patients become more religious or spiritual during this time. Some patients experience a change in values and are grateful to have encountered and conquered a life-threatening illness (Entonen & Wiren, 1992). Some patients state that they appreciate life more than they did prior to SCT and pay more attention to the small joys of life (Baier et al., 1987). One patient described the experience by stating that previously everything had been black and white and after the transplantation there was color in his life (Bach, Hijort, & Mathiesen, 1995). Faith in one's spiritual leader or God can support patients in their daily struggle (Boyd, 1994). Despite difficult, temporary or lasting impairment, a patient has the potential to adjust in the hope of a new and prolonged life (Haupt & Fleidner, 1992).

Psychosocial Aspects of the Care of Children Prior to the Transplantation

Depending on the age of the child having the transplantation, he or she will need to be included in the decision-making process (Karaiskou et al., 1997). In this process, contact with another family who already underwent the procedure might be helpful. The environment of the unit on which the transplantation will take place should be visited by the family, including the parents, the patient, the potential donor, and any other siblings. Open and honest answers to the childrens' concerns are mandatory. Children may want to know the length of admission. Seasonal events and holidays may help to pass time. A play therapist might be an asset to the multidisciplinary team.

Pot-Mees and Zeitlin (1985) interviewed parents of young patients within the first weeks of admission prior to transplantation. A second interview was conducted in order to look at the behaviors of the child, the behaviors of the siblings, and the parents' own mental states and marital relationships. The team evaluated the psychological state of the child prior to transplantation, focusing on the intellectual and self-perception of the child. During the treatment period, they evaluated the child's and parents' adjustment on a weekly basis. They found effects on the entire family from the moment a SCT was proposed. Most of the children appeared to be less influenced by the treatment option than their parents were. Anxiety, depression, periodic lack of cooperation, and developmental regression in the children, and social and financial difficulties within the families were found. An increase in psychosocial support was necessary.

Nilsson (1987) suggested that most parents are not influenced by the information given to them prior to the transplantation, but that they followed the recommendation of the doctor to offer the child the best treatment available. Parents do not feel as if they have a choice for their child. According to Pot-Mees and Zeitlin (1985), the patients lead a relatively normal life during the months prior to the transplantation with normal participation in school and family life. Only one child showed major behavioral problems. On the other hand, the parents reported signs of persistent distress and depression during this phase. The parents realized that they would be putting the child through a very stressful treatment that was the only possibility for cure. Feelings of doubt were evident despite their decision to proceed with the treatment.

To reduce feelings of isolation and frustration, communication with the referring physician and the treatment center are of great importance. Although many parents are not able to pay attention to their child's fear of dying, it is important that the child be able to express his or her fear of death to prevent distortion of an honest communication (Vecchi & Coppola, 1991).

The donor siblings can show considerable signs of distress and ambivalent feelings, and it is very important to communicate with them about their feelings, especially if the family is more occupied with the child that will undergo transplantation. Siblings who are neither the donor nor the sick child also showed mixed feelings. They may be relieved at not having to go to the hospital, while also experiencing feelings of rejection and being shoved aside, because they can do nothing to help their brother or sister.

Psychosocial Aspects of Care of Children During and After the Transplant Period

The admission of a child to the hospital changes the whole lifestyle of the family. In many countries one of the parents is admitted with the patient to give the child the opportunity to stay together with a significant person during the treatment (Pot-Mees & Zeitlin, 1985). This might reduce anxiety, although the feeling of fear is normal for both the patient and his or her parents (Nilsson, 1987). Patients also need assistance in maintaining as normal a life as possible for the other children at home (Dennis, 1989).

During the period of transplantation, a child is restricted in many activities of daily life. Many children have to stay in a cubicle or sterile tent for a long time during the aplastic phase. This limits their space to play. Food is also restricted at this phase, with only certain foods allowed in a sterile tent or isolation. However, the isolation procedures have been minimized over the years and many centers allow children to do many things differently, such as wear their own clothes. For children it is very important to have close eye or skin contact with friends, a significant caregiver, or other patients. All centers have developed one or more ways for young patients to have contact with friends (Hansson & Kerstin, 1990).

A way to communicate with children and to understand some of their inner feelings, joys, and fears is to have children draw (Monteiro de Barros & Pot-Mees, 1994). Spontaneous drawings can provide new insights into the care of children because they show not only the reality, but also unconscious feelings such as anxieties due to the unknown, anger, and isolation, particularly at the beginning of the treatment and before discharge. Feelings of insecurity and vulnerability can also be perceived in drawings by children. It is also important to see the change a child goes through, adapting to the situation and going through a process of surviving treatment for a life-threatening disease. Another theme that can be seen in drawings is the relationship between the children and persons close to them. For caregivers it is important to consider the personality of the child and his or her cultural background to correctly interpret and understand the drawings of the child's inner world.

Another interesting way to stimulate children during the transplant phase is with humor by clowns (Simonds, Beaussier, & Vissuzaine, 1994). Clowns should be a part of the team around the child. It is important to be sensitive to the changing mood on the unit and to be able to take into consideration the stage the child is in. Although children need their rest, clowns can be very helpful in initiating spontaneous laughter, singing, or even more serious emotions. Through their ability to create a magic environment, children can live in their own fantasies and dreams. Dissolving some of the stresses and tensions not only in children but also in their parents and to the staff is an important contribution to care.

Children younger than five years old tend to lose their self-help skills. Some children stop eating and drinking on their own, and some become incontinent again. Signs of loss of speech and mobility are often observed. Children between 5 and 16 show signs of boredom, frustration, depression, overdependency on their parents, and sometimes an increasing lack of compliance. The feeling of losing control over the situation can cause children to try to control the situation by refusing to eat or take medication.

Body image plays an important role not only for adults but also for children (Harbin & Richardson, 1991) after transplantation. Children develop a sense of differences in appearance in simple terms (beautiful and ugly) at the age of three or four when they start to socialize with other children in play groups or kindergarten. An alternative to the typical body image should be carefully attended to.

After transplantation, physical and mental development can be impaired (Vickers, 1994). Although most children have initially delayed growth patterns, girls or boys might need further growth hormone therapy. GVHD can influence food tolerance. Food intolerance is seldom a permanent impairment, but usually children stay on a hypoallergenic diet for some time, depending on the recovery of the immune system. Taking into consideration the wide variation of development in all children, children after a transplantation may show delays in development such as in crawling, walking, and talking (e.g., speech and language development) (Vickers, 1994). Parents have to be prepared for these impairments and be able to anticipate their children's needs and support them in further development.

Returning to school after such an intensive treatment might be a problem, depending on the age and stage of development of the child. Peykerli and colleagues (2002) evaluated 55 children (mean age 14.2 ± 3.1 years) and looked at reasons why children might not be able to return to school in a reasonable time. Reasons for not returning or returning late to school were chronic GVHD and severe immunosuppression, fear of being unsuccessful at school, and disrupted body image.

Siblings of Children Undergoing SCT

Pot-Mees and Zeitlin (1985) examined the adaptation difficulties of siblings of transplanted children. In their study, six out of 19 siblings showed signs of behavioral problems including enuresis, eating and sleep disturbances, disobedience, and problems at school. The researchers concluded that not only the patient but also the rest of the family needs special attention during the transplantation procedure.

Care for Parents of Children Undergoing SCT

The treatment period places tremendous pressure on the relationship of the parents, not only socially and emotionally, but also financially as they face extra out-of-pocket living and traveling costs (Hostrup, 1996; Vickers, 1994). Because the parents are usually separated over a longer period of time, they may keep in touch through many expensive phone calls. Sometimes a closer connection between the partners can be seen (Hostrup, 1996). It is important to realize that the parent who takes care of the situation at home may have the feeling of being left out, because immediate input regarding the care of the transplant child may not be possible. Many parents show a high rate of anxiety and distress. Parents have also complained of claustrophobic feelings because the space is limited. They may also suffer from sleep disturbance and increased mental and physical fatigue or exhaustion (Nilsson, 1987). To preserve the role of the parents of someone giving love and comfort, the parents should actively participate in the care for the child. They should not be involved in any painful treatment (Hansson & Kerstin, 1990), though they should be present when the child has to undergo a specific treatment. Support of a psychologist and sexual counselor may be necessary for the parents to live through the SCT experience and keep their relationship together.

Asian parents of children undergoing a transplantation can show difficulties with role changes (Pot-Mees & Zeitlin, 1985). In Asian families, the father is usually the decision maker but if the mother stays at the hospital with the child, she may be the one who makes important decisions for the child. This puts an additional pressure on the relationships of the partners and the whole family.

In addition to regular contacts with doctors and nurses to clarify questions and understand the procedure, strategies to support the child, siblings, and parents may include having the child visit with a psychologist for talking, drawing, or painting and play therapy (Hansson & Kerstin, 1990). Parents on the other hand, may need contact with a social worker that can help them work through their feelings and provide support. Next to a thorough preparation before discharge, Peykerli and colleagues (2002) suggest a need for continuing psychological support for school-age children, their siblings, and their parents.

Nurses Impact on QOL

Patients often ask nurses to assist them in obtaining the best possible quality in their lives. One of the goals of nursing, therefore, is to promote the strengths of patients and their surroundings and to optimize their abilities and improve their QOL (Fliedner, 1994). It is important to look at difficulties from the patients' perspective, their beliefs, feelings, judgments, and decisions, and not to assume we know what is best for them. Next to a firm knowledge base regarding transplantation, skills such as effective communication, confidence, and determination to pass the knowledge to others are mandatory (Boyd, 1994). Nurses working with oncology patients and patients who undergo a SCT can affect the QOL of patients and families by being concerned with QOL as part of the treatment. To prepare patients for changes in their lives after SCT, nurses should support them in reevaluating their value system and reassure them of the value of life itself (Fliedner, 1992). Nursing care based on knowledge and skill as well as sympathy and empathy can have a significant impact on the experience of the SCT patient.

Barbieri and colleagues (1998) describe the nurse's role and point out that the trusting relationship between patient and nurse must be based on the unconditional acceptance of the other, self-awareness and understanding of one's own actions and responses, and recognition of the difference between words and actions. The strong relationship between good clinical practice and technical skills including homogenous actions is just as important as the awareness of what the patient says in words and/or body language.

Patients expect nurses to possess excellent professional skills, as well as consideration of the individuality of a patient, and mental or other forms of support (Keskimäki et al., 1997). Some patients critique the care they receive while undergoing SCT. Keskimäki and associates (1997) found that patients were not sufficiently informed about nutritional aspects, consequences of SCT, hygiene, and other required activities. Patients' also felt socioeconomic consequences of the treatment were underestimated and not sufficiently described.

Nurses, working together with a multidisciplinary team, are the primary caregivers for patients and often share the most intimate, emotional aspects of their lives. A multidisciplinary approach to problems that might arise after SCT has to start prior to the transplantation procedure to prevent as many problems as possible or to treat them at an early stage. The multidisciplinary team must address all dimensions of QOL (Fradique et al., 1994) and look at the patient from a holistic point of view (Haupt & Fliedner, 1992).

Nurses often serve as advocates for patients and families who are too devastated to be their own advocates. Mental support of patients during and after SCT must be available. Nurses are often seen as the second most important supporter of the patient, next to the spouse and the family (Wiren, Hamalainen, & Entonen, 1993). The essence of SCT nursing should be seen as relief of the suffering of patients and their loved ones. "Being there" for the patient in the most private moments of suffering or joy is our responsibility, and it can be a contribution to the patient's QOL. Patients need to discuss the potential changes caused by the illness and its treatment and talk about social relationships and everyday matters. Wendel and associates (1991) found it important to give structured and clear information at the right time and in the right manner, based on the individual patient's needs (Rafi et al., 1999). Nurses, therefore, play a pivotal role in the multidisciplinary team by educating the patient in a structured manner (Desouza et al., 2000). Evaluations of nursing care can guide quality changes improving the care starting with the pretransplant information to the support and care of patients after SCT in the outpatient setting.

Asking patients what really concerns them, what their coping strategies are, and how they have dealt with side effects in prior treatment phases or other stressful times of life may help them remember these strategies at a later time, and they may use them again. Defining the concept of QOL for each individual patient will direct attention to appropriate interventions for enhancing QOL following transplantation (Fliedner, 1992). Some patients, such as those with chronic leukemia, have never had any experience with aggressive treatment regimens. Nurses may want to ask these patients prior to SCT how they have dealt with any signs of being sick so far, evaluate the resources of the patients, and help identify suitable coping strategies.

Based on regular assessments of sexuality, nurses can support patients and their partners who are experiencing sexual difficulties to find a new self-concept and redefine their sexual relationships. Nurses can assist by providing sexual health education, accurate information, and specific suggestions for problems. Continued periodic assessment can be helpful to adjust nursing care plans to enhance quality of intimacy after transplantation (Fliedner, 1993).

The mind–body relationship should be taken seriously, as medical care should not be limited to "mechanical engineering" (Yang, 1990). Nurses can help prevent harm by providing accurate and timely information about the known long-range complications of SCT (Haberman et al., 1993). Nurses can assist the patient in taking the first steps into the experience of life after SCT (Fliedner, 1994). Dannie (1988) emphasized the fact that careful outpatient care is as essential as inpatient care, especially within the first three months of discharge. It is also essential that nurses on the SCT unit provide nursing care in a consistent manner so that patients and families do not worry or become insecure (Hansson & Kerstin, 1990). Clear standard care protocols should be developed for any technical and physical procedure to provide consistent care for patients.

To promote continuity of care after discharge from the unit, a care coordinator should be appointed, either by the hospital (Verhoeven & Smiet, 1995) or funded by a project from the community (Jones, Burley, & Heron, 1995). The coordinator or liaison nurse is the important link between the different caregivers and quality of care provided. A careful assessment of the needs of patients and their close surroundings is crucial to establishing a care plan, monitoring the implementation of the planned interventions, and evaluating the care together with patients. Careful planning of the logistic conditions, such as using a rotating patient chart and communicating with community workers on a regular basis, is the most important factor contributing to the success of and continuity in care. Other tasks of the liaison nurse include psychological support, education, management, and communication. The nurse can function as a resource for information and support not only for patients but also for relatives and staff members inside and outside the hospital (Jones et al., 1995). The liaison nurse can offer to teach health care workers not familiar with the treatment in order to better serve patients and their families. After discharge from the hospital nurses can serve as consultants by answering the patients' many questions via the phone. A close collaboration including guidelines about when to contact the physician needs to be developed upon discharge form the hospital. Documentation of the information and instructions provided for outpatients is mandatory to ensure continuity of care.

Despite recent advances that allow for outpatient autologous and allogeneic treatments (Bracha et al, 1999; Leather et al., 1998; Svahn, 1999) or transplantation without isolation procedures (Stotts & Bouchard, 1997) it is essential that nurses realize that the nursing care remains the same. Outpatients need the same support and care as SCT inpatients. Some patients "shop around" to undergo SCT in an environment that fits their personal needs and expectations. Yet, all SCT patients need the same thorough education and care facilities prior to, during, and after this intensive treatment. During this treatment the informal caregiver, usually a family member, should not be forgotten. He or she requires the same education and care. In addition to previous concerns about SCT care, nurses now need to organize a 24 hour a day–7 day a week service to ensure continuity of care throughout the process (Leather et al., 1998).

Nurses must be aware that patients have to go through a normal process of adaptation and coping, which includes periods of depression and anxiety. But if patients cannot resolve these problems within a reasonable time, or the problems become too severe, interventions should be planned and incorporated into the care for patients after SCT. The multidisciplinary team should compare the patient's condition after transplantation with the situation prior to the transplantation when deciding on the most appropriate intervention. Nursing research on issues such as the effects of the treatment on patients and their social networks, and appropriate nursing interventions, is necessary in the near future.

REFERENCES

Aaronson, N. K. (1988). Quality of life: What is it? How should it be measured? *Oncology*, *12*(5), 69–74.

Amrane, F., & Legree, N. (1991). The leisures in L.A.F. room. *Proceedings of the 7th Meeting of the EBMT Nurses Group* (p. 83). Cortina d'Ampezzo, Italy.

Andersson, C. (1991). An active role of the relatives during the bone marrow transplant procedure. *Proceedings of the 7th Meeting of the EBMT Nurses Group* (pp. 17–18). Cortina d'Ampezzo, Italy.

Atlan, N., Kalayoglu-Besisik, S., & Sargin, D. (1999). The sexual relationship in hematopoietic stem cell transplantation survivors. *EBMT Nurses Group Journal*, *2*, 5–7.

Bach, K., Hijort, K., & Mathiesen, A. M. (1995). A method to improve nursing care and its effect on the rehabilitation of patients undergoing autologous bone marrow transplantation. *EBMT Nurses Group Journal*, *1*, 36–38.

Baier, E., Schmid, A., Werner-Dreissler, M., & Schuster, V. (1987). Life after BMT— Psychological aspects after discharge. *Proceedings of the 3rd Meeting of the EBMT Nurses Group* (pp. 63–69). Interlaken, Switzerland.

Barbieri, S., Ventura, O., Prati, R., Canepa, M., Nobili, A., Agresta, M., Vaserelli, A., & Lombardi, A. (1998). Experience: Nurses in the mirror. *EBMT Nurses Group Journal*, *2*, 6–8.

Baruch, J., Benjamin, S., Treleaven, J., Wilcox, A. H., Barron, J. L., & Powles, R. (1991). Male sexual function following bone marrow transplantation for hematological cancer. *Bone Marrow Transplantation*, *7*(2), 52.

Baumgartner, M. (1990). The problems and support of BMT patients in the laminar airflow unit: Observations of a nursing care team. *Proceedings of the 6th Meeting of the EBMT Nurses Group* (pp. 89–95). The Hague, The Netherlands.

Bilbrough, C. (1997). Pioneering a haematology support network. *EBMT Nurses Group Journal*, *1*, 16–21.

Boyd, C. (1994). Quality of life: Patient education for bone marrow transplant patients, Is it more effective if your patient is a health care professional? *EBMT Nurses Group Journal*, *1*, 16–20.

Braat, D. D. M. (2001). Fertility following bone marrow transplantation. *EBMT Nurses Group Journal*, *2*, 24–26.

Bracha, D., Raz, H., Sarelli, R., Grinberger, A., Rizel, S., Hardan, I., & Stemmer, S. M. (1999). Outpatient transplant: safe, feasible and well accepted by the patients. *EBMT Nurses Group Journal*, *2*, 10–12.

Bremmers, M., Verhoeven, M., & Raemakers, J. (2000). Zero twenty four-three six five one two one: Telephone consultation. *EBMT Nurses Group Journal*, *2*, 20–22.

Chabot, L. F., & Legaré, C. (1997). The implementation of a programme of foot massage to enhance patients and family coping during bone marrow transplant. *EBMT Nurses Group Journal, 2,* 18–21.

Charley, C. (1996). The patient's response to the peripheral blood stem cells programme. *EBMT Nurses Group Journal, 1,* 13–22.

Dannie, E. (1988). Out patient care of BMT patients. *Proceedings of the 4th Meeting of the EBMT Nurses Group* (pp. 35–41). Chamonix, France.

Dannie, E. (1991). Quality of life after bone marrow transplantation. *Proceedings of the 7th Meeting of the EBMT Nurses Group* (pp. 29–30). Cortina d'Ampezzo, Italy.

De Bruyn, I., Pol, M., Koppejan, M., Brand, I., Baeten, F., ter Beek, J., Postma, A., van Dommelen, M. L., de Heer Kloots, J., van Helden, C., Klein Heerenbrink, B., Nijhuis, L., Passies, A., Prompers, N., Ruisendaal, G. J., Schoenmakers, J., Speekenbrink, Y., Streppel, J., Willemse, A., Oosterveer, M. A. P. (2001). Ten years of psychosocial support for patient and family—Contact group bone marrow transplantation, The Netherlands. *EBMT Nurses Group Journal, 2,* 20–21.

Defendini, C., Midon, N., & Perrot, R. (1994). Preparing the patient for entering the air flow room. The support of a booklet. *EBMT Nurses Group Newsletter, 2,* 28–30.

Dennis, J. (1989). Preparation and support for the patient and family during displacement bone marrow transplantation. *Proceedings of the 5th Meeting of the EBMT Nurses Group* (pp. 9–15). Badgastein, Austria.

Desouza, S., Glogoski, G., Norcott, J. & Rennell, D. (2000). Is a multi-disciplinary pre-transplant assessment clinic useful in blood cell transplant? *EBMT Nurses Group Journal, 2,* 25–32.

Dillon, I. (1985). Psychological and emotional problems of patients undergoing bone marrow transplantation. *Proceedings of the 1st Meeting of the EBMT Nurses Group* (pp. 64–69). Bad Hofgastein (Salzburg), Austria.

Entonen, A., & Wirén, R. (1992). Adaptation to severe intestinal GVHD after BMT. *EBMT Nurses Group Newsletter, 2,* 15–17.

Evans, M. G. C., Barrett, A. J., & Horsler, H. (1988). Quality of life and late effects in 31 patients more than 4 years after BMT for leukemia. *Proceedings of the 4th Meeting of the EBMT Nurses Group* (p. 43). Chamonix, France.

Ferrell, B. R., Grant, M., Schmidt, G. M., Rhiner, M., Whitehead, C., Fonbuena, P., & Forman, S. J. (1992a). The meaning of quality of life for bone marrow transplant survivors. Part 1: The impact of bone marrow transplant on quality of life. *Cancer Nursing, 15*(3), 153–160.

Ferrell, B. R., Grant, M., Schmidt, G. M., Rhiner, M., Whitehead, C., Fonbuena, P., & Forman, S. J. (1992b). The meaning of quality of life for bone marrow transplant survivors. Part 2: Improving quality of life for bone marrow transplant survivors. *Cancer Nursing, 15*(4), 247–253.

Fliedner, M. (1992). Contribution to the panel discussion on quality of life. *EBMT Nurses Group Newsletter, 1*, 26–29.

Fliedner, M. (1993). Sexual satisfaction and functioning after BMT—A review of the literature. *EBMT Nurses Group Newsletter, 1*, 41–44.

Fliedner, M. (1994). Quality of life after BMT—A review of the literature. *EBMT Nurses Group Journal, 2*, 50–57.

Fradique, E., Heitor, M. J., & Costa, E. F. (1994). Quality of life after bone marrow transplantation. *EBMT Nurses Group Journal, 1*, 7–15.

Frank-Stromborg, M. (1992). *Instruments for clinical nursing research*. Boston: Jones and Bartlett.

Gloriod, A., Morel, N., Devillers, A., Guillaume, S., Tiberghien, P., Flesh, M., & Cahn, J. Y. (1992). Evaluation of anxiety and/or depression in patients undergoing allogeneic BMT for hematological malignancies. *EBMT Nurses Group Newsletter, 1*, 4–8.

Goldberg, L., Segal, J., Armeli, N., Sharon, R., & Akerling, S. (1992). The attitude of family members of patients toward the work demanded of them as care givers in the hospital. *EBMT Nurses Group Newsletter, 1*, 12–16.

Goldman, J. M. (1993). Bone marrow transplantation in Europe—Can the geographical differences be explained? *Journal of Internal Medicine, 233*, 311–313.

Goren, E. (1990). BMT and sexuality: In search of an extended nursing role. *Proceedings of the 6th Meeting of the EBMT Nurses Group* (pp. 123–129). The Hague, The Netherlands.

Gratwohl, A., Hermans, J., Goldman, J. M., & Gahrton, G. (1993). Bone marrow transplantation in Europe: Major geographical differences. *Journal of Internal Medicine, 233*, 333–341.

Haberman, M., Bush, N., Young, K., & Sullivan, K. M. (1993). Quality of life of adult long-term survivors of bone marrow transplantation: A qualitative analysis of narrative data. *Oncology Nursing Forum, 20*(10), 1545–1553.

Hansson, G., & Kerstin A. (1990). The psychological care of children undergoing bone marrow transplantation. *Proceedings of the 6th Meeting of the EBMT Nurses Group* (pp. 61–67). The Hague, The Netherlands.

Harbin, P., & Richardson, V. (1991). Body image—A pediatric BMT unit perspective. *Proceedings of the 7th Meeting of the EBMT Nurses Group* (pp. 43–46). Cortina d'Ampezzo, Italy.

Harris, J. L., & Hyde, H. L. (1993). A study to show the benefit of a rehabilitation programme following bone marrow transplantation. *EBMT Nurses Group Newsletter, 1*, 12–14.

Haupt, K., & Fliedner, M. (1992). Quality of life after bone marrow transplantation. *EBMT Nurses Group Newsletter, 2*, 31–33.

Haupt, K., & Keller, K. (1989). The written information for patient and donor. *Proceedings of the 5th Meeting of the EBMT Nurses Group* (p. 175). Badgastein, Austria.

Hirsch, I., Claisse, J. P., Tabani, K., & Gluckmann, E. (1994). Bone marrow transplantation with a matched unrelated donor: Quality of life a year after. *EBMT Nurses Group Journal, 1,* 52–53.

Holtkamp, M. J., Roodbergen, R., van der Wall, E., van Dam, F. S. A. M., Gualtherie van Weezel, L. M., Muller, M., & Rodenhuis, S. (1996). Nursing implications associated with changes in concentration and memory following multiple courses of high-dose chemotherapy with autologous peripheral blood stem cell transplantation. *EBMT Nurses Group Journal, 2,* 27–31.

Hostrup, H. (1996). Investigating the families' experience of the nursing care of children undergoing ABMT. *EBMT Nurses Group Journal, 2,* 19–23.

Hucklesby, E. (1992). Role of the relatives. *EBMT Nurses Group Newsletter, 2,* 22–25.

Ilves, L., Tuomarila, T., & Jussila, L. (1988). Patients after successful bone marrow transplantation (BMT) as volunteer supporting persons. *Proceedings of the 4th Meeting of the EBMT Nurses Group* (p. 81). Chamonix, France.

Ilves, L., Salovaara, H., Vepsäläinen, P., & Tuomarila, T. (1990). Experiences of help by voluntary supporting persons (SP) in the treatment of bone marrow transplant patients. *Proceedings of the 6th Meeting of the EBMT Nurses Group* (pp. 33–35). The Hague, The Netherlands.

Inder, A. (1990). Long-term effects of bone marrow transplantation at Christchurch Hospital. *Proceedings of the 6th Meeting of the EBMT Nurses Group* (pp. 81–86). The Hague, The Netherlands.

Jones, S. G., Burley, R. C., & Heron, D. (1995). The role of the community liaison nurse for the leukemia and transplant unit at the Christie Hospital. *EBMT Nurses Group Journal, 1,* 45–48.

Karaiskou, A., Malama, S., Sphigou, T., Alexopoulou, A., Loumidi, D., & Koutseli, V. (1997). Health care in a paediatric BMT unit: Illustrating two years experience of psychosocial support by the nursing staff. *EBMT Nurses Group Journal, 1,* 60–64.

Kelly, M. (1997). Sexuality: Do nurses address sexual issues in the bone marrow transplant patient? *EBMT Nurses Group Journal, 2,* 4–13.

Keogh, F., O'Riordan, J. M., McCann, S. R., & McNamara, C. (1995). Bone marrow transplantation: Assessing the need for psychological intervention. *EBMT Nurses Group Journal, 1,* 29–35.

Keskimäki, R., & Tammisto, M. (1994). Instructions after bone marrow transplantation for adults. *EBMT Nurses Group Journal, 1,* 49–51.

Keskimäki, R., Tammisto, M. & Uotinen, H. (1997). Quality of life after allogeneic or autologous bone marrow or peripheral blood stem cell transplantation. *EBMT Nurses Group Journal, 1,* 48–59.

Kersteman, J., & van de Loo, F. (1991). Using the video film for patient introduction. *Proceedings of the 7th Meeting of the EBMT Nurses Group* (p. 79). Cortina d'Ampezzo, Italy.

Kretzer, D. A., Morgan, T., & Swan, N. (1994). Adaptation of the mead model for nursing for use in a bone marrow transplant (BMT) unit. *EBMT Nurses Group Journal, 2,* 31–34.

Larsen, J., Stenstrup, K., & Lerche Olesen, S. (1989). The development of a means of communication information to prospective bone marrow transplant patients. *Proceedings of the 5th Meeting of the EBMT Nurses Group* (pp. 63–69). Badgastein, Austria.

Leather, M. J., Herrmann, R. P., Cannell, P. K., Buffery, S., & Seward, C. (1998). Nursing Challenges: Autologous transplantation patient treated at home. *EBMT Nurses Group Journal, 1,* 11–14.

Lenssen, P. (2000). Cancer-related fatigue. *EBMT Nurses Group Journal, 2,* 17–19.

Lienhart, V. (2001). Complementary therapies for nausea and vomiting. *EBMT Nurses Group Journal, 1,* 13–16.

Meeberg, G. A. (1993). Quality of life: A concept analysis. *Journal of Advanced Nursing, 18,* 32–38.

Molassiotis, A., Boughton, B. J., Burgoyne, T., & van den Akker, O. B. A. (1994). Psychological and physical difficulties in patients post BMT. *EBMT Nurses Group Journal, 1,* 2–6.

Monteiro de Barros, M. C., & Pot-Mees, C. (1994). Enhancing communication: Understanding drawings of bone marrow transplant children. *EBMT Nurses Group Journal, 1,* 56–57.

Morgan, G. (1991). Striking the balance between the need for ongoing research and optimum patient care. *Proceedings of the 7th Meeting of the EBMT Nurses Group* (pp. 49–50). Cortina d'Ampezzo, Italy.

Muir, A. (2000). Sexuality and bone marrow transplantation (BMT)—Considerations for nursing care. *EBMT Nurses Group Journal, 1,* 7–11.

Naylor, N. (1987). Patient's own story. *Proceedings of the 3rd Meeting of the EBMT Nurses Group* (pp. 78–88). Interlaken, Switzerland.

Neyens, M. (1987). Psychological approach of a patient in isolation. *Proceedings of the 3rd Meeting of the EBMT Nurses Group* (pp. 58–59). Interlaken, Switzerland.

Nilsson, U. (1987). Experiences and consequences for families whose child goes through a bone marrow transplantation. *Proceedings of the 3rd Meeting of the EBMT Nurses Group* (pp. 26–33). Interlaken, Switzerland.

Nogay, G., Bilgen, H., Anak, S., Yalman, N., Özgenç, S., Can, E., & Gedikoglu, G. (1998). Depression in the siblings of pediatric BMT patients. *EBMT Nurses Group Journal, 2,* 30–32.

Peykerli, G., Bilgen, H., Ozgenc, S., Can, E., Yalman, N., Anak, S., & Gedikoglu, G. (2002). "Back to School" after pediatric stem cell transplantation. *EBMT Nurses Group Journal, 1*, 14–17.

Planzer, M., & Baumann, D. (1987). Physiotherapy in Life-Islands. *Proceedings of the 3rd Meeting of the EBMT Nurses Group* (pp. 34–42). Interlaken, Switzerland.

Pot-Mees, C., & Zeitlin, H. (1985). Psychosocial aspects of a bone marrow transplantation for child and family: Some first observations. *Proceedings of the 1st Meeting of the EBMT Nurses Group* (pp. 29–34). Bad Hofgastein (Salzburg), Austria.

Pugh, J., & Toy, A. (1989). Sperm banking—A cause for concern. *Proceedings of the 5th Meeting of the EBMT Nurses Group* (pp. 171–173). Badgastein, Austria.

Rafi, H., Rieux, C., Pautas, C., Beaune, J., Kuentz, M., Bernaudin, F., Jabot-Lestang, L., Christophe, M. G., & Cordonnier, C. (1999). To what extent should we inform the patients before stem cell transplant. *EBMT Nurses Group Journal, 2*, 8–9.

Salovaara, H., Riitta, W., Ilves, L. & Kauppila, M. (1999). The coping of a patient after a bone marrow transplantation or a stem cell transplantation. *EBMT Nurses Group Journal, 1*, 20–26.

Saudubray, C., Tellaa, K., Feral, T., Moarau, G., & André, M. (1989). Project for a booklet for patients admitted for a bone marrow transplantation. *Proceedings of the 5th Meeting of the EBMT Nurses Group* (p. 165). Badgastein, Austria.

Simonds, C., Serge Beaussier, P., & Vissuzaine, A. (1994). Clowns in the bone marrow transplant unit: A challenge. *EBMT Nurses Group Journal, 1*, 54–55.

Slater, C., Bass, G. A., Boraks, P. A., Price, J., & Marcus, R. E. (1995). Patients' perceptions of information and support given with regard to fertility pre and post bone marrow transplantation. *EBMT Nurses Group Journal, 1995-1*, 39–41.

Spilker, B. (1990). Introduction. In B. Spilker (Ed.), *Quality of life assessments in clinical trials* (pp. 3–9). New York: Raven Press.

Stotts, M., & Bouchard, M. (1997). Allogeneic bone marrow and blood cell transplantation without protective isolation: A seven year retrospective review. *EBMT Nurses Group Journal, 1*, 13–15.

Svahn, B.-M. (1999). Homecare in allogeneic stem cell transplantation. *EBMT Nurses Group Journal, 2*, 17–18.

Toy, A. (1989). Outpatient care following bone marrow transplantation. *Proceedings of the 5th Meeting of the EBMT Nurses Group* (pp. 143–148). Badgastein, Austria.

Valdmaa, E., & Lundqvist, C. H. (1995). Support groups for relatives to patients with hematological malignancies. *EBMT Nurses Group Newsletter, 1*, 18–19.

Van den Brand, I. (2001). Life after bone marrow transplantation: The Paradox between cure and crippling. *EBMT Nurses Group Journal, 2*, 10–12.

van de Loo, F. M. P., & Mentink, C. H. (1987). Life after BMT: Psychological aspects after discharge. *Proceedings of the 3rd Meeting of the EBMT Nurses Group* (pp. 70–77). Interlaken, Switzerland.

Van Nierop, G. (1992). Ethical aspects of patient care in the laminar air flow unit. *EBMT Nurses Group Newsletter, 2,* 34–37.

Vecchi, R., & Coppola, A. (1991). Psychologic observations on the emotional involvement about death in young BMT patients. *Proceedings of the 7th Meeting of the EBMT Nurses Group* (pp. 77–78). Cortina d'Ampezzo, Italy.

Verhoeven, M. J. F. W., & Smiet, T. (1995). Continuity in nursing care: A necessity. *EBMT Nurses Group Journal, 1,* 42–44.

Vickers, P. (1994). Physical and psychological development of children following long-term isolation and matched or haploidentical mismatched bone marrow transplantation for one of the severe immunodeficiency disorders: A preliminary study. *EBMT Nurses Group Journal, 1,* 39–48.

Wendel, K., van Benthem, D., & Fliedner, M. (1991.) Psychological and psychiatric effects of BMT. *Proceedings of the 7th Meeting of the EBMT Nurses Group* (pp. 25–28). Cortina d'Ampezzo, Italy.

Wilke, S., Rudolf, G., Grande, T., Siegert, W., & Sowade, C. (1989). Dealing with interactional conflicts during a bone marrow transplantation in a psychotherapeutic liaison consulting service. *Proceedings of the 5th Meeting of the EBMT Nurses Group* (pp. 115–120). Badgastein, Austria.

Wirén, R., Hämäläinen, T., & Entonen, A. (1993). The BMT patient's mental support in our department. *EBMT Nurses Group Newsletter, 2,* 8–14.

Yang, W. (1990). The quality of life and the power to heal. *Proceedings of the 6th Meeting of the EBMT Nurses Group* (pp. 131–136). The Hague, The Netherlands.

Zhan, L. (1993). Quality of life: Conceptual and measurement issues. *Journal of Advanced Nursing, 17,* 795–800.

15

Fatigue and
Quality of Life
A Question of Balance

MARGARET BARTON-BURKE

Fatigue provides perhaps the perfect example of inquiry into quality of life.
—B. R. Ferrell (1995)

Fatigue and quality of life (QOL) are two illusive concepts in the field of nursing and nursing science. While both of these concepts are sources of multidimensional as well as multifactorial research, this research has been conducted in tandem, with only a few studies looking at the relationship between fatigue and QOL. Authors suggest that a combination of multidimensional and multifactorial mechanisms are likely to impact one's QOL (Barnett, 1997; Cella & Tulsky, 1990; Dow & Ferrell, 1994; Ferrans, 1990; Ferrans & Powers, 1985; Gotay, Korn, McCabe, Moore, & Cheson, 1992; Gough, Furnival, Schilder, & Grove, 1983; King et al., 1997; Pater et al., 1997; Vogelzang et al., 1997; Winningham, 1995; Winningham, 1999) as well as influence the sensation of fatigue (Camarillo, 1992; Lee, Lentz, Taylor, Mitchell, & Woods, 1994; Piper, Lindsay, & Dodd, 1987; Richardson, 1995; Smets, Garssen, Schuster-Uitterhoeve, & de Haes, 1993; Winningham, 1995; Winningham et al., 1994).

Richardson (1995) suggests that biological, psychological, social, and personal factors influence the onset, impact, expression, duration, and severity of the fatigue experience. Similar themes can be gleaned from the QOL literature. That is, writers from different disciplines (e.g., psychology, nursing, and medicine) propose that biological, psychological, social, and personal factors comprise an individual's QOL (Cella & Tulsky, 1990; Ferrans, 1990; Ferrell, 1995; Grant, Ackerman, & Rivera, 1994).

Additionally, the significant nexus between fatigue and QOL is the fact that both concepts are uniquely constructed by the meaning that the individual attributes to them. For example, early works (Bartley, 1965; Bartley & Chute, 1947) specified three distinct factors related to fatigue. First, it is a self-recognized state, second, it results from a directly experienced condition, and third, there is an inferred connection between ways an individual feels and the amount of exertion experienced. Although tools exist to measure fatigue, subjective reporting of the individual's perception is the most common way to currently assess fatigue in clinical populations. While Webb (1994) described QOL as an abstract concept that is neither a useful nor an accurate term for measuring what is essentially a subjective experience, she posited that in actual practice QOL assessment needs to incorporate not only objective measurement scales but also in-depth interviews that reflect the individual's experiences and idiosyncrasies.

The purpose of this chapter is to introduce the current knowledge about cancer-related fatigue (CRF) and attempt to develop linkages between CRF and QOL. The relationship between these two concepts will be explored through analysis of theory and research. Specific nursing practice interventions will be developed. Additionally this chapter presents reconstructed knowledge about CRF and QOL, thus building new knowledge about the subject matter.

Quotations are interspersed throughout the chapter in an effort to blend qualitative and quantitative perspectives of human science. The quote at the beginning of the chapter by Ferrell, a nurse scientist with extensive work in the area of cancer pain, illustrates the nature of the attention being given to fatigue and QOL.

Fatigue and Cancer—A Beginning Exploration

It's a different kind of tired than you could ever describe. . . . It used to be like it would be too much effort to lift your hands from your lap but it wouldn't be like you would want to go to sleep. . . . And it wouldn't be like sleeping would help. It wouldn't be like you had done too much exercising and you were worn out. It's different than anything that you could experience. . . . It's different from all kinds of stuff. It's just it's own kind of tiredness. . . . It's completely immobilizing.

—Ellie (From Barton-Burke, 2002)

Fatigue is a universal complaint associated with most disease and illness states. However, fatigue is a phenomenon that is also seen in healthy populations. As an illness phenomenon, fatigue affects one's ability to perform everyday activities and increases dependence on others, which ultimately affects the QOL of the fatigued individual. The quote above elegantly illustrates the fatigue experience from a personal perspective. Fatigue has important implications for cancer care and offers a unique nursing challenge.

Fatigue has been described as the most distressing symptom resulting from cancer and its treatment (Ehlke, 1988; Haylock & Hart, 1979; King, Nail, Kreamer, Strohl, & Johnson, 1985; Knobf, 1986; Piper, Lindsay, Dodd, Ferketich, Paul, & Weller, 1989; Rhodes, Watson, & Hanson, 1988). This symptom can and in many cases does have significant impact on the QOL of cancer patients.

A framework for thinking about cancer and the therapies associated with the treatment of the disease is presented in Figure 15-1. The framework depicts potential etiologies contributing to fatigue and consequently the impact of fatigue on quality of life for the person with cancer. These etiologies are known to potentiate the sensation of fatigue for the person with cancer. This figure illustrates both the physical and psychological nature of fatigue.

Cancer contributes both physically and psychologically to the fatigue experienced by persons with the disease. For example, it is thought that the accumulation of metabolites, changes in sleep patterns, and concomitant diseases are a few of the

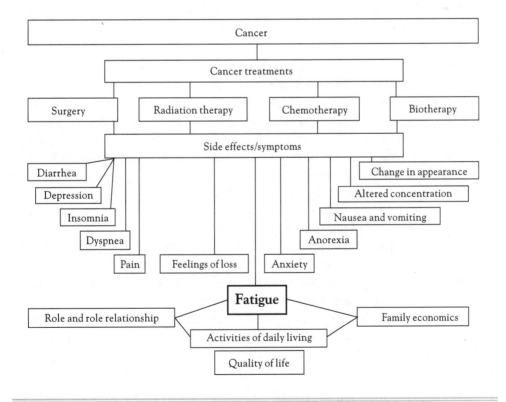

Figure 15-1. **The impact of cancer and its treatments on fatigue and quality of life.**
Source: Copyright 1995 by Margaret Barton-Burke. All rights reserved. Used with written consent of the author.

factors that contribute to the physiological nature of fatigue. Additionally, concerns about survival, daily activities including family concerns, and the stress of having a diagnosis of cancer add to the psychological and social nature of fatigue.

Cancer therapies such as surgery, radiation, chemotherapy, and biotherapy are associated with numerous symptoms and side effects and depending on the type and combination of treatments used, there can be many more symptoms and side effects than those illustrated in Figure 15-1.

Quality of Life—The Concept

Some of the factors that contribute to the quality of life are common to all human beings: they are inscribed in the genetic code of the human species and probably have not changed significantly since the Stone Age. Civilized and sophisticated as we may be, we have inherited from our distant ancestors the ability to derive some of our most profound satisfactions from the activities of daily life—when we eat, drink and love; dream, tell stories or enact imaginings in gesture and pictures; participate in community events where we are both spectators and actors.

—R. Dubos (1976)

Nurses have always focused on helping patients to maintain or regain an acceptable QOL despite the disease and its treatment. Dubos (1976) suggested that health professionals only discuss the concept of QOL from within an illness context. Rarely do health care providers attempt to understand QOL for the healthy person. Fatigue is one symptom that impacts QOL for healthy or ill persons. Recently, however, QOL for persons with cancer has become a major concern as more aggressive treatments become available and morbidity figures increase (Gotay et al., 1992). It is now evident to nurses and scientists that clinical trials must include instruments that capture the morbidity associated with treatments, including fatigue and its effects on the multiple domains of quality of life (Gotay et al., 1992).

Incorporating into treatment decisions the likely impact on QOL is especially important with cancer patients who typically receive toxic therapy. Usually nurses are the health care providers who give serious consideration to the symptom of fatigue because they are the provider who observes the impact of CRF on the patient and their families' lives. Interestingly, Smets and colleagues' (1993) review of the literature on fatigue and cancer revealed that the majority of published work has been authored by nurses.

Quality of life must be defined in the context of particular factors that affect a person's feelings about life. For persons with cancer it is logical to focus on the changes in QOL resulting from their disease or treatment, keeping in mind that deleterious changes may or may not be the result of physical symptoms.

Table 15-1. **Quality of Life Definitions—A Sampler**

A person's sense of well-being, satisfaction or dissatisfaction with life, or happiness or unhappiness. (Dalkey & Rourke, 1973)

A vague and ethereal entity, something that many people talk about, but which nobody very clearly knows what to do about. (Campbell, Converse, & Rodgers, 1976)

The satisfaction of needs. (Ferrans & Powers, 1985)

Patients' appraisal of and satisfaction with their current level of function compared to what they perceive to be possible or ideal. (Cella & Cherin, 1988)

A pragmatic, day-to-day, functional representation of a patient's physical, psychological, and social response to a disease and its treatment. (Schipper, 1990)

Individuals' overall satisfaction with life and their general sense of personal well-being. (Shumaker, Anderson, & Czajkowski, 1990)

Quality of life is a multidimensional construct including, at minimum, physical, social, and psychological domains as well as disease and treatment-related symptoms. Quality of life is a state of well-being that is a composite of two components: 1) the ability to perform everyday activities that reflect physical, psychological, and social well-being, and 2) patient satisfaction with levels of function, control of disease, and treatment-related symptoms. (Gotay et al., 1992)

Quality of life is purported to be the whole picture: 1) assessment of functional status, 2) disease and treatment-related symptoms, 3) psychological function, 4) social function, 5) patient satisfaction with care rendered, 6) degree of economic disruption that may occur, 7) impact of the treatment on body image and sexual function, and 8) spiritual and existential concerns. (Ganz, 1993)

Definitions and models of QOL abound, and Table 15-1 identifies a small sample of the many definitions of QOL that can be found in the scientific literature to date. Additional definitions are provided in Appendix 1. Of note is the explicit agreement across scholars that QOL is a multidimensional phenomena. Quality of life may be connected to the degree of satisfaction with present life circumstances, adequate self-esteem, a purpose in life, and minimal anxiety. Additionally, the concept of QOL may be connected to a complex network of support, positive personal attitudes, adequate physical functioning, and perceived well-being.

Finally, a simplistic example for understanding QOL can be found in a mathematical equation similar to that created by Cella and Cherin (1988). Table 15-2 depicts the equation with an individual's actual experience as the numerator and the individual's expectation of the experience as the denominator; the sum represents an indication of the individual's QOL. Nurses working with persons diagnosed with cancer may find it helpful to consider this mathematical equation as patients describe and discuss the impact of fatigue on their QOL.

Table 15-2. **Quality of Life Equation**

$$\frac{\text{Individual's actual experience}}{\text{Individual expectation of experience}} = \text{Quality of life}$$

Source: Adapted from Cella & Cherin, 1988.

Interestingly, only a few published studies (Berger, 1993; Camarillo, 1992; Cella & Bron, 1999; Ferrell, Grant, Dean, Funk, & Ly, 1996; Lovely, Miaskowski, & Dodd, 1999; Rhodes, Watson, & Hanson, 1988) describe the relationship between fatigue and QOL for the person with cancer. These studies highlight the lack of knowledge about fatigue and its relationship to other symptoms, energy levels, livelihood, relationships, roles, and leisure activities.

Quality of life is implicit in the oncology nursing research literature on fatigue. Decreases in both physical and mental functioning from fatigue have been reported by numerous investigators (Aistars, 1987; Blesch et al., 1991; Cimprich, 1990; Ehlke, 1988; Pickard-Holley, 1991; Piper, Lindsay, & Dodd, 1987; Potempa et al., 1986). Both Aistars (1987) and Winningham (1992) suggested that fatigue associated with cancer must be managed, or impaired functional status with decreased quality of life may result.

Theories Undergirding the Knowledge of Fatigue

As a group [fatigue] theories present concepts but do not provide explicit testable hypotheses. Further theory development is particularly needed in better integrating the physiological mechanisms into the current models that can provide rationale for interventions. Additionally feedback mechanisms and/or interactions between key constructs in these models should be established (ex: the relationship between pain and fatigue where fatigue can be the cause and the result of pain). We also recommend that theory should focus in areas where nursing can make a difference in outcomes, i.e., activity/rest, sleep, symptom management, psychological and environment.

—Excerpt from the transcript of the Oncology Nursing Society
State-of-the-Knowledge Conference, November 19–22, 1992, Park City, Utah

People reason (or theorize) for two purposes: (1) to reach conclusions about the world in order to describe, explain, and predict phenomena in it and (2) to achieve action in order to bring about the changes they consider desirable.

Fatigue has been identified as one of the most common and disturbing symptoms of cancer and its treatment. The reported incidence of fatigue in patients receiving active treatment for cancer, including surgery, radiation therapy, chemotherapy, and biotherapy, has exceeded 90 percent (Blesch et al., 1991; Nail & Winningham, 1993). Fatigue is a phenomenon that has important implications for theory-building, research, and practice in oncology nursing. Clinically, individuals may discontinue treatment because of fatigue, practitioners may limit doses of various forms of treatment due to fatigue, and individuals with cancer may attribute impairment of QOL to fatigue (Piper, Rieger, Brophy, Haeuber, Hood, Lyver, & Sharpe, 1989; Quesada, Talpaz, Rios, Kwizrock, & Gutterman, 1986). Despite the prevalence of fatigue in cancer patients, as well as its impact, its mechanisms are poorly understood and lack theoretical descriptions, explanations, or predictors.

In part, the myriad of definitions of fatigue in the literature lack clarity, cohesiveness, and consistency. Table 15-3 provides a select list of fatigue definitions from the literature. Although there is no general agreement regarding a definition for

---

Table 15-3. Definitions of Fatigue—A Selected List

Fatigue is a decrease in physical performance. (Grandjean, 1968)

A state of increased discomfort and decreased efficiency resulting from expenditures of energy reserve. (Hart & Frell, 1982)

A subjective sense of weariness or tiredness resulting from exertion or stress or as a condition of impaired efficiency resulting from prolonged mental and/or physical activity or from an attitude of boredom or from disgust with monotonous work. (Varricchio, 1985)

Subjective feelings of generalized weariness, weakness, exhaustion, and lack of energy resulting from prolonged stress that is directly or indirectly attributable to the disease process. (Aistars, 1987)

Fatigue is a human response to the experience of having cancer and to undergoing treatment for cancer. (Nail & King, 1987)

Fatigue is defined as a subjective feeling of tiredness that is influenced by circadian rhythm. It can vary in unpleasantness, duration, and intensity. When acute, it serves a protective function; when it becomes unusual, excessive, or constant (chronic), it no longer serves this function and may lead to the aversion to activity with the desire to escape. (Piper, Lindsay, & Dodd, 1987)

An overwhelming sense of exhaustion and decreased capacity for physical and mental work regardless of adequate sleep. (Kim, McFarland, & McLane, 1989)

A condition characterized by the subjective feeling of increased discomfort and decreased functional status related to a decrease in energy. (Pickard-Holley, 1991)

A state of decreased capacity for physical or mental work, the perception of which arises from a complex interaction of somatic and psychologic factors. (Winningham, 1992)

Fatigue is a subjective phenomenon related to indicators of fatigue such as energy expenditure, sleep disturbances, attentional deficits, decreased endurance, somatic complaints, and weakness. The subjective experience impacts objective performance. (Winningham et al., 1994)

fatigue, there is consensus that fatigue is a multifactorial and a multidimensional phenomenon.

Conceptual definitions form the basis for both theoretical thinking and research about fatigue and are linked to the philosophical nature of the discipline from which theory and research arise. Fatigue theories can be found in the disciplines of psychology (Grandjean, 1968), physiology (Gibson & Edwards, 1985), ergonomics (Bhambhani, Eriksson, & Steadward, 1991; Bohle & Tilley, 1993; Brunier & Graydon, 1993; Cabon, Coblentz, Mollard, & Fouillot, 1993; Carson, 1994; Gratz & Boulton, 1994; Harma, Ilmarinen, Knauth, Rutenfranz, & Hanninen, 1988a, 1988b; Kecklund & Akerstedt, 1993; Oginska, Pokorski, & Oginska, 1993; Reynolds, 1994; Scholz, Millford, & McMillan, 1995; Stiles, 1994), nursing (Aistars, 1987; Cimprich, 1990; Lee et al., 1994; Milligan & Pugh, 1994; Piper et al., 1987; Potempa et al., 1986; Pugh & Milligan, 1993; Winningham, 1992), and medicine (Christen, Stage, Galbo, Christensen, & Kehlet, 1989).

There are currently ten theories in the literature offering theoretical explanations of fatigue. These theories can be found in Table 15-4 and fall into one of two paradigms, health or illness.

Three fatigue theories in the paradigm of health include Grandjean's General State of Fatigue Theory (1968), the science of ergonomics, and Edwards' Theory of Neuromuscular Fatigue (Gibson & Edwards, 1985). All three theories consider fatigue as a phenomenon that occurs in healthy individuals.

Grandjean states that "the term fatigue is often used with different meanings and is applied in such a diversity of contexts that it has led to a confusion of ideas" (Grandjean, 1968, p. 427). Grandjean, a psychologist, presented general fatigue from

Table 15-4. Theories Undergirding Explanations of Fatigue

Health Paradigm (Discipline)

Grandjean's (1968) General State of Fatigue Theory (Psychology)
Ergonomics (Ergonomics)
Edwards' (Gibson & Edwards, 1985) Theory of Neuromuscular Fatigue (Physiology)

Illness Paradigm (Discipline)

Aistars' (1987) Organizing Framework (Nursing)
Lee and colleagues' (1994) Multidimensional Model of Fatigue (Nursing)
Potempa's (1986) General Fatigue Model (Nursing)
Pugh and Mulligan's (1993) Childbirth Fatigue Framework (Nursing)
Cimprich's (1990) Attentional Fatigue (Nursing)
Piper, Lindsay, and Dodd's (1987) Integrated Fatigue Model (Nursing)
Winningham's (1992) Psychobiologic Entropy Hypothesis (Nursing)

a physiological standpoint. In Grandjean's General State of Fatigue Theory, the reticular activating system is the key to an individual's fatigue. He makes a logical case for explaining fatigue from a neuropsychological perspective, and although his model is outdated, his description of symptoms is useful and referred to even today.

Ergonomics is the science that seeks to adapt work or working conditions to the worker. It can also be thought of as the study of people adjusting to their environments. Scientists from this discipline examine worker fatigue as it relates to the industrial environment (e.g., fatigue in assembly line workers, fatigue and tiredness associated with computer use). Theoretical descriptions, explanations, or predictions based on the science of ergonomics seem inappropriate to use as a model for persons with cancer.

In Edwards' Theory of Neuromuscular Fatigue, he proposed that both central and peripheral mechanisms of the central nervous system are involved in the fatigue experience. This theory offers a logical chain of reasoning to explain fatigue from a physiological perspective. However, it does not explicate the relationship of the immune system and other factors such as psychosocial or environmental factors, which may be involved in the fatigue experience.

Fatigue theories within the illness paradigm include Aistairs' Organizing Framework for Fatigue (1987), Lee and colleagues' Multidimensional Model of Fatigue (1994), Potempa's General Fatigue Model (1986), Pugh and Mulligan's Childbirth Fatigue Framework (1993), Cimprich's Attentional Fatigue (1990), Piper, Lindsay, and Dodd's Integrated Fatigue Model (1987), and Winningham's Psychobiologic Entropy Hypothesis (1992). The discipline from which these descriptive and explanatory theories arise is nursing. Lee and associates (1994) and Potempa and colleagues' (1986) work treated fatigue as a general phenomenon, while Pugh and Mulligan's (1993) framework focused on the fatigue associated with childbirth. The remainder of the illness paradigm fatigue theories relate directly to persons with cancer.

Lee and colleagues (1994) proposed that fatigue is a subjective response to environmental demands that exceed resources, while Potempa and colleagues posited that psychological, physiological, pathophysiologic, and personality factors mediate the perception of fatigue. Potempa and colleagues suggested that environmental factors also influence this perception. Their conceptualization of fatigue was based on a balance between energy conservation and energy expenditure. If one's energy is kept in balance, then fatigue is not experienced. However, if an individual does not maintain energy reserves, or energy reserves become depleted, as in chronic illness, the individual experiences chronic fatigue.

Pugh and Mulligan (1993) offered a framework to explain fatigue in a specific population. This theory identified physiological, psychological, and situational factors that may cause fatigue and influence performance factors during labor and delivery. It has several commonalities with other models but is specific to the child-birth experience rather than the cancer experience.

In oncology, Aistars' (1987) Stressor Model examined physiological, psychological, and situational stressors and fatigue. This model helped explain the difference between tiredness and fatigue. It may be useful clinically since Aistairs hypothesized that prolonged stress causes fatigue. This occurs physiologically by activating the reticular activating system and the sympathetic nervous system, resulting in a release of stress hormones. Ultimately, these hormones lead to a depletion of energy stores in the body. This theory tends to describe and explain cancer-related fatigue; however, it does not guide practice or research. Furthermore, it does not explain the relationship between the stressors and the response.

Cimprich's theory of attentional fatigue was based on attentional theory developed by James, Posner, and Kaplan (Cimprich, 1990). Two kinds of attention (directed attention and involuntary attention) are central to Cimprich's conceptualization. Directed attention reflects a controlled process that supports purposeful activities of daily life and requires mental efforts to sustain. Multiple factors, including informational, affective, and behavioral, increase the requirements for directed attention when dealing with a life-threatening illness. If the demands exceed the attentional capacity, the person is at risk for fatigue. The fatigue of directed attention leads to impairment in purposeful activities. The model also is prescriptive and contains a conceptual basis for alleviating attentional fatigue, including nursing components to conserve directed attention (Cimprich, 1990). Richardson (1995) suggested that the application of theoretical frameworks addressing components of fatigue, such as Cimprich had done, may enhance understanding of fatigue in persons with cancer.

In oncology nursing, Piper's Integrated Fatigue Model (Piper et al., 1987; Piper, 1991) and Winningham's Psychobiologic Entropy Hypothesis (Winningham, 1992) both offer a broader interpretation and a holistic perspective of fatigue for the person with cancer. This perspective distinguishes the discipline of nursing from other disciplines.

Piper's Integrated Fatigue Model (Piper et al., 1987; Piper, 1991) presents a thorough and complex framework for explaining the fatigue of cancer. The manifestations as well as the etiologies of fatigue are considered in Piper's work. The model has been developed over time specifically for individuals with cancer. Figure 15-2 emphasizes the complex nature of the phenomenon.

This theory has many strengths, including (1) offering a comprehensive approach to looking at cancer-related fatigue, (2) blending knowledge about fatigue from several disciplines, (3) grounding in the clinical phenomenon, and (4) its use in assessing the fatigued individual. However, Figure 15-2 depicts a static theory, lacking specific interactions, theoretical statements, propositions, and outcomes. The

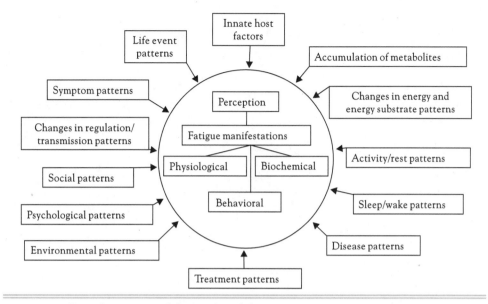

Figure 15-2. **Piper's integrated fatigue model.**

Source: Reprinted from the *Oncology Nursing Forum* with permission from the Oncology Nursing Press, Inc. Piper, B., Lindsey, A., & Dodd, M. 1987. Fatigue mechanisms in cancer patients: Developing nursing theory. *Oncology Nursing Forum* 14(6), 17–23.

lack of theoretical links between categories points to the need for continued development of this theory. A significant theoretical and scientific outgrowth of Piper's Integrated Fatigue Model is the Piper Fatigue Scale, a measurement tool based on this model. Finally, this model is clinically relevant and it could be developed into a comprehensive assessment tool for fatigue.

Winningham's (1992) Psychobiologic Entropy Hypothesis proposes a model in which any symptom that decreases activity can increase perceptions of fatigue, decrease functional status, promote disability, and result in decreased QOL. Winningham, a nurse physiologist, developed this theory to explain fatigue, particularly in the cancer patient, through an explanation of fatigue as a symptom that can be influenced by the disease, treatment, and subsequent symptoms (side effects) of cancer.

Figure 15-3 highlights the various factors that contribute to fatigue in the person with cancer; additionally, fatigue is conceptualized as both a primary and secondary phenomenon. Winningham hypothesized that if fatigue cannot be alleviated, then another fatigue can occur secondary to the primary fatigue.

This model differs from other nursing theories in that it focuses on activity and energetics, thereby offering a different paradigm. Theoretically, propositional statements are offered by Winningham (1992) and can be found in Table 15-5. Additionally, Winningham proposed an energetic continuum and a fatigue-inertia spiral,

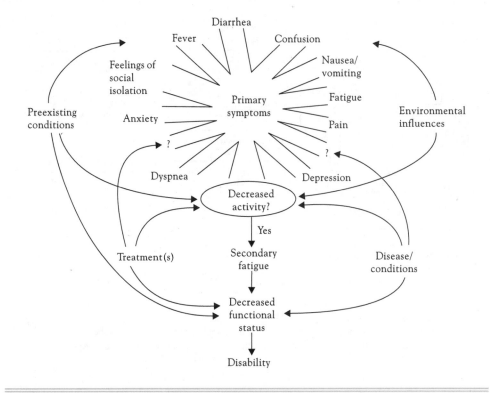

Figure 15-3. **Winningham's psychobiologic entropy hypothesis.**
Source: Copyright 1992, 1993 by Maryl L. Winningham. All rights reserved. Used with written consent of the author.

Table 15-5. **Propositions of the Winningham Psychobiologic Entropy Hypothesis**

- Too much as well as too little rest promotes fatigue.
- Too much as well as too little activity promotes fatigue.
- A dynamic balance between rest and activity minimizes fatigue; an imbalance between the two promotes fatigue.
- Any symptom or condition that contributes to diminished daily activity will contribute to increased perceived fatigue and decreased capacity for functioning.
- Any treatment or intervention that provides relief of a symptom that contributes to decreased activity may also mitigate fatigue *provided* the intervention does not have a sedating or catabolic effect.

Figure 15-4. **Energetic continuum of the Winningham psychobiologic entropy hypothesis.**

Figures 15-4 and 15-5. Winningham (1992) contended that there is a range of fatigue extending from fatigue-inertia to energy-vigor, as well as a spiraling phenomenon related to fatigue.

Winningham's Psychobiologic Entropy Hypothesis suggests a systems theory with feedback mechanisms; however, all feedback loops have not been explicated to date. A feedback loop, which is clearly visible in the model, relates to primary fatigue. If primary fatigue is ablated, there should be no progression to a secondary fatigue. Conversely, if primary fatigue progresses to secondary fatigue, eventually the patient will experience a decrease in functional status, and disability will ensue.

The model considers environmental factors and preexisting conditions as contributors to cancer-related fatigue, but to what extent these factors influence fatigue is unclear. This theory may be clinically useful for assessment and management of fatigue, although its usefulness in oncology nursing has not been determined at this

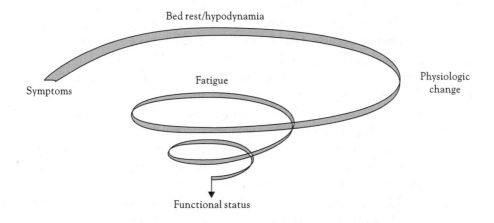

Figure 15-5. **Fatigue-inertia spiral of the Winningham psychobiologic entropy hypothesis.**

time. Neither Winningham's nor Piper and colleagues' theories have been tested empirically to date.

The dearth and disparity in the literature regarding theoretical descriptions, explanations, and predictors about the phenomenon of CRF supports the need for further work in theory development for oncology nursing practice, CRF, and QOL.

Nursing Research Related to Fatigue, Cancer, and Quality of Life

Fatigue is a common problem for many patients with cancer. However, it should be viewed not only as a symptom, but also as a profound experience that affects all aspects of a patient's life and has a great impact on quality of life.

—G. E. Dean and B. R. Ferrell (1995)

Research issues related to the subject of QOL are dealt with elsewhere in this book. This portion of the chapter will focus on research related to fatigue, cancer, and QOL. As mentioned earlier in this chapter, there are few published studies describing the relationship between CRF and QOL (Berger, 1998; Camarillo, 1992; Cella & Bron, 1999; Lovely, Miaskowski, & Dodd, 1999; Ferrans, 1990; Ferrell et al., 1996; Piper, Lindsey, Dodd, Ferketich, Paul, & Weller, 1989; Ream, 1996). An overview of the issues related to fatigue research will be presented, and studies that combine fatigue and QOL will be highlighted.

An increasing number of articles in the research literature critically analyze the subject of fatigue and the person with cancer. Combining the review by Richardson (1995) with articles by Irvine, Vincent, Bubela, Thompson, and Graydon (1991); Potempa (1993); Smets and associates (1993); and Winningham and colleagues (1994), one gleans the essence of the research conducted in the area of fatigue, as well as the strengths and weaknesses of this literature.

Fundamental to all research is the conceptualization of the phenomenon under scrutiny. It becomes important to the research that definitions of fatigue be both conceptual and operational. This is vital to one's understanding when comparing research results. However, terms to describe fatigue and definitions of the concept are used interchangeably. In the research that has been conducted, definitions of fatigue vary from terms used to denote a physical sensation or experience (Haylock & Hart, 1979; Kobashi-Schoot, Hanewald, van Dam, & Bruning, 1985; Kogi, Saito, & Mitsuhashi, 1970; Pearson & Byars, 1956; Rhoten, 1982) to those meaning a mental concept such as lack of concentration or deficits in cognitive functioning (Cimprich, 1990, 1993, 1995).

In addition to researcher-constructed definitions, the person with cancer also constructs definitions of fatigue. These definitions are usually descriptive and qualitative, for example:

Monica: . . . it's almost as if the gravity force is pulling me down to earth. It's like a rock. It just pulls. That's how I explain it.

Annie: It's an effort to move.

Monica: It's just like a gravity.

Ellie: I can't watch television.

Annie: It's hard to read. I can't read and that's my passion. I love to read.

Monica: You can't concentrate.

Annie: And I find if I don't take some time that I'm so debilitated. So Monday morning I cancelled my morning activities, spent 2½ hours in bed. I can't even tell you how unlike me that is. But it was either that or get so debilitated that then I'm snapping at my children and I'm totally like . . . (From Barton-Burke, 2002)

In published research the meaning attributed to fatigue by both researcher and subject is rarely made clear to the reader. Many times both the conceptual and operational definitions are inconsistent, or one may be missing from the research. Exploratory research by Glaus, Crow, and Hammond (1996); Krishnasamy (1996); Pyritz (1996); and Ream (1996) are attempts to clarify and define the concept of fatigue.

Fatigue is often operationalized as the subjective feeling of tiredness and lack of physical energy, but fatigue is also a concept with several dimensions of expression and multiple influencing factors. These include, but are not limited to, physical and cognitive dimensions; activity, hydration, nutrition, or motivational factors; and acuity or chronicity of the fatigue. Smets and colleagues (1993) posited, "which of these aspects describes the fatigue experience of cancer patients best is currently unknown" (p. 220).

Fatigue must be considered a multidimensional and multifactorial construct that should be measured as such, but this is not always reflected in the choice of measurement strategies (Irvine et al., 1991; Potempa, 1993; Richardson, 1995; Smets et al., 1993; Winningham et al., 1994). Tools used to measure fatigue have been unidimensional, comprised mostly of single items in a general symptom checklist (McCorkle, 1987; McCorkle & Young, 1978; Pearson & Byars, 1956; Rhoten, 1982), or multidimensional self-report questionnaires, with limited reliability and validity testing (Kobashi-Schoot, Hanewald, van Dam, & Bruning, 1985; Kogi, Saito, & Mitsuhashi, 1970; Piper, Lindsay, Dodd, Ferketich, Paul, & Weller, 1989).

Objective physiologic measures, such as muscle function, hemoglobin and hematocrit values, and anaerobic metabolism and energy expenditure, have not been routinely used for research related to fatigue. Other clinical measures such as CA 125 (Pickard-Holley, 1991) and tumor necrosis factor (TNF) (St. Pierre, Kasper, & Lindsay, 1992) offer some insight into CRF as a physical phenomenon with links to tumor-related byproducts.

Varricchio (1985, 1995) submitted that no standard exists for overall fatigue measurement. In addition to definitional considerations, objective correlates have not been identified and agreed on, and the subjective nature of fatigue cannot be ignored (Varricchio, 1995). Valid, reliable, psychometrically sound scientific instruments available to measure fatigue in the cancer population include Piper, Lindsay, Dodd, Ferketich, Paul, and Weller (1989); Smets, Garssen, Bonke, and de Haes (1995); and Schwartz (1998b). Glaus (1993, 1994) reported the development and use of a Visual Analogue Fatigue Scale in her research.

Most of the research on fatigue in cancer patients has not clearly identified specific correlates of fatigue. It is not clear how the direct effects of cancer, symptoms related to cancer, effects of cancer treatment, and the strain of dealing with cancer interact to generate or exacerbate fatigue (Irvine et al., 1991; Irvine et al., 1994; Loge & Kaasa, 1998; Pickard-Holley, 1991; Richardson, 1995). Additional confounding or intervening variables, such as the time of day fatigue is measured, baseline energy levels, changes in fatigue patterns over time, and circadian rhythms, are not addressed in the cancer-related fatigue literature.

Many patients with cancer identify fatigue as a frequent and significant side effect. To date, few sufficiently rigorous studies have registered systematically the number of cancer patients experiencing fatigue, taking into account the stage of the disease process and the extent of the problem.

Most studies reporting fatigue as a side effect of cancer treatments have limitations in that they include subjects presently under treatment as well as those who have completed treatment. In addition, subjects are interviewed only once, so it is impossible to establish any fatigue patterns. Many studies include patients with a variety of tumors, treatments, sites of treatments, and stages of disease; and no comparison groups are used (Irvine et al., 1991; Nail & King, 1987; Richardson, 1995; Smets et al., 1993). While several correlates of fatigue have been postulated, research to date has failed to verify consistent relationships among fatigue, sleep deprivation, anemia, and/or psychological distress (Irvine et al., 1991). No longitudinal studies nor studies on pediatric populations reporting CRF are found.

The majority of research on cancer-related fatigue has been conducted on Caucasian populations with small samples from single institutions. Studies are needed that target ethnically diverse populations from multiple settings.

However, in an effort to study the epidemiology of fatigue, a nationwide survey of 419 patients, 197 U.S.-based oncologists, and 200 caregivers (family members and friends who aid in the care of cancer patients' course of therapy (Vogelzang et al., 1997). Cancer patients, oncologists, and caregivers documented that fatigue had profound effects on patients, including their ability to work, meet family needs, and cope with disease. The study concluded that 78% of cancer patients' experience fatigue during the course of their disease; 53% responded that they experienced fatigue on most days, if not every day. Eight of ten physicians surveyed believed that fatigue was overlooked and undertreated, yet despite this prevalence, less than half of all physicians and cancer patients discussed it, and even fewer were treating it. Physicians believed that pain is the more debilitating and prevalent side effect, while patients say that fatigue affects their lives three times more than pain.

From this same study it could be implied that fatigue affects QOL since 61% of cancer patients in this survey said that fatigue adversely affected their ability to work, while 51% reported that they are unable to do their usual activities because of fatigue. The majority of patients claimed that fatigue affects their everyday lives. Almost 57% were unable to enjoy life fully because of fatigue and 31% said fatigue affected their hope of successfully fighting their cancer. Approximately 16% of patients surveyed said that treating their fatigue was as important as treating the cancer itself. Forty-two percent said that fatigue negatively affects their ability to take care of their families, while 29% said that they had difficulty just getting out of bed, and another 24% were fatigued to a point where they could not even eat.

Pater and colleagues (1997) examined factors affecting the level of fatigue among cancer patients participating in clinical trials and found that patients reporting the greatest amount of fatigue were females with ovarian or lung cancer who had metastatic disease and poor performance status. These data corroborate empirical evidence and the scientific literature in which the population reported to be most at risk for fatigue is younger women, that is women with breast cancer or ovarian cancer (Jamar, 1989; Irvine, Vincent, Graydon, Bubela, & Thompson, 1994; Pickard-Holley, 1991; Vogelzang, et al., 1997).

Additional findings (Pater et al., 1997) of patients treated with prophylactic antiemetics experience significantly less fatigue than did those not receiving this treatment. Efficient symptom management can decrease the experience of fatigue (Barnett, 1997; Buchsel, Barton-Burke, & Winningham, 2000; Gaston-Johansson, Fall-Dickson, Bakos, & Kennedy, 1999; Groopman, 1998; Jacobsen et al., 1999; Winningham, 1995, 1999). These findings suggest that optimal and organized management of one symptom may reduce the intensity of another symptom.

Despite the prevalence and disturbing nature of fatigue associated with cancer treatments, its complex nature and measurement difficulties have limited research efforts (Irvine et al., 1991). Its prevalence and impact require that cancer care researchers devote more time to assessing this common phenomenon with methodologically sound studies. Serious research efforts must be concentrated in this area to provide an empirical base for clinical practice (Richardson, 1995).

In conclusion, a few studies describing patient experiences with fatigue and the relationship between fatigue and quality of life have been published. These studies highlight the lack of knowledge about fatigue and its relationship to other symptoms, energy levels, livelihood, relationships, roles, and leisure activities.

The study by Rhodes and associates (1988)is a descriptive, retrospective study of symptoms and self-care behavior in chemotherapy patients. Investigators reported that tiredness and weakness were the symptoms that most interfered with self-care activities. This article was one of the first to suggest an association between CRF and QOL.

Camarillo's (1992) work, cited extensively throughout this chapter, stemmed from her unpublished graduate research on the meaning of fatigue. In this research Camarillo used Piper and colleagues' (1987) fatigue framework for conceptualization of fatigue. She applied her findings to the quality of life domains of physical, psychological, social, and spiritual care.

In a pilot study utilizing the Piper Fatigue Scale (Piper, Lindsay, Dodd, Ferketich, Paul, & Weller, 1989) and the Ferrans (1990) Quality of Life Index-CA version, Berger (1993) determined that as levels of perceived fatigue increased, there was a significant decrease in reported QOL among individuals receiving outpatient chemotherapy. These findings were the basis for Berger's doctoral research.

European author Ream (1996) reported in a qualitative study that patients describe aspects of fatigue that impact on everyday living and QOL. Study results suggested that both personal and disease attributes contribute to the perceptions of CRF, and that two concepts, control and commitment, are influential in managing fatigue.

Ferrell and colleagues (1996) concluded from secondary analysis of data collected from several studies that "fatigue is a force that affects all dimensions of QOL rather than being just an isolated physical symptom" (p. 1546).

Cella and Bron (1999) reviewed the use of epoetin alfa in the treatment of anemia. These researchers found anemia contributed to reduced QOL but no further conclusion could be drawn. Lovely and colleagues (1999) researched the relationship between fatigue and QOL in patients with glioblastoma multiforme. They found that patients with glioblastoma multiforme experience increases in fatigue after radiation therapy. These increases in fatigue are associated with decreases in almost all aspects of patients' QOL.

Fatigue—A Clinical Symptom

> Annie: Sometimes deep breathing or even taking 15 minutes to lay down all
> help.
>
> Monica: Power naps.
>
> Ellie: I have a chair that I sit in and I stare into space.
>
> Annie: Stare into space or something like that.
>
> Ellie: . . . I didn't used to be like this.
>
> (From Barton-Burke, 2002).

Despite the paucity of knowledge regarding the scientific underpinnings of CRF and the research limitations, it can be concluded that fatigue is a prevalent problem among persons with cancer. However, fatigue is a clinical symptom requiring intervention, and there is a dearth in the literature of research-based interventions for CRF. Most CRF interventions rely on empirics—clinical practices that work despite the lack of research supporting them.

The model in Figure 15-6 depicts the scope of interventions for cancer-related fatigue. In this example it is applied to fatigue; however the model may be used with any cancer-related symptom. The model is similar to other QOL models in the inclusion of classical QOL domains, it is different in that the foundation of the model is the physical dimension of care or the person with cancer. After the physical dimension has been addressed, care can be extended to the psychological, social, spiritual/existential, and economic dimensions. Care needs can arise in one or all

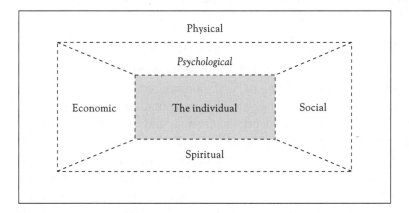

Figure 15-6. **The nature of care in oncology nursing.**

dimensions depending on the requirements of the individual or the family. The care model presupposes not only medical and nursing interventions, but also a multidisciplinary approach to relevant clinical symptoms.

Physical Care

Fatigue precedes, accompanies, and follows most malignancies and treatment (Woo, Dibble, Piper, Keating, & Weiss, 1998). If an individual has a concomitant illness, such as cardiac, respiratory, or renal disease, these factors may contribute to the fatigue experience.

Interventions following cancer therapies are based on the incidence of fatigue related to a given treatment. Most individuals with cancer undergo surgery for diagnosis or treatment. Despite the high incidence of postoperative fatigue observed in clinical practice, little research exists examining causes, correlates, and interventions for postoperative fatigue (Winningham et al., 1994).

The majority of CRF research has been conducted on individuals receiving radiation and chemotherapy. While more is known about the prevalence, duration, and patterns of fatigue in patients receiving radiation therapy than other treatments (Barrere, Trotta, & Foster, 1993; Haylock & Hart, 1979; Irvine et al., 1991; Kobashi-Schoot et al., 1985; Nail & King, 1987; Piper, Rieger et al., 1989; Richardson, 1995), the prevalence of fatigue related to the administration of chemotherapy may occur at rates approximating 75 to 100 percent (Smets et al., 1993).

Biotherapy, particularly interferons, interleukin-2, tumor necrosis factor, and colony stimulating factors, expose persons with cancer to exogenous and endogenous cytokines. Fatigue is the dose-limiting toxicity of this cancer treatment (Piper, Rieger et al., 1989; Quesada et al., 1986). It has been suggested that the fatigue of biotherapy may be more intense, protracted, and debilitating than that of the other three major treatment interventions (Piper et al., 1989). In addition, the mechanisms of biotherapy may differ completely from those of other interventions.

Additional factors related to CRF include conditions such as malnutrition, cachexia, and weight loss, along with the accumulation of cell destruction end products and toxic metabolites. Infections, anemia, and drug therapy (pain medication, concomitant drugs such as antiemetics, and over-the-counter drugs) have been implicated in CRF, while inactivity and bedrest may contribute to sleep deprivation and consequently fatigue (Berger & Farr, 1999). Most of these factors contribute to fatigue by having the potential to decrease energy stores within the body.

Anemia is frequently mentioned as a possible factor in CRF (Maxwell, 1984). This condition is probably a factor when hemoglobin levels are low. Research (Irvine et al., 1991; Piper et al., 1987; Smets et al., 1993) has failed to show a correlation between fatigue and anemia, however. A systematic, methodologically sound study has not been conducted to date.

Interventions should be grounded in a comprehensive assessment of the individual's fatigue. To date no clinical tools exist that offer the possibility of a comprehensive assessment. However, if one extrapolates from the pain assessment model currently used in clinical practice, a comprehensive fatigue assessment could be developed and would include

- An assessment of hydration, nutritional status, lab values (hemoglobin and hematocrit), and other contributing factors such as diarrhea
- A fatigue diary that also monitors pain, nausea and vomiting, sleep, mood, appetite, and medications
- An assessment of fatigue using a 0–10 scale (0 being no fatigue, 10 being the most)
- An assessment of onset, duration, cause (if applicable), and response to the fatigue

Nursing interventions should be focused on energy conservation, work simplification and modification, and optimal rest. Tables 15-6 and 15-7 give examples of specific interventions. In addition to promoting effective sleep, interventions should provide for hydration, nutrition, and the management of associated side effects.

Finally, exercise has been shown to be an effective research-based intervention (Graydon, Bubela, Irvine, & Vincent, 1995; Mock et al., 1994; Mock et al., 1997; Schwartz, 1998a, 2000; Schwartz, Thompson, & Masood, 2002; Winningham, 1991; Young-McCaughan & Sexton, 1991). Exercise has been reported to decrease fatigue and increase feelings of vigor. Due to limitations in these studies, no firm conclusions can be drawn, yet the results are promising enough to warrant further research.

Psychological

Validating a patient's symptoms and acknowledging their medical bases may be valuable in helping the patient to cope during therapy. Symptoms identified as physiological generally are more acceptable to patients than those considered to be psychological. Therefore, physiological symptoms are more likely to be reported than psychological symptoms, which may be associated with feelings of guilt.

There is evidence to suggest that psychological distress is a potentially important variable to consider when caring for the person with CRF. Anxiety, confusion, anger, stress, and worry have all been associated with fatigue (Knobf, 1986; McCorkle & Young, 1978; Piper et al., 1987).

The goals in the psychological sphere of care are to address the negative impact of psychological stressors and to learn to modify or avoid them. Interventions may

Table 15-6. **Work Simplification—Teaching Sheet**

Energy is the capacity for doing work.

Work and moderate exercise are good for almost everyone. Your physical ability depends on many things, such as your age, health, and body build. Other factors such as your experience doing the work, the weather, and your state of mind can affect your capability/capacity to work.

The following are important tips to simplify your ability to work or exercise:

1. **Work Rate.** A slow, steady rate of work, with short rest periods, will get the job done without exhausting you. You may find that you can safely do a job that would usually be too hard to finish by doing it at a slower pace.

   REMEMBER, if you double your work speed, you will use two or three times the energy each minute.

   REMEMBER that fast walking takes 1½ times more energy than slow walking.

   REMEMBER that walking up stairs takes seven times more energy than walking on level ground.

2. **Rest.** Frequent short rest periods are a must whether at work or at home.

   REMEMBER, short rest periods are of more benefit than fewer long rests.

3. **Distribution of the Work Load.** Avoid straining and do not try to do a two-person job yourself.

   REMEMBER that peak loads for short periods may call for more energy at one time than you have.

4. **Weather.** In hot weather, sunlight increases strain on the body, so keep in the shade.

   REMEMBER that you cannot do as much work on a hot, humid day as you can on a cool one.

   REMEMBER that the heart must supply a large amount of blood to the skin to cool the body in hot weather.

5. **Physical Condition.** Simple walking has been found to be a safe, practical form of exercise if you are experiencing fatigue or lack of energy.

   REMEMBER that it is important to keep in good physical condition through regular, moderate activity.

6. **Weight.** Keep your weight within normal limits.

   REMEMBER that excess weight overworks the lungs and heart.

7. **Age.** If you are in good health, your ability to do work at age 50 will be about 70 percent of your ability at age 25. Your ability to do work at age 70 will be about 50 percent of your ability at age 25.

   REMEMBER, an older person cannot work as hard as a younger person.

8. **Emotions.** Worries, fears, and tensions will prevent you from relaxing during rest.

   REMEMBER that emotional stress can increase your feelings of fatigue and lack of energy.

IN ORDER TO PROTECT YOURSELF AND AVOID ENDANGERING OTHERS, ASK YOUR HEALTH CARE PROVIDER TO TELL YOU IF CERTAIN ACTIVITIES SHOULD NOT BE DONE.

Source: Adapted from Beyer Memorial Hospital, Ypsilanti, MI; Occupational Therapy, Whittier Rehabilitation Hospital, Haverhill, MA. Reprinted with permission.

Table 15-7. **Conserve Your Energy—Teaching Sheet**

In General. The easier way of doing your work should be more pleasant because it takes less time and energy. This should eliminate feelings of fatigue and lack of energy.

REMEMBER to always walk slowly and control your breathing.

REMEMBER to sit for as many activities as possible.

REMEMBER to use slow, smooth flowing movements. Rushing will increase your discomfort. Think about what you are going to do next.

REMEMBER to take frequent rests. This may help your fatigue and leave you ready to go on with other activities.

REMEMBER to organize your activities and try to do them in the same manner all the time. Repetition of the same methods will make you more proficient in them. You will save time and energy.

REMEMBER to consider when the best time is for each activity. If morning is the most difficult time for you, do as much as you can the evening before. For example, wash in the evening.

REMEMBER, don't carry equipment if you can wheel or push it in or on a cart.

REMEMBER to use shortcuts whenever possible AND eliminate unnecessary tasks.

Bathing and Showering. Carry all the materials you need to the bathroom. Make only one trip. Place all items within easy reach and at waist level. Less energy is used if all necessary materials are placed on a wheeled table and pushed to the bathroom. Work slowly. Rest frequently.

REMEMBER to sit to undress, bathe, dry, and dress.

REMEMBER to use a moderate water temperature.

REMEMBER to use items such as long-handled sponges or a kitchen towel to wash your back. Other assistive devices such as a handheld shower head or soap-on-a-rope may be helpful.

Dressing. Gather all necessary items and place them within easy reach.

REMEMBER to complete above-the-waist dressing by choosing front-opening and/or loose-fitting garments. Fasten underclothes at the front of the body.

REMEMBER to complete below-the-waist dressing by using a cross-leg method to put on socks, underwear, trousers/pants, and shoes—in that order. Pull both underpants and trousers/pants to the knees, then stand only once. Pull to the waist and fasten.

REMEMBER to take frequent rests as you need them. Avoid overexertion, fatigue, and loss of energy. Allow plenty of time to dress and avoid rushing.

REMEMBER to gather all soiled clothes while seated.

Grooming. Keep all necessary items together within easy reach.

REMEMBER to sit and rest both elbows on a counter or tabletop while doing tasks, for example, rolling hair, applying makeup, combing hair, shaving, and brushing teeth.

REMEMBER that if brushing teeth is a chore, use an electric toothbrush.

REMEMBER to use different types of mirrors for your needs.

REMEMBER that short hair is easy to care for or have help in styling your hair, either at a salon or by a family member at home.

Kitchen Activities. Place the things you have to work within easy reach. Keep them in the same

continues

Table 15-7. **continued**

---

place all the time.

REMEMBER to slide things, do not lift them. Have a rolling table to wheel items.

REMEMBER to unclutter your storage area so that you can easily reach and find what you need. Disorganized storing of kitchen equipment and food is the cause of many needless steps and a waste of energy.

REMEMBER to use a stepladder for obtaining objects from high shelves or when cleaning a cupboard or cabinet. Request assistance from family members to obtain out-of-reach items and when cleaning.

REMEMBER to prepare food for two or more meals at one cooking session. Refrigerate or freeze the additional meals for another time. When possible, cook one-bowl, one-dish meals.

REMEMBER to use ready-mixes and frozen, dehydrated, and packaged foods; they save energy. Energy is saved by cooking the items and cutting them afterwards. An egg slicer serves to slice soft, cooked items such as carrots.

REMEMBER to use electrical appliances for chopping, grinding, grating, mixing, blending, cutting, or opening cans.

REMEMBER to use Teflon pans to eliminate time and energy spent on cleaning up. Soak your dishes after you use them. Drain dishes instead of towel drying.

Activities of Daily Living. Do the tasks requiring the most exertion when you have the most energy. By planning the day well, you may feel less fatigue. Frequent short rests before you get tired are better than long rests after you get tired. For example, if you intend to socialize in the evening, plan to rest in the afternoon to avoid getting too tired to enjoy yourself. Finally, learn to consider environmental surroundings. Avoid working outdoors during extremely hot or cold weather.

REMEMBER to alternate easy activities with difficult ones and take rests in between to avoid fatigue.

REMEMBER to sit down to work whenever possible. Pace all work to your own speed. Working in a relaxed, steady pace is optimal and saves energy.

REMEMBER to try to regulate your workload so that a similar level of energy is used from day to day. Distribute tedious tasks throughout the week.

REMEMBER to assign tasks and responsibilities within your family or to co-workers if possible.

Source: Adapted from Whittier Rehabilitation Hospital, Occupational Therapy Department, Haverhill, MA. Reprinted with permission.

include providing anticipatory guidance or education regarding the likelihood of experiencing fatigue and the fatigue patterns associated with particular treatments. Prioritizing activities of daily living may help the fatigued individual to regain some control. Behavioral interventions such as relaxation, guided imagery, or stress management and the use of antianxiety agents may be taught and may aid in reducing psychological distress (Ream & Richardson, 1999).

Psychological disorders are seen in almost half of all hospitalized and ambulatory cancer patients, with the majority of patients (68 percent) showing adjustment disorders with depressed or anxious mood. Major depression may be seen in roughly 5 to 15 percent of cancer patients—higher than the prevalence in the general population (6 percent), but probably no higher than seen in comparably ill patients with other diagnoses (Pies, 1996). Caution should be used when relating depression to fatigue, since depressive symptoms vary along a continuum of severity in patients with cancer. These symptoms range from no depression at all in more than 40 percent of patients with cancer, to mild, moderate, or severe symptoms in the remainder (Pies, 1996). If the health care provider suspects clinical depression, referral is the appropriate intervention.

Finally, by determining an individual's attentional ability and whether attentional fatigue is operational, Cimprich's (1993) experimental intervention may be appropriate. Her study aimed at increasing subjects' participation in activities thought to maintain or restore directed attention. The intervention included setting aside a minimum of 30 minutes, three times a week, for simple restorative activities such as walking or sitting in a natural environment, tending plants, gardening, or bird-watching.

Social

Social issues can aggravate or relieve CRF by altering the individual's social sphere. Meyerowitz, Sparks, and Spears (1979) studied 50 postmastectomy patients receiving adjuvant chemotherapy and found that 96 percent of the patients reported having fatigue and noted a decrease in general work-related levels of activity. Jensen and Given (1991) found CRF in both individuals with cancer and their caregivers.

Jamar (1989) described several important aspects of fatigue in women with ovarian cancer. In addition to physical problems, 75 percent of the women reported that activities had to be given up or changed. Social factors such as living arrangements and help with needs at home showed a significant relationship to fatigue level. The highest levels of fatigue were among single parents and those without help at home.

Oversolicitous help from family and friends may contribute to the individual's feeling of helplessness. By discussing family members' and friends' assistance, the health care team can reduce patients' feelings of helplessness that may contribute to CRF.

Goals for intervention should be based on usual social roles and cultural values and mores. Interventions may include evaluating patient and family dynamics as well as support systems, and informing the patient and the family of community resources and referring to these resources as necessary.

Cimprich's (1993) research showed higher rates of returning to work and of engaging in newly initiated, purposeful activities. These findings provide a basis for further testing of the efficacy of attention-restoring interventions in people with CRF.

Spiritual/Existential and Economic

The two areas of limited knowledge and research are the spiritual/existential and economic spheres of care. Non-research-based intervention for spiritual and existential care could include exploring the meaning of the fatigue and cancer experience for the individual. Encouraging open communication about spiritual concerns and praying, if appropriate, may bring comfort to the person with CRF.

From an economic perspective, CRF may result in job absenteeism. The implications may be that financial resources become limited, individuals are forced into disability programs, and jobs or insurance is lost. Additionally, financial barriers may block access to care or needed treatment.

CONCLUSION

Cancer-related fatigue remains a difficult symptom to manage and an illusive concept to study, but it is a real phenomenon to the individual with CRF and a constant reminder of cancer. A significant discrepancy can exist between a health care provider's perception of an individual's CRF and the individual's own perception. Ongoing assessment of CRF can offer valuable information for determining the best therapeutic, prophylactic, and palliative interventions, and research must test their feasibility.

Although many disciplines have examined CRF, there is no agreement on definition, causality, indicators of effect, nor are there remedies, treatments, and prescriptions. It is clear that further investigation is needed on this subject by multidisciplinary teams of researchers.

As individuals with cancer, and their families, focus on managing their disease, their normal lives, including jobs, homes, friends, pursuits of interest, as well as, the basic activities of daily living remain important to them. Fatigue often disrupts the patient's ability and desire to accomplish valuable role functioning thereby diminishing one's perceived QOL. The dearth and disparity in the literature regarding theoretical descriptions, explanations, and predictors of the CRF phenomenon support the need for further work in the arena of CRF and QOL (Barton-Burke, 1998).

REFERENCES

Aistars, J. (1987). Fatigue in the cancer patient: A conceptual approach to a clinical problem. *Oncology Nursing Forum, 14*(6), 25–30.

Aronson, L. S., Teel, C. S., Cassmeyer, V., Neuberger, G. B, Pallikkathayil, L., Pierce, J., Press, A. N., Williams, P. D., & Wingate, A. (1999). Defining and measuring fatigue. *Image: Journal of Nursing Scholarship, 31*(1), 45–50.

Barnett, M. (1997). Fatigue. In S. Otto (Ed.), *Cancer Nursing* (pp. 669–678). St. Louis, MO: Mosby.

Barrere, C., Trotta, P., & Foster, J. (1993). The experience of fatigue in women undergoing radiation therapy for early stage breast cancer. *Oncology Nursing Forum, 20*(2), 335.

Bartley, S.H. (1965). *Fatigue: Mechanism and management.* Springfield: Charles C. Thomas.

Bartley, S. H., & Chute, E. (1947). *Fatigue and impairment in man.* New York: McGrawHill.

Barton-Burke, M. (1998). Cancer-related fatigue: A holistic view. *Progress in Palliative Care, 6*(5), 153–159.

Barton-Burke, M. (2002). *Breast cancer experience: Women's reflections years after diagnosis.* College of Nursing Dissertation, University of Rhode Island.

Berger, A. (1993). Measurement of fatigue and quality of life in cancer patients receiving chemotherapy [Abstract 54]. *Oncology Nursing Forum, 20*(2), 311.

Berger, A. (1998). Patterns of fatigue and activity and rest during adjuvant breast cancer chemotherapy. *Oncology Nursing Forum, 25,* 51–62.

Berger, A.M., & Farr, L. (1999). The influence of daytime inactivity and nighttime restlessness on cancer-related fatigue. *Oncology Nursing Forum, 26*(10), 1663–1671.

Bhambhani, Y. N., Eriksson, P., & Steadward, R. D. (1991). Reliability of peak physiological responses during wheelchair ergometry in persons with spinal cord injury. *Archives of Physical Medicine and Rehabilitation, 72*(8), 559–562.

Blesch, K. S., Paice, J. A., Wickham, R., Harte, N., Schnor, D., Purl, S., Rehwalt, M., Kopp, P., Manson, S., Coveny, S., McHale, M., & Cahill, M. (1991). Correlates of fatigue in people with breast or lung cancer. *Oncology Nursing Forum, 18*(1), 81–90.

Bohle, P., & Tilley, A. (1993). Predicting mood change on night shift. *Ergonomics, 36*(1–3), 125–133.

Brunier, G. M., & Graydon, J. (1993). The influence of physical activity on fatigue in patients with ESRD on hemodialysis. *Association of Nephrology Nursing Journal, 20*(4), 457–462.

Buchsel, P. C., Barton-Burke, M., & Winningham, M. L. (2000). In M. L. Winningham, & M. Barton-Burke. Treatment: An overview (pp. 153–169). *Fatigue in cancer: A multidimensional approach.* Sudbury, MA: Jones & Bartlett Publishers.

Cabon, P., Coblentz, A., Mollard, R., & Fouillot, J. P. (1993). Human vigilance in railway and long-haul flight operation. *Ergonomics, 36*(9), 1019–1033.

Camarillo, M. A. (1992). The oncology patient's experience of fatigue. *Quality of Life—A Nursing Challenge, 1*(2), 39–44.

Campbell, A., Converse, P. E., & Rodgers, W. L. (1976). *The Quality of American Life*. New York: Sage.

Carson, R. (1994). Reducing cumulative trauma disorders: Use of proper workplace design. *American Association of Occupational Health Nursing, 42*(6), 270–276.

Cell, D., & Bron, D. (1999). The effect of epoetin alfa on quality of life in anemic cancer patients. *Cancer Practice, 7*(4), 177–182.

Cella, D. F., & Cherin, E. A. (1988). Quality of life during and after cancer treatment. *Comprehensive Therapy, 14*(5), 69–75.

Cella, D. F., & Tulsky, D. S. (1990). Measuring quality of life today: Methodological aspects. *Oncology, 4*(5), 29–38.

Christen, T., Stage, J. G., Galbo, H., Christensen, N. J., & Kehlet, H. (1989). Fatigue and cardiac and endocrine metabolic response to exercise after abdominal surgery. *Surgery, 105*, 46–50.

Cimprich, B. (1990). Attentional fatigue in the cancer patient. *Oncology Nursing Forum, 17*(2), 218.

Cimprich, B. (1993). Development of an intervention to restore attention in cancer patients. *Cancer Nursing, 16*(2), 83–92.

Cimprich, B. (1995). Symptom management: Loss of concentration. *Seminars in Oncology Nursing, 11*(4), 279–288.

Dalkey, N., & Rourke, D. (1973). The delphi procedure and rating quality of life factors. In *The Quality of Life* (p. 210). Washington, DC: Environmental Protection Agency.

Demetri, G. D., Kris, M., Wade, J., Degas, L., & Cella, D. (1998). Quality of life benefits in chemotherapy patients treated with epoetin alfa independent of disease response or tumor type: Result from a prospective community oncology study. *Journal of Clinical Oncology, 16*, 3412–3425.

Dow, K. H., & Ferrell, B. R. (1994). Long-term cancer survival: A quality of life model. *Quality of Life—A Nursing Challenge, 3*(4), 81–86.

Dubos, R. (1976). The state of health and the quality of life. *The Western Journal of Medicine, 125*(1), 8–9.

Ehlke, G. (1988). Symptom distress in breast cancer patients receiving chemotherapy in the outpatient setting. *Oncology Nursing Forum, 15*(3), 343–346.

Ferrans, C. E. (1990). Development of a quality of life index on patients with cancer. *Oncology Nursing Forum, 17*(3), 15–21.

Ferrans, C. E., & Powers, M. J. (1985). Quality of life index: Development and psychometric properties. *Advances in Nursing Science, 8*(1), 15–24.

Ferrell, B. R. (1995). Fatigue and quality of life. *Quality of Life—A Nursing Challenge, 4*(1), 1.

Ferrell, B. R., Grant, M., Dean, G. E., Funk, B., & Ly, J. (1996). "Bone tired": The experience of fatigue and its impact on quality of life. *Oncology Nursing Forum, 23*(10), 1539.

Ganz, P. (1993). *American Cancer Society National Conference on Clinical Trials.* Atlanta, GA: The American Cancer Society.

Gibson, H., & Edwards, R. H. T. (1985). Muscular exercise and fatigue. *Sports Medicine, 2*(2), 120–132.

Glaus, A. (1993). Assessment of fatigue in cancer and non-cancer patients. *Supportive Care in Cancer, 1*(6), 305–315.

Glaus, A. (1994). Fatigue and cancer—indivisible twins? A comparison between cancer patients, patients with disease other than cancer and healthy people. *Pflege, 7*(3), 183–197.

Glaus, A., Crow, R., & Hammond, S. (1996). A qualitative study to explore the concept of fatigue/tiredness in cancer patients and in healthy individuals. *European Journal of Cancer Care, 5*(Suppl. 2), 8–23.

Gotay, C. C., Korn, E. L., McCabe, M. S., Moore, T. D., & Cheson, B. D. (1992). Quality of life assessment in cancer treatment protocols: Research issues in protocol development. *Journal of the National Cancer Institute, 84*(8), 575–579.

Gough, I. R., Furnival, C. M., Schilder, L., & Grove, W. (1983). Assessment of the quality of life of patients with advanced cancer. *European Journal of Cancer & Clinical Oncology, 19*(8), 1161–1165.

Grandjean, E. (1968). Fatigue: Its physiological and psychological significance. *Ergonomics, 11*(5), 427–436.

Grant, M., Ackerman, D., & Rivera, L. M. (1994). Impact of dietary counseling on quality of life in head and neck patients undergoing radiation therapy. *Quality of Life Research, 3,* 77–78.

Gratz, R. R., & Boulton, P. (1994). Health considerations for pregnant childcare staff. *Journal of Pediatric Health Care, 8*(1), 18–26.

Graydon, J. E., Bubela, N., Irvine, D., & Vincent, L. (1995). Fatigue-reducing strategies used by patients receiving treatment for cancer. *Cancer Nursing, 18*(91), 23–28.

Groopman, J. E. (1998). Fatigue in cancer and HIV/AIDS. *Oncology, 12*(93), 335–347.

Harma, M. I., Ilmarinen, J., Knauth, P., Rutenfranz, J., & Hanninen, O. (1988a). Physical training intervention in female shift workers: The effects of intervention on fitness, fatigue, sleep, and psychosomatic symptoms, Part 1. *Ergonomics, 31*(1), 39–50.

Harma, M. I., Ilmarinen, J., Knauth, P., Rutenfranz, J., & Hanninen, O. (1988b). Physical training intervention in female shift workers: The effects of intervention on the circadian rhythms of alertness, short-term memory, and body temperature, Part 2. *Ergonomics, 31*(1), 51–63.

Hart, L., & Frell, M. I. (1982). Fatigue. In C. M. Norris (Ed.), *Concept clarification in nursing* (pp. 251–261). Rockville, MD: Aspen.

Haylock, P., & Hart, L. (1979). Fatigue in patients receiving localized radiation. *Cancer Nursing, 2*(6), 461–467.

Irvine, D., Vincent, L., Bubela, N., Thompson, L., & Graydon, J. (1991). A critical appraisal of the research literature investigating fatigue in the individual with cancer. *Cancer Nursing, 14*(4), 188–199.

Irvine, D., Vincent, L., Graydon, J. E., Bubela, N., & Thompson, L. (1994). The prevalence and correlates of fatigue in patients receiving treatment with chemotherapy and radiotherapy. *Cancer Nursing, 17*(5), 367–378.

Jacobsen, P. B., Hann, D. M., Azzarello, L. M., Horton, J., Balducci, L., & Lyman, G. H. (1999). Fatigue in women receiving adjuvant chemotherapy for breast cancer: Characteristics, course, and correlates. *Journal of Pain and Symptom Management, 18*(4), 233–242.

Jamar, S. (1989). Fatigue in women receiving chemotherapy for ovarian cancer. In S. Funk, E. Tornquist, M. Champagne, L. Archer Copp, & R. Wiese (Eds.), *Key aspects of comfort: Management of pain, fatigue and nausea.* New York: Springer.

Jensen, S., & Given, B. (1991). Fatigue affecting family care givers of cancer patients. *Cancer Nursing, 14*(4), 181–187.

Kecklund, G., & Akerstedt, T. (1993). Sleepiness in long distance truck driving: An ambulatory EEG study of night driving. *Ergonomics, 36*(9), 1007–1017.

Kim, M. J., McFarland, G. K., & McLane, A. M. (1989). *Pocket guide to nursing diagnosis.* St. Louis, MO: C.V. Mosby.

King, C. R., Haberman, M., Berry, D. L., Bush, N., Butler, L., Dow, K. H., Ferrell, B. R., Grant, M., Gue, D., Hinds, P., Kreuer, J., Padilla, G., & Underwood, S. (1997). Quality of life and the cancer experience: The state-of-the-knowledge. *Oncology Nursing Forum, 24*(1), 27–41.

King, K. B., Nail, L. M., Kreamer, K., Strohl, R. A., & Johnson, J. E. (1985). Patients' descriptions of the experience of receiving radiation therapy. *Oncology Nursing Forum, 12*(4), 55–61.

Knobf, M. (1986). Physical and psychologic distress associated with adjuvant chemotherapy in women with breast cancer. *Journal of Clinical Oncology, 4*(5), 678–684.

Kobashi-Schoot, J. A. M., Hanewald, G. J. F. P., van Dam, F. S. A. M., & Bruning, P. F. (1985). Assessment of malaise in cancer patients treated with radiotherapy. *Cancer Nursing, 8*(5), 306–313.

Kogi, K., Saito, Y., & Mitsuhashi, T. (1970). Validity of three components of subjective fatigue feelings. *Journal of Science and Labour, 46*(5), 251–270.

Krishnasamy, M. (1996, August 12). An *exploration of the nature and impact of fatigue as experienced by patients with advanced cancer: Searching for a nursing intervention.*

Presented at the 9th International Conference on Cancer Nursing, Brighton, England.

Lee, K. A., Lentz, M. J., Taylor, D. L., Mitchell, E. S., & Woods, N. F. (1994). Fatigue as a response to environmental demands in women's lives. *Image: Journal of Nursing Scholarship, 26*(2), 149–154.

Loge, J. H., & Kaasa, S. (1998). Fatigue and cancer—prevalence, correlates and measurement. *Progress in Palliative Care, 6*(2), 43–47.

Lovely, N., Miaskowski, C., & Dodd, M. (1999). Relationship between fatigue and quality of life in patients with glioblastoma multiforme. *Oncology Nursing Forum, 26*(5), 921–925.

Maxwell, M. (1984). When the cancer patient becomes anemic. *Cancer Nursing, 7*, 321–326.

McCorkle, R. (1987). The measurement of symptom distress. *Seminars in Oncology Nursing, 3*(4), 248–256.

McCorkle, R., & Young, K. (1978). Development of a symptom distress scale. *Cancer Nursing, 1*, 373–378.

Meyerowitz, B., Sparks, F., & Spears, I. (1979). Adjuvant chemotherapy for breast carcinoma: Psychosocial implications. *Cancer, 43*(5), 1613–1618.

Milligan, R. A., & Pugh, L. C. (1994). Fatigue during the childbearing period. *Annual Review of Nursing Research, 12*, 33–49.

Mock, V., Barton Burke, M., Sheehan, P., Creaton, E. M., Winningham, M. L., McKenney-Tedder, S., Schwager, L. P., & Liebman, M. (1994). A nursing rehabilitation program for women with breast cancer receiving adjuvant chemotherapy. *Oncology Nursing Forum, 21*(5), 899–908.

Mock, V., Dow, K. H., Meares, C. J., Grimm, P. M., Dienemann, J. A., Haisfield-Wolfe, M. E., Quitasol, W., Mitchell, S., Chakravarthy, A., & Gage, I. (1997). Effects of exercise on fatigue, physical functioning, and emotional distress during radiation therapy for breast cancer. *Oncology Nursing Forum, 24*(6), 991–1000.

Nail, L. M., & King, K. B. (1987). Fatigue. *Seminars in Oncology Nursing, 3*(4), 257–262.

Nail, L. M., & Winningham, M. L. (1993). Fatigue. In S. L. Groenwald, M. H. Frogge, M. Goodman, & C. H. Yarbro (Eds.), *Cancer nursing principles and practice* (3rd ed.) (pp. 608–619). Boston, MA: Jones and Bartlett.

Oginska, H., Pokorski, J., & Oginska, A. (1993). Gender, aging, and shiftwork intolerance. *Ergonomics, 36*(1–3), 161–168.

Pater, J. L., Zee, B., Palmer, M., Johnston, D., & Osoba, D. (1997). Fatigue in patients with cancer. Results with National Cancer Institute of Canada Clinical Trial Group studies employing the EROTC QOL C-30. *Supportive Care in Cancer, 5*(5), 410–413.

Pearson, P. G., & Byars, G. F. (1956). The development and validation of a checklist measuring subjective fatigue. (Report no. 56–115). School of aviation. USAF: Randolph AFB, Texas.

Pickhard-Holley, S. (1991). Fatigue in cancer patients: A descriptive study. *Cancer Nursing, 14*(1), 13–19.

Pies, R. (1996). Psychotropic medications and the oncology patient. *Cancer Practice, 4*(3), 164–166.

Piper, B. F. (1991). Alterations in energy: The sensation of fatigue. In S. B. Baird, R. McCorkle, & M. Grant (Eds.), *Cancer nursing—A comprehensive textbook* (pp. 894–908). Philadelphia: W. B. Saunders.

Piper, B. F., Lindsay, A. M., & Dodd, M. J. (1987). Fatigue mechanisms in cancer patients: Developing nursing theory. *Oncology Nursing Forum, 14*(6), 17–23.

Piper, B., Lindsay, A., Dodd, M., Ferketich, S., Paul, S., & Weller, J. (1989). Development of an instrument to measure the subjective dimension of fatigue. In S. Funk, E. Tournquist, M. Champagne, L. Copp, & R. Wiese (Eds.), *Key aspects of comfort: Management of pain, fatigue and nausea* (pp. 199–208). New York: Springer.

Piper, B. F., Rieger, P. T., Brophy, L., Haeuber, D., Hood, L. E., Lyver, A., & Sharpe, E. (1989). Recent advances in the management of biotherapy-related side effects: Fatigue. *Oncology Nursing Forum, 16*(6), 27–34.

Potempa, K. (1993). Chronic fatigue. In J. Fitzpatrick & J. Stevenson (Eds.), *Annual review of nursing research* (pp. 57–75). New York: Springer.

Potempa, K., Lopez, M., Reid, C., & Lawson, L. (1986). Chronic fatigue. *Image 18*(4), 165–169.

Pugh, L. C., & Milligan, R. (1993). A framework for the study of childbearing fatigue. *Advances in Nursing Science, 15*(4), 60–70.

Pyritz, D. (1996, August 12). *Uncovering the cancer patient's experience of fatigue.* Presented at the 9th International Conference on Cancer Nursing, Brighton, England.

Quesada, J., Talpaz, M., Rios, A., Kwizrock, R., & Gutterman, J. (1986). Clinical toxicity of interferons in cancer patients: A review. *Journal of Clinical Oncology, 4*(2), 234–243.

Ream, E. (1996, August 12). *Exploration of the concept of fatigue in patients with cancer.* Presented at the 9th International Conference on Cancer Nursing, Brighton, England.

Ream, E., & Richardson, A. (1999). From theory to practice: Designing interventions to reduce fatigue in patients with cancer. *Oncology Nursing Forum, 26*(8), 1295–1303.

Reynolds, C. (1994). Electromyographic biofeedback evaluation of a computer keyboard operator with cumulative trauma disorder. *Journal of Hand Therapy, 7*(1), 25–17.

Rhodes, V. A., Watson, P. M., & Hanson, B. M. (1988). Patients' descriptions of the influence of tiredness and weakness on self-care abilities. *Cancer Nursing, 11*(3), 186–194.

Rhoten, D. (1982). Fatigue and the post surgical patient. In C. M. Norris (Ed.), *Concept Clarification in Nursing* (pp. 277–300). Rockville, MD: Aspen.

Richardson, A. (1995). Fatigue in cancer patients: A review of the literature. *European Journal of Cancer Care, 4,* 20–32.

Richardson, A., Ream, E., & Wilson-Barnett, J. (1998). Fatigue in patients receiving chemotherapy. Patterns of change. *Cancer Nursing, 21,* 17–30.

Schipper, H. (1990). Guidelines and caveats for quality of life measurement in clinical practice and research. *Oncology, 4,* 15–24.

Scholz, J. P., Millford, J. P., & McMillan, A. G. (1995). Neuromuscular coordination in squat lifting, I: Effect of load magnitude. *Physical Therapy, 75*(2), 119–132.

Schwartz, A. L. (1998a). Patterns of exercise and fatigue in physically active cancer survivors. *Oncology Nursing Forum, 25*(3), 485–491.

Schwartz, A. L. (1998b). The Schwartz cancer fatigue scale: Testing reliability and validity. *Oncology Nursing Forum, 25*(4), 711–717.

Schwartz, A. L. (2000). Daily fatigue patterns and effect of exercise in women with breast cancer. *Cancer Practice, 8*(1), 16–24.

Schwartz, A. L., Thompson, J. A., & Masood, H. (2002). Interferon-induced fatigue in patients with melanoma: A pilot study of exercise and methylphenidate. *Oncology Nursing Forum, 29*(7), E85–E90.

Shumaker, S. A., Anderson, R. T., & Czajkowski, S. M. (1990). Psychological tests and scales. In B. Spiker (Ed.), *Quality of life assessments in clinical trials* (pp. 95–113). New York: Raven Press.

Smets, E. M., Garssen, B., Bonke, B., & de Haes, J. C. (1995). The multidimensional fatigue inventory (MFI): Psychometric qualities of an instrument to assess fatigue. *Journal of Psychosomatic Research, 39*(3), 315–325.

Smets, E. M. A., Garssen, B., Schuster-Uitterhoeve, A. L., & de Haes, J. C. J. M. (1993). Fatigue in cancer patients. *British Journal of Cancer, 68*(2), 220–223.

Stiles, D. D. (1994). Video display terminal operators . . . technology's biopsychosocial stressors. *American Association of Occupational Health Nursing Journal, 42*(11), 541–547.

St. Pierre, B., Kasper, C. E., & Lindsay, A. M. (1992). Fatigue mechanisms in patients with cancer: Effects on tumor necrosis factor and exercise skeletal muscle. *Oncology Nursing Forum, 19*(3), 419–425.

Varricchio, C. G. (1985). Selecting a tool for measuring fatigue. *Oncology Nursing Forum, 12*(4), 122–127.

Varricchio, C. G. (1995). Measurement issues in fatigue. *Quality of Life—A Nursing Challenge, 4*(1), 20–23.

Vogelzang, N. J., Breitbart, W., Cella, D., Curt, G. A., Groopman, J. E. & Horning, S. J. (1997). Patient, caregiver, and oncologist perceptions of cancer-related fatigue. Results of a tripart assessment survey. *Seminars in Hematology, 34*(3 Suppl 2), 4–12.

Webb, P. (1994, November 24). *Quality of life, quality of care in oncology.* Report from an interdisciplinary round table meeting held in conjunction with the 19th Congress of the European Society of Medical Oncology (ESMO), Lisbon, Portugal.

Winningham, M. L. (1995). Fatigue: The missing link to quality of life. *Quality of Life Research, 4,* 2.

Winningham, M. L. (1999). Fatigue. In C. Yarbro, M. Frogge, & M. Goodman (Eds.). *Cancer symptom management,* 2nd ed. (pp. 58–76). Sudbury, MA: Jones and Bartlett Publishers.

Winningham, M. L., & Barton-Burke, M. (2000). *Fatigue in cancer: A multidimensional approach.* Sudbury, MA: Jones & Bartlett Publishers.

Winningham, M. L. (1991). Walking program for people with cancer: Getting started. *Cancer Nursing, 14*(5), 270–276.

Winningham, M. L. (1992, March 12). *The energetics of activity, fatigue, symptom management & functional status: A conceptual model.* Presented at the 1st International Symposium on Symptom Management, San Francisco, California.

Winningham, M. L. (1995). Fatigue: The missing link to quality of life. *Quality of Life—A Nursing Challenge, 4*(1), 2–7.

Winningham, M. L., Nail, L. M., Barton-Burke, M., Brophy, L., Cimprich, B., Jones, L. S., Pickhard-Holley, S., Rhodes, V., St. Pierre, B., Beck, S., Glass, E. C., Mock, V. L., Mooney, K. H., & Piper, B. (1994). Fatigue and the cancer experience: The state of the knowledge. *Oncology Nursing Forum, 21*(1), 23–36.

Woo B., Dibble, S. L., Piper, B. F., Keating, S. B. & Weiss, M. C. (1998). Differences in fatigue by treatment methods in women with breast cancer. *Oncology Nursing Forum, 25*(5), 915–920.

Young-McCaughan, S., & Sexton, D. (1991). A retrospective investigation of the relationship between aerobic exercise and quality of life in women with breast cancer. *Oncology Nursing Forum, 18*(4), 751–757.

Patient Perspectives

Cancer Survivorship
Quality for *Life*

SUSAN A. LEIGH • ELLEN L. STOVALL

From Patienthood to Survivorship

Much of the change within our health care system is directly related to the miracles and advances of modern medicine. While the development of sophisticated therapies now offers new hope to people who are diagnosed with cancer, the providers of this potentially *miraculous* health care are challenged to maintain a focus on the individual concerns of the people under their care. In the midst of complex technology, elaborate delivery systems, complicated protocols, managed care, and fiscal regulations, it is easy to become trapped in the pace, chaos, and frustration of change and to lose sight of the individuality of peoples' needs.

Historical Perspective

The primary focus of cancer care over the past few decades has obviously been the eradication of the disease. Objective, quantitative measurements (e.g., blood counts, tumor regression, or length of survival) became relevant parameters of success once effective therapies were available. Attending physicians usually made care decisions based solely on information related to the disease, treatment, and potential for response. Physical survival—staying alive!—became the utmost goal, while concerns about the quality of that survival remained a luxury. Qualitative concepts of care, though, were hardly novel.

Prior to the explosion of technology and scientific advances in health care, the World Health Organization (1948) defined health as "a state of complete physical, mental, and social well-being and not merely the absence of disease or infirmity" (p. 29). Science and technology may have changed the course of treating and *curing* a select group of cancers, but nurses, mental health professionals, and patients themselves changed the course of *caring* for people with cancer. Objective measurements and observations remain important but, when used alone, give an incomplete picture of the overall impact of the disease.

As the quality of survival is in the eye of the beholder, patient autonomy is of paramount importance. Many researchers and clinicians now recognize the importance of the *patient perspective*, especially when monitoring fatigue, pain, and psychosocial distress (Clark, 1994). Thus, issues affecting quality of life (QOL) are gaining recognition as major components of the cancer care equation.

Defining Quality of Life

Who Defines Quality of Life?

No matter how many ways QOL is defined, it all boils down to individual perspectives of personal experiences. An individual's answer to the question "What does QOL mean to you?" is highly subjective and personal and can change depending on the specific situation, including time frame, mood, location, family dynamics, and many other variables. The important point is that, no matter how subjective the question may be, it must be asked in order to assess the total patient experience. Frank (1991) writes:

> *What happens when my body breaks down happens not just to that body but also to my life, which is lived in that body. When the body breaks down, so does the life. Even when medicine can fix the body, that doesn't always put the life back together again.* (p. 8)

Incorporating QOL assessments into everyday practice is no longer a luxury, but rather an important and necessary component of cancer care. As the delivery of care becomes more complicated for the professional caregiver, so does the experience of receiving care for anyone diagnosed with cancer. Complex therapies lead to complicated choices, and the decision making that accompanies these choices warrants a more knowledgeable and assertive health care consumer.

Cancer Survivors' Bill of Rights

For many categories of cancer, the potential for extended survival has increased so dramatically that patients are compelled to become more informed about their disease and treatment options. An early example of informed consumerism is illustrated in the Cancer Survivors' Bill of Rights (Table 16-1) (Spingarn, 1988). Published by

Table 16-1.   The Cancer Survivors' Bill of Rights

The American Cancer Society presents this Survivors' Bill of Rights to call public attention to survivor needs, to enhance cancer care, and to bring greater satisfaction to cancer survivors, as well as to their physicians, employers, families, and friends:

1. **Survivors have the right to assurance of lifelong medical care, as needed. The physicians and other professionals involved in their care should continue their constant efforts to be:**
   — sensitive to the cancer survivors' lifestyle choices and their need for self-esteem and dignity;
   — careful, no matter how long they have survived, to have symptoms taken seriously, and not have aches and pains dismissed, for fear of recurrence is a normal part of survivorship;
   — informative and open, providing survivors with as much or as little candid medical information as they wish, and encouraging their informed participation in their own care;
   — knowledgeable about counseling resources, and willing to refer survivors and their families as appropriate for emotional support and therapy which will improve the quality of individual lives.

2. **In their personal lives, survivors, like other Americans, have the right to the pursuit of happiness. This means they have the right:**
   — to talk with their families and friends about their cancer experience if they wish, but to refuse to discuss it, if that is their choice, and not to be expected to be more upbeat or less blue than anyone else;
   — to be free of the stigma of cancer as a "dread disease" in all social relations;
   — to be free of blame for having gotten the disease and of guilt for having survived it.

3. **In the workplace, survivors have the right to equal job opportunities. This means they have the right:**
   — to aspire to jobs worthy of their skills, and for which they are trained and experienced, and thus not to have to accept jobs they would not have considered before the cancer experience;
   — to be hired, promoted, and accepted on return to work, according to their individual abilities and qualifications, and not according to "cancer" or "disability" stereotypes;
   — to privacy about their medical histories.

4. **Since health insurance coverage is an overriding survivorship concern, every effort should be made to assure all survivors adequate health insurance, whether public or private. This means:**
   — for employers, that survivors have the right to be included in group health coverage, which is usually less expensive, provides better benefits, and covers the employee regardless of health history;
   — for physicians, counselors, and other professionals concerned, that they keep themselves and their survivor-clients informed and up-to-date on available group or individual health policy options, noting, for example, what major expenses like hospital costs and medical tests outside the hospital are covered and what amount must be paid before coverage (deductibles);
   — for social policy makers, both in government and in the private sector, that they seek to broaden insurance programs like Medicare to include diagnostic procedures and treatment which help prevent recurrence and ease survivor anxiety and pain.

Source: Adapted from Spingarn, 1988. Used with permission.

the American Cancer Society in 1988, this proclamation was written *by* a cancer survivor *for* cancer survivors (Spingarn, 1988). The author, Natalie Davis Spingarn, insisted that the consumer voice be heard and not be modified by the medical establishment. Spingarn addressed individual, interpersonal, and social rights to greater care and satisfaction throughout the cancer experience and illustrated a shift from passive patienthood to a more proactive survivorship.

A Shift toward Survivorship

The concept of survivorship was initially introduced to the field of oncology in 1986 with the founding of the National Coalition for Cancer Survivorship (NCCS) (Leigh & Logan, 1991). Events preceding the initial organizational meeting included a combination of dramatic advances in cancer therapy and an increasing population of cancer survivors, along with changing social trends that saw the development of resource and support networks for patients and their family members.

New therapies to treat cancer elevated the hopes and expectations of surviving this disease. Access to information about scientific breakthroughs became readily available to the general public, and awareness about cancer prevention, early detection, second opinions, and treatment options increased. Many types of cancer shifted from being considered almost certain acute disease to a more expected chronic disease, while some patients were actually considered cured. This new sense of hope contributed to changes in how decisions were made and who made them.

Historically, the cancer patient's agenda was more often than not set by health care providers, specifically physicians. Eventually, patients decided to exercise more control over all aspects of cancer care that affected their lives, especially those in the frequently neglected psychosocial realm. Thus, a proliferation of support groups, hotlines, resource materials, and patient networks emerged and gave birth to a new social movement that began to inform and empower people with cancer.

This movement remained undefined until NCCS emerged and its leadership began writing about a new concept called survivorship. Life with and after cancer was described as more than black and white, patient versus survivor, cured or not cured. It was seen as a multitude of events and feelings that changed and continued beyond the actual treatment phase. For many people affected by cancer, life after therapy was about not just how long one lived, but how well one lived.

Mullan (1990) initially described survivorship as the act of living on, a dynamic concept with no artificial boundaries. Carter (1989) further described this theme as a process of *going through*, suggesting movement through phases. From these models, survivorship came to be viewed as a continual, ongoing process with a focus on quality of life concerns rather than a stage or outcome of survival (Leigh, 1994). Survivorship is not just about long-term survival, which is how the medical profession generally defines it. Rather, when viewed from the perspective of someone diagnosed with this disease, it can be defined as *the experience of living with, through, or beyond cancer* (Leigh & Logan, 1991). From this point of view, survivorship begins at the moment of diagnosis and continues for the remainder of life (Mullan, 1990).

Defining Survivors

Other semantic discrepancies revolve around who can be considered a cancer survivor. When cancer was considered incurable, the term *survivor* applied to the family members whose loved one died from the disease. This terminology was used for years by the medical profession and insurance companies. When potentially curative therapy became a reality, physicians selected the five-year parameter to measure survival. Freedom from disease and biomedical longevity became the standard of success when the outcome was measurable and quantifiable.

Quantitative Model: Medical

Even as the five-year landmark has been modified as a parameter for describing survival, medical professionals still seem inclined to categorize anyone receiving therapy or not completely free of disease as a *patient*, and everyone who is not under treatment or with no evidence of disease as a *survivor*. Many survivors, though, feel that a conscious and deliberate attempt must be made to resist the urge to pigeonhole the terms *cancer survivor* and *cancer survivorship* by using a calculus based on years out of treatment or disease-free survival. Quantitative definitions fail to give recognition to the strenuous efforts of people who are not cured of their disease, require maintenance therapy or periodic changes in treatment modalities, and remain alive for over five years. Other survivors experience late recurrences, are diagnosed with second malignancies, or develop delayed effects of treatment, requiring further therapy. Additionally, many survivors with poor prognoses struggle day to day attempting to beat the odds and overcome pessimistic expectations about life expectancy.

Qualitative Model: Consumer

While the expectation for survival may hold different meanings for all involved, it is the survivors themselves who define survivorship and give meaning to their struggles. Quantity of life means nothing without QOL that has some significance and purpose to the person living through the experience. A truly patient-centered measure of success would utilize QOL parameters, with or without measurements of longevity. To help make this transition, health care providers can look for ways to eliminate the use of words and descriptions that:

1. *Erect unnecessary boundaries* around the person with cancer (e.g., "He's not a survivor; he's not five years posttreatment yet.")
2. *Utilize terms of clinical measurement* in order to have a label for someone off-treatment (e.g., "She's not cured yet; she's only been in remission for three years.")
3. *Impose limitations on hope or take hope away from someone* when few treatment options exist (e.g., "Why do you insist on calling her a survivor? This is her third recurrence and you need to face the reality that she's going to die.")

The act of defining the word *survivor* is one of empowerment, as noted by Gray (1992) in "Persons with Cancer Speak Out." Over the past decade, the language of cancer has evolved to the point where the term *cancer victim* is the oddity and *cancer survivor* is more the norm. While it is arguable that the term *patient* somehow belongs in the science and practice of medical and psychosocial oncology, few will disagree that the term *survivor* evokes a more powerful image.

As the concept of the empowered survivor has encouraged a shift from paternalism to partnership, cancer support and advocacy organizations around the country have enlarged the language of survivorship to include other qualitative descriptives of this population. Many survivors favor powerful labels (e.g., veteran, victor, advocate, activist, or warrior) (Leigh, 2001). Others dislike the use of warlike metaphors and prefer a gentler label (e.g., thriver, graduate, blessed, or triumpher). And some who may be living with recurrent or metastatic disease have an extreme dislike for the term survivor and express anger about oversimplifying survivorship while emphasizing only positive aspects of recovery (Mayer, 1998). Although this may all sound confusing or insignificant to some readers, an important point is that survivors themselves should be able to identify their own issues and define themselves rather than relying on the agendas and descriptives of the health care community (Leigh, 1994).

Cancer survivors are hardly the only ones adding to this labeling confusion. Due to the current rise in managed care, survivors are also called *clients, consumers,* or *customers.* These labels reflect the influence of business in our current health care marketplace. But this new influence is not without its problems. A most unfortunate addition to this cadre of labels has been a long-term survivor's use of the term *beggar* when describing herself within her health maintenance system.

None of these descriptives is necessarily right or wrong. As the potential for surviving cancer expands, so must the language describing this expansion. Whether utilizing quantitative or qualitative descriptives, survivors and practitioners simply need to define these terms within the context they are used. Thus, the term *survivor* in this chapter reflects the NCCS definition: "from the time of its discovery and for the balance of life, an individual diagnosed with cancer is a survivor" (Mullan, 1990).

Stages of Survival and Quality of Life

Obviously, cancer survivors have different issues and concerns depending on their circumstances along the survival continuum. In the classic article "Seasons of Survival: Reflections of a Physician with Cancer," Mullan (1985) was the first to propose a model of survival that includes acute, extended, and permanent stages. QOL issues are of paramount importance in all of these stages. It must be noted that cancer survivors can die in any of the three stages, and QOL issues are just as important during the dying process as during survival. This chapter will not address death and dying as a separate entity.

Acute Stage

The acute (or immediate) stage of survival begins at the time of the diagnostic workup and continues through the initial courses of medical treatment. The survivor is commonly called a patient during this stage, and initially the primary focus is on physical survival: "How long will I live?" "Will I be cured?" "Will I lose my hair?" Usually, without any prior training, those who are ill are required to make sophisticated medical decisions about therapy at a time of intense vulnerability, fear, and pressure. Inexperienced in navigating the complicated culture of medicine or advocating for themselves, many people continue to rely on their physicians to make treatment-related decisions for them. Others, though, are not so quick to surrender the decisions about their lives to any one person. They are asking for information, explanations, second opinions, and more effective communication in an attempt to understand the choices and decisions before them.

Many supportive care services are more available for patients in the acute stage. Access to the medical team, counselors, patient support networks, resource libraries, hotlines, and family support systems help survivors navigate this stage. In order to improve chances for *quality* survival, advocating for oneself becomes as important as effective therapy. But the picture changes, sometimes dramatically, once treatment ends.

Extended Stage

If the disease responds during the initial course of therapy, the survivor will move into the extended (or intermediate) stage of survival. This stage is often described as *watchful waiting*, *limbo*, or *remission* as survivors monitor their bodies for symptoms of disease recurrence. Uncertainty about the future prevails as medical-based support systems are no longer readily available, and survivors must learn to deal with the unknowns by themselves: "How many times a day should I examine myself?" "Is this symptom a sign of recurrence, or is it normal?" "Why do I still feel tired/fearful/depressed?" Recovery entails dealing with the physical and emotional effects of treatment, while re-establishing social roles can be challenged by ignorance and discrimination. The quality of one's life after cancer becomes a major concern.

While no longer a patient, the person may not feel entirely healthy and may have difficulty feeling like a survivor. Ambiguity defines this stage as survivors find themselves afloat in a mixture of joy and fear—happy to be alive and finished with treatments, yet afraid of what the future may hold.

The need for continued supportive care during this transitional stage has been highlighted as early as the 1980s (Leigh, 1994; Mullan, 1990; Welch-McCaffrey, Loesher, Leigh, Hoffman, Meyskens, 1989). Community and peer networks often replace institutional support, and recovery entails regaining both physical and psychological stamina. Time frames for curing the body and healing the spirit are very individualized, and may or may not happen in harmony. Survivors must continue to advocate for themselves, often within the context of a group or recovery program, but may also begin advocating for others through support networks.

Permanent Stage

As a certain level of trust and comfort gradually returns, survivors enter the permanent (or long-term) stage of survival. This is roughly equivalent to what the medical establishment calls *cure* or *sustained remission*. While most survivors experience a gradual evolution from a state of "surviving to thriving," as described by Dow (1990), others must deal with the chronic, debilitating, or delayed effects of therapy. QOL becomes a major focus of long-term survival: "I guess I shouldn't complain about my infertility. After all, I'm alive." "How will I get health insurance if I lose this job?" "Will I get cancer again?" Although many of these long-term survivors have no physical evidence of disease and appear to have fully recovered, all remain at risk for recurrence of the original disease or for the development of other malignancies.

Meanwhile, the life-threatening experience of cancer is never forgotten. In many ways, survival enhances appreciation for life, while at the same time reminding survivors of their vulnerability. The metaphor of the Damocles syndrome illustrates this dichotomy: Dressed in royal fineries and surrounded by good food and fine wine, Damocles could not eat or drink, as he imagined that the thin thread holding the sword above his head might break at any moment (Koocher & O'Malley, 1981). How individual survivors interpret this metaphor of life will influence the quality of their survival.

For many long-term survivors, a lack of guidelines to ensure or enhance disease-free survival is a major concern. Pediatric oncology is far beyond adult oncology in the systematic follow-up of long-term survivors so that potential pitfalls can be identified early and interventions instituted. Adults, on the other hand, often feel burdened by what Siegal and Christ (1990) called the *glorification of recovery*, whereby survivors are praised for overcoming diversity and sometimes scolded for complaining. The identification of real problems can be hampered when survivors appear healthy. No one wants to believe that something may be wrong, either physically, emotionally, or socially (Siegal & Christ, 1990; Smith, 1981). Symptoms of distress, both biomedical and psychosocial, must be taken seriously. In this age of cost-containment and managed care, long-term survivors need continued access to appropriate specialists more than ever, yet they are often denied referrals when the seriousness of their complaints are misunderstood, minimized, or considered too expensive.

As the population of long-term cancer survivors increases, attention to survival issues needs to be encouraged. Even if the disease is eradicated, the psychosocial sequelae of surviving a life-threatening experience must be recognized as barriers to a full recovery. Advocacy at national levels must continue to direct attention to these issues by involving survivors in politics and in guiding public policy.

Survivorship-Related Advocacy

While many health care providers see themselves as advocates for their patients, the idea of advocacy often intimidates survivors because they do not understand it. At a basic level, though, advocacy has little to do with public policy or politics. It means "active support on behalf of . . ." (Stovall & Clark, 1996, p. 276). Thus, physicians, nurses, and social workers act on behalf of their patients. Lawyers act on behalf of their clients. Members of the clergy act on behalf of their congregations. But more important, survivors and their families need to learn how to act on behalf of themselves in order to ensure quality survival from their perspectives. The NCCS model of advocacy is three-tiered: advocacy for self, advocacy for others, and advocacy for community.

For Self

When survivors act on behalf of themselves, it becomes self-advocacy. Although one may feel paralyzed, inarticulate, and extremely vulnerable when first diagnosed with cancer, this state does not last forever. It is imperative that survivors and their supporters overcome their state of inertia, develop plans of action, and make decisions that will affect both the quality and quantity of their lives. Effective communication with medical personnel and family members is the first step toward effectual self-advocacy.

Other examples of self-advocacy include (a) asking appropriate questions, (b) seeking second opinions, (c) accessing understandable information about treatments, and (d) requesting culturally relevant support. These examples will all lead to a feeling of empowerment.

Other reasons for encouraging self-advocacy include:

1. Gaining a sense of stability and control during unpredictable times
2. Building confidence in the face of insurmountable challenges
3. Seeking out others in the same situation for peer support
4. Improving chances for better and longer survival
5. Diminishing feelings of hopelessness and helplessness

By transforming apprehensions and anxieties into productive energy, survivors not only obtain up-to-date and accurate information, but also become more adept at advocating for themselves and others.

For Others

Many survivors who have recovered from their disease or are coexisting with cancer as a chronic illness have a need to "give something back" and assist their fellow survivors. Having learned how powerful it was to arm themselves with the nonmedical tools of survival—such as information gathering, effective communication, and peer support—there is a willingness to share the road maps of survival that may not have been readily available to them. This is the *veteran–rookie connection*—the experienced traveler paving the way for the newly diagnosed. This model of mutual aid is the foundation of the survivorship movement and is poignantly illustrated by a survivor who had just been diagnosed with Hodgkin's disease:

> I would need to find the *right* doctor and the *right* medical facility to meet my new, critical needs. And yet I was paralyzed. I needed to find someone immediately who knew my terror; someone I could talk with on a personal—rather than clinical—level; someone who had "been there." I needed to find a survivor. (Morrison, 1983, p. B5)

Most survivors are more than willing to talk to other survivors about cancer, usually enhancing the QOL for both parties. The veteran survivor feels good about being helpful, and the rookie survivor gains much needed support. Two cancer veterans may support each other when no one else seems to understand the occasional or continuing trauma of surviving a once-fatal disease. Some survivors use their personal experiences in other ways, including:

1. Starting or joining support groups
2. Manning local cancer hotlines
3. Speaking publicly and raising awareness about cancer to religious and civic groups and to the media
4. Encouraging community libraries and bookstores to update their cancer resources
5. Teaching medical students, health care professionals, and the business community about the many facets of surviving cancer
6. Raising funds for cancer research or support
7. Sitting on program, funding, or research committees as patient advocates
8. Helping to create community resource/retreat/healing centers

While many survivors feel a need to remain attached to the cancer community, many others do not. They exhibit no visible scars or problems. For them, cancer is past history and private. Yet, some survivors fear discrimination at work or in social settings if their medical history is known. Anticipated rejection can keep the most vocal survivor silent and can greatly diminish the quality of that person's life. Obviously survivors who do not fear recrimination are still needed to advocate on behalf of those who do.

For Community

With the rapid growth of cancer-related advocacy over the past decade, especially on a national level, many successes can be reported. This type of advocating often focuses on national agendas and public policy. For example, advocates representing pediatric oncology have raised awareness about the increasing population of adult survivors of childhood cancers, many who now have chronic health problems, are unable to find affordable insurance, or suffer discrimination in school or in the workplace. These young survivors are not only outspoken but extremely effective when recommending changes in health policy.

Another potent example of a national initiative is illustrated by the work of breast cancer advocates. In less than three years during the early 1990s, a well-organized, informed, articulate, and sometimes angry group of women challenged the United States government to earmark millions of dollars from the Department of Defense to be used for breast cancer research. And it worked! While highly controversial, this was unprecedented in the history of research funding and exemplifies the power of the masses.

When problems surrounding cancer care are identified, *anyone* can tell his or her story to the media. *Anyone* can write to politicians. And many survivors can and are testifying before legislative bodies in an effort to change public opinion and public policy about cancer.

Quality Cancer Care

As the United States moves away from a health care system of predominantly fee-for-service insurance plans to those under managed care, national cancer advocacy organizations must be on the alert to issues affecting oncology. Because of this trend, in 1995 NCCS surveyed health care providers, scientists, government officials, and professional and advocacy organizations about the critical issue of quality cancer care. Besides addressing the strengths and weaknesses of the old and new systems, NCCS (1995) called for several fundamental issues to be reflected in standards and guidelines for reliable measurements of care. These are presented in Table 16-2.

In our current climate of managed care, disease-repair, and bottom-line system of cost containment, care is time and time is money. Convincing the "powers that hold the purse strings" to finance programs and projects that focus on QOL becomes one of our major challenges.

In today's medical and political climate, the concept of QOL is called an endangered species by Ferrell (1993), and "may be lost during health care reform and amidst what [she has] termed the 'dehumanization' of cancer" (p. 1471). The Texas Cancer Council responded to this growing concern by outlining ten Ethical Principles for Cancer Care (Table 16-3) as a moral basis for delivering comprehensive care to people with cancer. The complete work includes practical guidelines for action so that these principles can be put into practice.

CONCLUSION

The impact of the cancer experience permeates all aspects of one's life and must be measured in terms of both quantity *and* quality. Although the lives of many cancer survivors have been saved or extended, they have also been permanently altered. Survivors themselves must identify their needs, voice their concerns, and advocate for needed social changes and continued support throughout the continuum of cancer care. Only after acknowledging the full spectrum of survivorship can survivors truly celebrate and appreciate quality of life *for* life.

Table 16-2. **Special Considerations in Measuring Quality Cancer Care**

1. The diversity of the diseases called "cancer," some of which are encountered infrequently by any one provider.
2. The need for specialized care, particularly in the acute stage.
3. The need for standards that measure care across the continuum of survivorship, from prevention and screening, through early diagnosis and treatment, to long-term follow-up and palliative care.
4. The dramatic impact on the quality of available care due to geographic setting and socioeconomic status.
5. The situations where little effective care is available or is of an investigational nature.
6. The more costly nature of state-of-the-art treatment which occasionally offers only small benefits over established treatments.
7. The consideration of improvements in quality of life as significant end points that must be added to increased longevity.

Source: Adapted from NCCS, 1995. Used with permission.

Table 16-3. **Ethical Principles for Quality Cancer Care**

I. Since cancer affects a person's entire sense of well-being, cancer care cannot be equated with or limited to prevention, early detection, and treatment of bodily disease. To deal with the effects of cancer, this care should address humans as whole persons with biological, emotional, social, economic, informational, moral, and spiritual needs.

II. Benefiting persons with cancer is the highest priority of health-care professionals. Individuals fully benefit when they receive personalized, comprehensive, coordinated, and culturally sensitive care.

III. Patients are to be respected as autonomous, self-governing persons with the right to express their needs and emotions and make informed decisions in their own best interests.

IV. To make informed decisions, patients must be provided with information that is understandable, sufficient, and applicable to their circumstances.

V. Effective communication is essential in order to benefit persons with cancer and respect their autonomy. This communication rests on trust, concern, mutual respect, honesty, and self-awareness.

VI. Terminally ill patients are to receive continued health care, support, respect, and assurance.

VII. Collegial teamwork is essential for attending to the total human dimensions of cancer care.

VIII. Teamwork is sustained by caregiver collegiality, which is based on a mutual understanding of and respect for the individual and professional contributions of colleagues.

IX. The ability of health-care professionals to care for patients and those close to the patient depends on caregivers attending to their own personal, psychological, social, moral, and spiritual needs.

X. Basic, clinical, and psychosocial research is integral to improving cancer prevention, early detection, diagnosis, treatment, long-term follow-up, and the personal dimensions of cancer care. All research should contribute to, not detract from, beneficial and respectful care of individuals with cancer.

Source: Vanderpool, H. Y. (Ed.). *The human dimensions of cancer care: Principles and guidelines for action.* The Texas Cancer Council and Institute for the Medical Humanities, The University of Texas Medical Branch at Galveston, 1994. Copyright 1994 Texas Cancer Council. Used with permission.

REFERENCES

Carter, B. (1989). Going through: A critical theme in surviving breast cancer. *Innovations in Oncology Nursing, 5*, 2–4.

Clark, E. J. (1994). Parameters for conducting quality of life research. In B. Rabinowitz, E. J. Clark, & J. Hayes (Eds.), *Demystifying oncology research: A handbook for psychosocial and nursing practitioners* (pp. 21–24). State of New Jersey Commission on Cancer Research, Trenton, NJ.

Dow, K. H. (1990). The enduring seasons in survival. *Oncology Nursing Forum, 17*, 511–516.

Ferrell, B. R. (1993). To know suffering. *Oncology Nursing Forum, 20*, 1471–1477.

Frank, A. W. (1991). *At the will of the body*. Boston: Houghton Mifflin.

Gray, R. E. (1992). Persons with cancer speak out: Reflections on an important trend in Canadian health care. *Journal of Palliative Care, 8*, 30–37.

Koocher, G., & O'Malley, J. (Eds.). (1981). *The Damocles syndrome: Psychosocial consequences of surviving childhood cancer*. New York: McGraw Hill.

Leigh, S. (1994). Cancer survivorship: A consumer movement. *Seminars in Oncology, 21*, 783–786.

Leigh, S. (2001). Preface: The culture of survivorship. In C. H. Yarbro (Ed.), *Seminars in Oncology Nursing, 17*(4), 234–235.

Leigh, S., & Logan, C. (1991). The cancer survivorship movement. *Cancer Investigation, 9*, 571–579.

Mayer, M. (1998). *Advanced breast cancer: A guide to living with metastatic disease*, 2nd ed. Sebastopol, CA: O'Reilley & Assoc.

Morrison, J. (1983, March 9). Perspective: The survivor as advocate. *The Washington Post*, p. B5.

Mullan, F. (1985). Seasons of survival: Reflections of a physician with cancer. *New England Journal of Medicine, 313*, 270–273.

Mullan, F. (1990). Survivorship: An idea for everyone. In F. Mullan & B. Hoffman (Eds.), *Charting the journey: An almanac of practical resources for cancer survivors* (pp. 1–4). Mount Vernon, NY: Consumers Union.

National Coalition for Cancer Survivorship (NCCS) (1995). *Briefing paper: Quality cancer care*. Silver Spring, MD: NCCS.

Siegal, K., & Christ, G. H. (1990). Hodgkin's disease survivorship: Psychosocial consequences. In M. J. Lacher & J. R. Redman, Jr. (Eds.), *Hodgkins' disease: Consequences of survival* (pp. 383–399). Philadelphia: Lea & Febiger.

Smith, D. W. (1981). *Survival of illness*. New York: Springer.

Spingarn, N. D. (1988). *The Cancer Survivors' Bill of Rights*. Atlanta, GA: The American Cancer Society.

Stovall, E., & Clark, E. J. (1996). Survivors as advocates. In B. Hoffman (Ed.), *A cancer survivor's almanac: Charting your journey* (pp. 273–280). Minneapolis, MN: Chronimed Publishing.

Welch-McCaffrey, D., Loescher, L. J., Leigh, S. A., Hoffman, B., & Meyskens, F. (1989). Surviving adult cancer. Part 2: Psychosocial implications. *Annals of Internal Medicine, 3,* 517–524.

World Health Organization (1948). World Health Organization Constitution. In *Basic Documents* (p. 29). Geneva, Switzerland: WHO.

Chapter

17

Quality of Life
Stories by Patients and Families

Quality of Life
As a Survivor of Childhood Cancer

MARGARET GUNTHER LEE

Cancer is an amazing thing. It can cause you to realize how precious life is while at the same time, tearing you apart inside. Whether you are the patient or the caregiver, one cannot walk away the same after dealing with such a life-threatening illness. As a patient, I know that my experience with cancer has had a profound effect on my life physically, emotionally, socially, and spiritually.

I was diagnosed with Philadelphia Chromosome Positive Acute Lymphocytic Leukemia at the age of 12. Upon my diagnosis in June 1992, I faced two and a half years of weekly chemotherapy as well as many procedures, medications, and two weeks of cranial radiation. These years brought new challenges, suffering, and victory that I had never experienced before. As a Christian, I found the strength to face the hardships and challenges that my cancer brought in my relationship with the Lord.

During these years I was constantly reminded of the battle that was going on within my body. I often asked myself, "Is this really happening?" and wondered "Why me?" I felt so different from other kids my age. While they were worried about clothes, social events, and the opposite sex, I was concerned with staying in remission, keeping up in school, and how sick I would get from my next chemo. During this time, the hospital was my comfort zone. Here, there were many other kids who, like me, had no hair and were sick from chemo. However, these individuals had a spark inside them to press on, to endure the fire, and to make it through another day.

After getting used to the "cancer routine," it became a way of life for my family and me. I enjoyed seeing my doctors and nurses and my port-o-cath was my best friend. During these years I spent so much time at the hospital that I referred to it as my "second home." However, this new way of life was not easy. I was often physically tired and sick, especially after receiving chemo, and I missed anywhere from one day to a week of school after treatment each week. While the doctors, nurses, and other staff at the hospital worked diligently to restore my physical quality of life, my social quality of life declined. So many people were there to support me and pray for me, but as the months went by and it was obvious that I was not going to "Get Well Soon," some of my friends dropped by the wayside. I learned from experience that any serious illness will show you who your true friends are. While I did lose some very special friends during these years, I made many new friends at the hospital. Talking with others at the hospital who had cancer was so helpful to me. Often, these individuals were the only people who could understand how difficult it was to undergo countless treatments and procedures.

After completing treatment in November 1994, I was drained of energy and was finishing out the first semester of my ninth grade year at home. At the age of 14 I was excited about the days to come and the energy that I would be getting back. However, six weeks after I finished treatment I learned that my cancer had returned. Still exhausted, I was not sure that I was up for any more treatment. The next blow came when my doctor told me that my chance of survival with the only treatment option available, a bone marrow transplant, was only 20%.

Here is where the importance of quality of life comes into play. From an outsider's perspective, you probably would not understand why a 14-year-old cancer patient would refuse treatment. However, do not ever assume that you know what is best until you have been faced with the decision yourself. Chemotherapy and all the other treatment regimens that a cancer patient faces are often more difficult and more thoroughly draining than anything one will face here on earth. This was my mindset as I faced this relapse. However, I chose to have the bone marrow transplant and soon began chemo and a rigorous schedule of treatment to hopefully achieve remission once again.

There was no quality of life in those months before my transplant. Preparation for the bone marrow transplant was so much harder than my leukemia treatment. However, I survived the rigorous treatment and received my sister's bone marrow four months after the news of my initial relapse. I was in the hospital for a total of seven and a half weeks, during which I incurred many devastating side effects, some of which required ICU care on the ventilator. Wheeling out of the hospital for the first time in seven and a half weeks was truly amazing. Surrounded by my parents, my brother, and my sister, I marveled at the beauty of the sky, the trees, and the birds that I had only viewed through a distant hospital window for so many weeks. God was so good to me. I know that it is solely by His grace that I was even able to leave the hospital.

Even though I was able to return home in June, I still had a very long road ahead of me. Because my immune system was still weak, I spent the next year primarily at home and wore a hepa-filter mask when I went out in public. The side effects from my two and a half years of treatment and from my bone marrow transplant were really affecting me. I began to experience severe headaches for 80 to 90% of each day. In addition, my energy level began to decrease. In December 1995, one year after I had relapsed, I developed shingles directly above and behind my right eye. This launched a round of extreme pain due to post-herpetic neuralgia and a lifetime of eye problems from the damage from the shingles and the radiation treatments I had received. Years of cancer treatment and a bone marrow transplant, which were meant to restore my health, had left me with very little physical and social quality of life. With continual pain, extreme loneliness, and other daily struggles, I often wondered why the Lord had even brought me through the transplant. However, the Lord reminded me that He had a very special purpose and plan for my life here on earth.

Throughout the years, the support of my family has had a profound impact on my quality of life. They have always been right behind me 110% throughout my treatment. Both of my parents sought to be involved in my treatment, whether it was taking me to the hospital each week, standing beside me during my procedures, or staying with me when I was an inpatient. They were right there supporting me as I finished chemo as well as when I relapsed and had to decide whether or not I would receive any more treatment. We cried together, laughed, and grew together during these difficult years.

During 1996, my parents and I began searching for the reason why my energy level continued to decrease. After months of seeing doctors, having many tests, and changing medication dosages, my parents and I still did not have an answer as to why I was so exhausted. I spent much of my day around the house in bed or doing very low energy tasks. In addition, I continued my studies through a homebound program, doing my best to stay caught up in school.

In November 1996, I saw an endocrinologist who suggested that my fatigue might be due to low growth hormone levels. A few weeks later I underwent a series of inpatient tests. My growth hormone levels were indeed lower than the normal level, but I chose not to begin growth hormone shots due to the possible chance of relapse. However, by June I had no quality of life; I was bedridden with exhaustion and only "existed." My doctor suggested that I go in for growth hormone testing again. The test results showed that my growth hormone levels had decreased significantly. At this point, my quality of life was so poor that I was willing to risk the small possibility of relapse from growth hormone replacement if I could have several good months or years of life. So on June 13, 1997, I began the daily injections. Around

August of that same year I began to have a little more energy. As time went on and we increased the dosage I gained even more energy. I cannot express how much these shots have affected my quality of life. I continually thank the Lord for the brilliant individuals who determined how to produce growth hormones. Many people do not understand how I can give myself a shot everyday, but they have never experienced the extreme unending and debilitating exhaustion that I lived with for so long.

As my energy improved, I was able to take one or two classes a semester at my high school and complete the rest of my classes through the homebound program. I spent much of my time studying, as I was driven to do well in school. When I relapsed I had taken a semester off from school and was now in class with the grade below me. The combination of only attending one or two classes at school as well as not knowing many people in my new class was difficult. My social quality of life continued to decline, and I experienced severe loneliness. Since I was at home so much, I was extremely thankful to have siblings with whom I could interact. My sister, Catherine, and I had become very close, especially after she donated the bone marrow for my transplant. I considered Catherine to be my best friend and my link to the outside world.

Looking back, I can see that my doctors and nurses did everything in their power for so many years to bring me through my treatment. However, after being in my hospital bubble for so many years, I was not prepared to go back into the real world. I was left hanging, trying to figure out how to be a teenager. I felt so different; I had dealt with struggles and issues no child or teenager should ever have to face and I had watched countless friends die. This had really changed my priorities and my outlook on life and had caused me to become an adult at age 12.

Outwardly, I struggled to fit in with a group of people from whom I had been disconnected during my years of treatment. Entering my treatment as a petite girl, the extensive chemotherapy, steroids, and radiation had stunted my growth leaving me at four feet eleven inches tall. I was often mistaken for a 12-year-old, offered a kid's menu, or teased about my height. However, I have learned to laugh at the many comments that people feel compelled to make about my height. In addition, I know that one day I will appreciate looking much younger than I actually am.

After graduating from high school in May 1999, I chose to attend Union University that Fall. Still struggling with headaches, much eye pain, and a less than normal energy level, I only took 11 hours my first semester. Attending college was a tremendous milestone in my life. The Lord brought me through so much and improved my quality of life through the years, but my family and I did not know if I would be able to handle the demands of college. However, driven to succeed, I finished my freshman year with 28 credit hours.

Going to college allowed me to step out of a world where everyone knew that I had had cancer. It also allowed me to meet many new people and make new friends.

I remember standing in the hall one day before class thinking, "I actually feel comfortable standing around with a large group of people my age." During my junior high and high school years, I spent so much time with adults that I felt more comfortable with these more mature individuals. So, another milestone was reached; I had a greater social quality of life and was comfortable interacting with my peers.

I am now 22 years old and a senior at Union University where I am a psychology and family studies double major. Today I have a wonderful quality of life with plenty of energy, minimal pain, great friends, and a God who continues to amaze me. I hope to use my skills, both from school and from my life experiences, to work in missions after I graduate. Looking back, I can thank the Lord for allowing me to have cancer. I feel that I have grown so much as an individual in all qualities of life. I know that my experience with cancer has made me who I am today. While I do not know what my quality of life will be like a year from today or even a week from today, for me, this does not really matter. I do not know what the future holds, but I know the One who holds the future.

A Journey through Cancer

MICHAEL C. SULLIVAN

"No way would I let them nuke me or dump toxic waste into my bloodstream if I ever got cancer!" Such was my macho litany when discussions arose of people fighting cancer. The summer of 1987 provided me with a reality check and an ongoing discovery of my own values and strengths—which continues to this day. Along the way, I discovered the true meaning of love, enhanced my spirituality, and came to know what friendship *really* is.

In June of 1987 I injured my back moving a large booth container while closing our exhibit area at a trade show in Washington, DC. I flew home in agony. I called a friend who was a neurosurgeon, and he scheduled a CAT scan and appointment. At that appointment, we determined the back problem was going to resolve itself without surgery. Having become very aware of my body during this painful episode, I had noticed a lump in my left inguinal area and asked him about it. My doctor was unsure of what it was, and suggested that I should see a surgeon. The next morning I received a call in my office from the surgeon. He wanted to schedule an appointment. Cool, a doctor calling *me* for an appointment—rather than the other way around. We agreed to meet the following Monday. At that time, after poking and prodding, he said that we couldn't be sure of anything without minor surgery to either fix the hernia (which I was convinced was the problem) or to "biopsy" the lump. The procedure was scheduled for Friday, the first day of the longest three days of my life. (Biopsies should be illegal on Fridays! You can't get the information before Monday or Tuesday.)

Interestingly, when we came home from the outpatient center on Friday, and I went to bed, we saw something new in the actions of Max, our golden retriever. Before, when we wanted Max to get on the bed, it required extensive coaxing (if not an engraved invitation) to convince him it was okay. This day, however, Max immediately joined me on the bed and rested his large head and front paws on my leg, just below the dressing over the incision site. My wife Lynne came in to check the dressing and site; but when she reached for the area, Max firmly pushed her hand away with his nose. *He* was going to take care of the old man! (Later, he relented and allowed her to do her ministrations.)

Tuesday we got the dreaded news: LYMPHOMA! (non-Hodgkin's). The fact that my wife worked at an NCI-designated Comprehensive Cancer Center was the first of many blessings I experienced during my journey. (At first, it didn't seem to be a blessing, however, with her background in critical care nursing, she could only relate my cancer to her experiences with the terminally ill patients who she had cared for.) We were devastated.

One of the benefits of being married to a nurse is that the compulsiveness, assertiveness, and perfectionism of the profession spills over into the personal life as well. Starting Tuesday afternoon, and continuing throughout my journey, Lynne was "on top" of arranging, scheduling, monitoring, and following up on every specialist I was to see and every procedure I was to undergo. Actually, my role in this journey was easy—I just sat (or lay) back and appreciated whatever was my fate for that day, and that I had gotten through *one* more day.

Initially, we decided that since my lymphoma was a low-grade "indolent" type, we could not pursue a "cure." Shortly thereafter, however, the cancer center added a new radiation oncologist to the staff. He was an expert in a new "inverted Y" type of radiation therapy. Since my disease was rated as a Stage II, we decided to "shoot the works" with a course of radiation.

The doctor may have been a technical expert, but his understanding of patient concerns and fears left a lot to be desired. He refused to prescribe an antiemetic because he didn't want to "create a self-fulfilling prophesy"! Naturally, after the first 140 rads to my abdomen, I came home and threw up. It took Lynne almost three hours to get a prescription filled for compazine—while I retched and reconsidered my decision to undergo therapy.

Eventually, I became somewhat used to the Monday through Friday nausea and vomiting. The nausea and vomiting became a part of my life. I learned that the compazine tablets and suppositories, if taken around the clock, slightly ameliorated these symptoms, as did eating immediately after arriving home. After that first treatment, I asked the radiation oncologist to decrease the dose. At a lower dose (120 rads per treatment), I tended to better tolerate the therapy. Because my symptoms were less intense with the lower dose, the radiation oncologist wanted to raise the dose back to

140 rads. I adamantly refused his efforts to persuade me that a higher dose was better for me. Later, I found out that he wrote on my chart that I was a noncompliant patient.

Throughout the eight weeks of radiation, Max provided me with unconditional love and attention. If the truth be known, Max was often in the way. He was so concerned with my vomiting that he stayed *very* close with his nose near my face. He stayed with me for the first 20 minutes or so after I arrived home, always placing his body between me and Lynne, preventing her from caring for me. We quickly realized that Max had his own routine and concerns for my care. Whenever I could, I walked Max twice a day, discussing my thoughts and feelings with him. I really think he understood.

I was disturbed by the constant fatigue I experienced during radiation. The fatigue affected my ability to carry out routine activities—the walks with Max were slower and shorter, weekends were spent taking *long* naps, and driving to work was a major effort. All my efforts were aimed at getting through each day. I didn't have the energy for any extra activities.

Throughout the radiation, I had the false impression that when radiation was completed, my life would return to normal. But that wasn't the case. I was discouraged and depressed. I wanted to feel better. I wanted to be normal. It took several months to regain some energy. In fact, my energy and stamina are less now than before the radiation.

In 1989 my lymphoma recurred. I had several enlarged axillary nodes and one under the jaw. It was disquieting, to say the least, but easily managed with an oral agent (Chlorambusol®). Taking an oral agent that had no side effects allowed Lynne and me to maintain a normal life style—notwithstanding the continued nagging fear of recurrence.

In July 1992 my cancer came back with a vengeance. That same week, we discovered that Max had an inoperable liver tumor, with metastatic pleural effusions that caused labored breathing. His symptoms came on so suddenly! The quality of his life was diminished—he wasn't able to take walks, eat, or rest comfortably. We had Max put to sleep a few days after he was diagnosed. I still miss him. (It was not a good summer.) Luckily, a two-year-old golden retriever, Trigger, was in need of a good home, and we adopted him. He stepped right into Max's footsteps in boosting my spirits, exercising me, and showering me with unconditional love.

After a discussion with my oncologist, I decided to have a bone marrow transplant. (Although my marrow had been harvested shortly after diagnosis, he decided that I should have a peripheral stem cell transplant instead.) Preparatory to the procedure, I had to undergo a course of CHOP. During this chemotherapy, I would schedule my business trips for the weeks between treatments. On Monday I would go to the hospital to have a blood test, then go on to the airport for my flight. I had a small insulated bag in which I carried my Neupogen®, syringes, needles—and later, when I had my central line in, the catheter care items. The flight attendants would give me ice to keep the Neupogen® cool, and I would get ice at the hotel to continue the cooling task. Each morning I would give myself a shot and tend to my catheter care. (We discovered that old 35-mm film containers were perfect receptacles for the needles.) As cumbersome as it all may seem, my little "freedom kit" allowed me a return to normalcy by permitting me to return to my peripatetic travel schedule.

The transplant is still a hazy memory to me. With the agreement of my physicians, I stayed "zonked" on Ativan® and left the daily decisions on care to Lynne. I had a difficult time with the ablative chemotherapy. That, coupled with a stubborn fever, makes me grateful now for my decision to take an amnesiac. During the first two weeks, Lynne was at my bedside. Her every 20 minute mouth care resulted in my being the first patient in the unit to have no mouth sores at all. Engraftment was a long, slow process because the radiation to my pelvis had diminished marrow production in the radiated area. I waited for over 40 days before my AGC climbed above 500. I was astounded by the fatigue I experienced! Reading the morning paper was an all-day effort—and seldom completed. TV was of little interest, except for *Jeopardy* and *Wheel of Fortune*. Surprisingly, though, I did not feel bored. Between trying to read the paper, listening to tapes, and going over my many cards and letters, I seemed to have a pretty full day. Every day Lynne would arrive at 6:30 A.M. to help with my shower and breakfast. She would stay until rounds and then go to work—after reviewing my plan of care for the day with my nurse. At 6:30 P.M. she would arrive again and stay until I nodded off around 10 P.M.

Finally, I got to go home, and that certainly raised my spirits. But, again, I was astounded at my lack of stamina and overwhelming fatigue. The week after my arrival home, Lynne had to go to a conference in Florida. I was sure I could handle everything on my own. That idea, naturally, was disposed of and replaced with a plan to have her father stay with me. The concept was further refined by her mother, who was convinced that the "boys" would fail miserably at attempted bachelorhood. She joined Lynne's dad, and the three of us had a great time! (Although we all kept forgetting that I should wear a mask at the grocery store!) The time was special, because I was able to interact with them on subjects other than my disease and care. There were some good laughs—beginning the first night when Lynne's dad flew out of bed after being awakened by Trigger's wet muzzle in his ear!

Although I have had another recurrence posttransplant, my spirits and hopes are up! I have faced the dreaded "C-word" and survived—and will continue to do so. However, I was shaken by a very good friend's diagnosis of non-Hodgkin's lymphoma. His doctor was never able to get Ken into remission. In the brief span of 18 months, Ken's health declined. He died the day I flew to Florida to be with him.

Why Ken? Why not me? These are questions that keep running through my head. Every experience on this journey has given me a much stronger appreciation for the fragility and preciousness of life. Not only will I never again hunt for sport, but also I won't even step on bugs when Trigger and I are out on our walks!

I have adjusted to a life without the stamina I had before my treatments. It was difficult to accept the fact that my mountaineering days are over. It took me several years before I finally was willing to give away my backpacking and rock-climbing gear.

Lynne is a nurse researcher who focuses on quality of life issues. As I prepared this article, I thought a lot about that subject. What *is* quality of life? When I was sick, quality of life was being as symptom-free as possible. It was being able to live as normal a life as possible. It was enduring the various procedures and forms of treatment with the least amount of difficulty and loss of dignity. It was the knowledge that I had an excellent health care team. It was the complete support and prayers of family, friends—and even strangers—to help pull me through the experience. I am so very fortunate, because the good Lord provided me with these excellent resources.

Now that I'm through the process, I realize that quality of life has an all new meaning. As a cancer survivor, I feel that I must repay that gift of survival with a life of quality. I owe a great deal to a lot of people—many to whom I'll probably never be able to express sufficient gratitude for their contribution to my survival. I feel an obligation to contribute something in return for this extra time that has been given to me. How do I do this? I believe that I have an obligation to ensure that other cancer survivors are provided with support, encouragement, and prayer. All cancer survivors and their families and friends receive a terrifying education. *Now,* I have the opportunity to be the educator. I can also help health care personnel understand that I—and all cancer survivors—have had a life before cancer and will have a life after cancer. I believe that we must remind our doctors and nurses to listen to our stories, and learn what is important to us.

Shortly after my peripheral stem cell transplant, a friend—who, by the way, had kept me inundated with cards, calls, and good wishes—was diagnosed with breast cancer. Lynne and I were able to help guide Rosemari through her battle with cancer by sharing our own experiences and tips for care. Just being there to take her to chemotherapy, or spending time with her so she was not alone, was an opportunity to repay those who had done the same for me.

We must also ensure that newly diagnosed patients understand the importance of gaining and maintaining some control over their treatment—and, thus, over their disease—and their lives. I was lucky—I had my favorite nurse at my bedside throughout the process. But it doesn't require a nurse or medically trained family member to realize that we *do* need that modicum of control over a situation that has the potential for spinning us out of control so easily.

All of us who have been treated for cancer are fortunate in having a caring and understanding staff to meet our needs. But what many people forget (both laypeople and health professionals) is the fact that cancer doesn't just strike the patient—it strikes the entire family. Spouses and loved ones should not be forgotten in the support process.

In 1981, shortly after Lynne and I began dating, her family had a picnic at a local park. As an only child who had little contact with aunts or uncles, I was unprepared to walk into a gathering of nearly a hundred assorted relatives of her clan! However, that clan was a tremendous support to me as I've wended my way through this nine-year journey. Also, my parents, family, friends, neighbors, and fellow church members were of immeasurable value and contributed significantly to the positive outcomes of my treatments. No words, however, can fully express the awe, respect, and, of course, the love I feel for my bride. She was—and is—the reason I am here now. I live because of her. I live *for* her. Lynne is the *quality* of my life!

(*Author note:* Michael has died since writing this piece.)

Life's Presents

LYNNE M. RIVERA

On that fateful day in July 1987, I did not realize that my life would change so dramatically. For several months following Mike's diagnosis of cancer, I felt that my life was falling apart. I felt out of control. Eventually, I have come to realize that Mike's cancer has changed my life in many positive ways.

Life is fragile and temporary, but grand! How many times in a day do I think about how fortunate I am to have had Mike alive and healthy to share another day with me? We were very fortunate to have the resources that provide us with the physicians, the nurses, and the medical technology that continued to give us another chance at remission.

Nine years and three recurrences later, I realized that every day was a gift from God. This was not to say that my life was perfect and without the usual deadlines and little frustrations. Believe me, there were still days when I would like to twitch my nose and make a troublesome colleague, friend, family member, or husband disappear from sight; or maybe they would have liked me to disappear. However, every day *was* special and enhanced by the love of family and friends, and the love and companionship of my wonderful husband (who finally succumbed to cancer).

A Personal Perspective of Quality of Life

ANONYMOUS PATIENT

Having cancer at 35 years is an especially traumatic experience since it occurred very suddenly, and it is a rare type of oral cancer usually found in males over 45 who have a history of smoking or drinking. I was in good health at the time, and I did not smoke or drink. My career was starting to take off, as I was getting good reviews of my work as a consultant. A new relationship was going okay also. Then it happened. When diagnosed, I thought that it was sure death. My experience with cancer from family history was that if you have cancer, you die. Mother, grandmother, grandfather, great uncle, all had cancer and died a short while after diagnosis. I cried and was in a state of shock for days. A few days later, I had the surgery and then went home. A few weeks later, I returned to work. At first, I was disoriented at work, but within six months, my work was better than before. I was stronger, more confident, and took more risks. Later, I left my job due to political reasons, boredom, lack of opportunity (I kind of topped out), and my relationship ended (she had feelings for another man). I moved to a nearby city in search of another job/career and a relationship.

There are some themes that emerged for me six months to a year after the surgery and continue to be driving yet divergent forces guiding my life. The most upfront theme is the continuous awareness of vulnerability, both physically and emotionally, a vulnerability that I had not felt before. The cancer could reoccur at any time; my life could be shortened at any time. Stronger values emerged or became more prominent for me. First, the defense mechanism of denial does not work very well for me anymore. I do not hide things well from myself or others. I am pretty much aware of things as they are, for better or worse. Being honest with oneself becomes the norm. This can be good and bad. Good, in that I do not waste time and energy on things that will get me nowhere. Bad, in the sense that I am constantly hit with reality head on, with no time for escape or assimilation. I see things in life quite clearly for the most part. I see through the deception and the facades. I think I have always been this way, but now it is more pronounced.

Another thing that happened for me is the emerging conflicting feelings, that things that were important in the past are not as important now. But, in a sense, things important in the past are even more important now. Let me explain. Let's take career. I do not really care anymore what I do for a living. I do not have dreams of being a success in business, climbing the corporate ladder, etc. (this development has been in motion for a while, but has intensified after the cancer). My self-worth is not based as much on work as it was in the past. On the other hand, things that I value in work, that I feel I need in order to feel good about myself in work are now more pressing than ever to find. Being paid for my value, being respected as a person, being respected as a professional, doing something I believe in, is ethical and makes a difference—these are the things that are important. A tough combination of things to find in the workplace in America in the 1990s. When I work, I need these things more than ever. Also, in terms of a relationship, the need for someone that thinks and lives like me is more needed than ever. A "soulmate" is very critical at this time in my life. Along with the need for a "soulmate" is the high level of vulnerability that I feel. Vulnerability due to financial instability, the various losses I have experienced, the physical vulnerability.

I have always been an introspective person to some extent. But, the cancer experience has forced me to examine myself internally more intensely and extensively than ever before. When you have cancer, there is nowhere to hide, no place to escape to, to postpone self-examination. Life hits you between the eyes, each and every day. The awareness of possible reoccurrence, this time not being so lucky to be alive and healthy, comes to your mind and guides your thoughts and actions each and every day. Risking everything and anything for some sense of peace, inner power, contentment, and the feeling of doing the right thing is the mode of living that guides me each and every day. I have always felt this way, but now I feel compelled to act this way, even though the fears, doubts, and anxieties are still there to confront me in regards to relationships and career, aging, family, finances, etc. Feel the fear and do it anyway, I guess is the motto.

I have also felt that I live outside the mainstream of society. But now, I feel an even stronger alienation from society's values and norms and ways of doing things. I have been fighting this internally; I would like to be one of the many. But gradually, internally, I am accepting that this will never happen because of who I am and, in large part, for what the cancer experience has forced me to face.

The cancer experience makes you feel and think and act in a way that says there is nothing to lose. When your life has been threatened and continues to be threatened every day—you live, what more is there to lose? That is the ultimate loss, isn't it? But, if you are still here on earth, it seems important to keep finding yourself and being honest with yourself. I feel constantly driven to take paths that will help me to become a stronger me, a more content me. These paths are scary and I want to turn back or avoid or deny them. But then, the force comes again, putting a sign in front of you saying that you cannot settle for less. I may not be here much longer. I cannot put it off. I do not want any regrets at the end of my life. The pain of dealing with cancer and that life is terminal is traumatic enough. To have regret and not be able to do anything about it, when your energy is drained and you're sick and in pain, would be more horror than I could imagine. I want to feel when I am on my deathbed that I have done it all, I have tried it all, I have explored the world and me and me with others, and I have learned a lot and shared a lot and accomplished a lot, and now I am ready to go to wherever it is we go.

Since my last story, I have experienced a recurrence of tongue cancer. Time passed quickly as life moves on. Now I am considered cured. Has my life changed much?

I did start my own business doing what I really enjoy doing. I put forth much energy to get it up and running. I did fairly well with it, although the economy has been on the decline and it has turned into a struggle to get business. I have developed a great relationship with my wife and best friend. I am continuing my business in a new location and things have gone okay. I have aged and I feel that I am on a good path with my life although it is still scary pursuing a career in organizational development, which is helping employees to communicate better with each other and managers to lead better. I like the fact that I help surface unresolved conflicts that employees may have with each other or with their manager. My goal to get the truth with is elusive and hidden. Maybe I am an idealist, but I believe that people can work well with each other and have some joy in the workplace. After all, we spend so many of our waking hours at work. We need to have some feeling of fulfillment from what we do for so much of our waking hours. Cancer is not staring me in the face right now, but I am a changed person forever. Having cancer makes you used to experiencing continuous feelings of anxiety, which is what we have in the workplace today. But hopefully, I can help others live with the uncertain times and know that it is okay to feel uncertain, to feel anxious, to feel that you are not sure where you are going.

Oncology and Spirituality: A Spouse's Story

ANONYMOUS SPOUSE

This is the first anniversary of the discovery of her malignant tumor. I offer a silent prayer of thanks to God with quiet relief that she is doing well and that we as a couple are able to celebrate this date, even though the beast still stalks her. With ambivalence I stare at the refrigerator magnet: "National Cancer Survivors Day, A Celebration of Life." The brightly colored words and dancing image mock me, for my gratitude is contingent and my hope is qualified.

The event of 12 months ago are terribly vivid. Memory replays them in slow motion in distinct contradiction to the racing emotions that accompany the mental narrative. Her surgeon's intervention was direct, quick, and effective, like his New York City street speech and manners. His style reassured her—no easy task—and that was sufficient for me. He performed the excision, and no other treatment was required. Behind large doors deep in the bowels of the hospital, the shadow on the radiologist's image was erased in the last surgery of the night. We had allowed for the worst possibilities, but she would be spared the wretched therapies of chemo and radiation. For us, it was a Passover event, as real as the Biblical story of the deliverance of the people of Israel from the bondage of the pharaoh's slavery. The dark angel did not visit our house. The dread of our adolescent children's fears would remain only anticipatory. We all went home and began living in our collective recovery.

We began a series of cycles. For two months and three weeks, the credo of "no bad news is good news" put her cancer in perspective and sustained us. We were appreciative for a competent clinician/researcher and for nurses whose competencies included caring. We were humbly mindful of our access to good health care, and acutely aware of the maldistribution of resources in this country. The support of friends and faith was precious. We enjoyed the sweet, dull routines of our former lives. And then, at the end of three months, her follow-up appointment with the surgeon climaxed the cycle. In the outpatient waiting area, we were never alone. As intrusive and discomforting as a drunk staggering onto a crowded bus, the figure of anxiety sat prominently between us. Wondrously, the surgeon's prognosis of encouragement dispelled the uninvited specter, and we began the cycle anew. The prayers of thanks were offered again, but this continuing encouragement now weighs upon her and, domino-like, on me.

She feels guilty that she is doing as well as she is. She does not suffer the physical afflictions of others who carry the diagnosis of cancer. Others are more stigmatized in their flesh and blood and bones, literally bearing the stigmata of disease or treatment. Does a survivor who thrives deserve the sympathy or attention offered to those who have been more authentically victimized? She takes the measure of her fears and contrasts them to the fears of those whose prognoses are truly frightening, and then lays hers aside. The effect on me is inhibiting: my dance for joy is performed solo and in private. And yet I know there is more at work in her.

Abused sexually as a child, she never expected to fall in love and marry, or give birth to two dear children, or work as a professional and contribute to her community. The first days of the diagnosis threatened her with losing all. She discovered then that she could be profoundly content with her life, that at long last there was a legacy of which she could be proud. Regardless of the future, she had found God's blessing for her. I was touched, surprised, and cried.

We go on now, like Sarah and Abraham, in faith and into a land unknown, uncertain of the future and sure that we are sustained, nevertheless. Fear commingles with hope; and guilt, with gratitude. She is fiercely resilient and tenacious in her vulnerability. The cancer is not living her; God is, and we are both blessed.

Conclusion

Chapter

18

Nursing and Patient Perspectives on *Quality of Life*

PAMELA S. HINDS • CYNTHIA R. KING

In this closing chapter, impressions and recommendations regarding nursing and patient perspectives on quality of life (QOL) during illness-related experiences will be summarized. These impressions and recommendations have application for theory, research, and practice. For future research, clinical, educational, and administrative efforts to sufficiently reflect the nursing and patient perspectives on QOL, most, if not all, of the recommendations need to be incorporated. The purposeful combining of the two perspectives in this text and in this chapter is not to deny the unique aspects of each, but to emphasize their conceptual commonalities and the link between the two that directly influences care given to patients. The link represents the merger of nurses' knowledge of disease, health, human development, and respect for patients with the perceptions, values, and preferences of patients. This merger influences care, the patients' response to their care, and ultimately the outcomes of the care. A second reason for combining both perspectives in the same text is to promote even further the commitment of nurses to solicit from patients their views on QOL and to do so in a way that convinces patients that their perspectives are heard, respected, and integrated into their care.

More than two dozen definitions and descriptions of QOL are contained in this text. This implies that nursing as a discipline has found multiple though differing conceptualizations to be useful. Most of these are not derived directly from patients but from available literature and clinical observations. The latter two sources are valid and valuable, but the direct participation of patients in defining their QOL adds to the validity and value of the existing definitions. Given the varying and diverse conceptualizations being used, it is important to state clearly the definition of QOL being used in any future work and to include a brief rationale for the selection of that conceptualization (see Table 18-1). Efforts to develop consensus definitions that best

Table 18-1	QOL—Related Recommendations for Future Research or Projects to Ensure That Nursing and Patient Perspectives Are Sufficiently Reflected

1. Solicit from patients their views on their QOL.
2. Include an explicit definition of QOL.
3. Provide a rationale for the definition of QOL included.
4. Use a definition of QOL that corresponds with the scope of the research or project.
5. Match the breadth of the conceptualization (global or focused) of QOL with a measurement approach.
6. Specify the domains of QOL and their definitions.
7. Provide a rationale for the domains of QOL included.
8. Distinguish the essential characteristics of QOL from variables that influence or are associated with QOL.
9. Make explicit the QOL model being used, including its domains, associated variables, and underlying assumptions.
10. Reflect the dynamism of QOL in the model used.
11. Avoid measuring QOL at a single point.
12. Avoid relying solely on a single, global item to measure QOL.
13. Solicit patient QOL ratings at true change points and not just at stable points during and after care.
14. Use established measures (those with known psychometric properties) of QOL.
15. Avoid using a standardized weighting system for the domains of QOL so that true change will not be obscured.
16. Quality of life at end-of-life needs to include the perspectives of patients and their significant others.

convey QOL for defined groups need to continue, but until such agreements on definitions are achieved, the conceptual basis for QOL needs to be explicitly stated. The incomplete conceptual analysis of QOL is most notable in pediatric populations (see Chapter 7), in situations in which the family rather than the individual is the unit of analysis (see Chapter 10), and in survivor populations (see Chapter 16). Rather than include a definition of QOL in their work, some authors imply a definition by the scale or scales used to measure QOL. It is inaccurate to assume that the term QOL evokes a shared understanding among nurses or other health care professionals.

It seems equally inaccurate to assume that patients share a common conceptualization of the term QOL until this has been documented or refuted through systematically solicited input from patients. The contributors to this text who are patients have offered the following key characteristics of QOL in the cancer experience:

1. A profound sense of personal vulnerability
2. An inability to deny that which is frightening
3. Changing perceptions of what is important in life
4. A desire to make a difference in the lives of others
5. A need to be respected by others
6. A loving connection with a special person
7. Learning to tolerate feeling alienated from a societal norm or value
8. A greater appreciation of daily activities
9. A need to be taken seriously
10. A profound sense of spirituality.

More specifically for health care providers, these contributors have indicated a desire to be honestly involved in decisions about their care without risk of being labeled "difficult" or "noncompliant." The contributors have also conveyed that key characteristics of QOL can change in importance during and after treatment for cancer. The essential characteristics of QOL offered by patients are somewhat different from those described by nurses and other professionals, although the difference may be strictly semantic. Nevertheless, the need remains for a direct comparison of these differences and more direct solicitations of QOL definitions from patients at the point of diagnosis of a life-threatening illness to cure or from diagnosis to death (see Table 18-1).

Although achieving consensus definitions of QOL is a priority, such definitions may legitimately differ by breadth and specificity according to the scope of the research or project. A broad, global definition will provide valuable flexibility when cultures or other large groups are being compared (see Chapter 4). The broad conceptual approach will need to be matched by an equally broad measurement approach (or use of global measures of QOL). Such a matched conceptual and measurement approach will likely yield findings that will invite us as nurses to view groups of patients and other individuals in new ways, or to further refine our previous impressions and understandings. This is the benefit of comparing groups on a similar basis— using a consensus definition of QOL. In contrast, a consensus definition and conceptualization that is narrowly focused can be matched with an equally focused measurement approach, for example, QOL in 7- to 12-year-old pediatric oncology patients experiencing pain. The benefit of the narrowly focused approach is that findings may translate more readily into direct care practices tailored for the studied group. The recommendations here are to use a consensus definition that corresponds to the scope of the research or project, and to match the breadth of the conceptualization with a corresponding measurement approach (see Table 18-1).

Whether the conceptual/measurement approach is broad and global or narrow and focused, the essential domains (along with the conceptual definitions of QOL and the attributes of QOL) need to be specified. The rationale for considering the essential domains also needs to be included (see Table18-1). At present, four domains are most commonly included in the nursing literature: physical functioning, emotion/psychological functioning, social functioning, and disease/treatment-related symptoms. However, the definitions of these domains vary across studies and projects. Current work in nursing with the domains of QOL indicates that the one or more domains that represent what is of greatest meaning to a patient or group at the time of measurement are those that most accurately convey QOL (see Chapter 8). Which domains convey meaning may vary by patient or by time and events. Padilla and Kagawa-Singer (Chapter 6) and Taylor (Chapter 5) suggest that the domain of spirituality used by some researchers may be the domain that most sensitively measures meaning. Although not yet confirmed by research data, this is an example of a rationale for considering spirituality an essential domain of QOL.

The careful effort put into clarifying the conceptual nature of QOL, including its essential characteristics and domains, will also benefit efforts to distinguish these from external sources of influence on QOL, such as antecedent and mediating variables (see Chapter 4). Distinguishing the features or characteristics that comprise QOL from the variables that affect QOL will further nurses' understanding of what QOL is for patients and what can be done to positively influence their QOL during care for cancer (Table 18-1). This effort will also result in a specification of relationships between QOL and other variables, or model-building, thus contributing to our theoretical understanding of this construct.

Models that seek to convey the context and the characteristics of QOL in the lives of patients receiving care related to cancer will need to reflect the dynamism of QOL over time and events, and the influence of both internal and external factors on QOL. Such dynamism could be conveyed by a feedback loop in the model or some other feature that would prevent the misrepresentation of QOL as occurring in linear, sequential fashion. The recommendation is that a model of QOL be specified or depicted in future work, that the underlying assumptions be made explicit, and that the dynamism of QOL be conveyed (Table 18-1).

Both patient and nursing perspectives indicate that QOL changes in degree or intensity and is time- and event-dependent. Not yet established is whether the intensity is also disease- and treatment-dependent. This change can be in an overall, general sense or in a particular domain or characteristic of QOL. Such change (or lack thereof) needs to be documented. Considering the dynamism of QOL, multiple measurement points with the same respondents, or a cross-sectional approach with very carefully delineated and justified measurement points, will be required. Measuring QOL at a single point will not suffice for full understanding of the nature of QOL, nor will it contribute information that could be used to guide clinical care (see Table 18-1).

Similarly, it is anticipated that as advances continue in the treatment of cancer, as the number of cancer survivors increases, and as supportive care improves, QOL may change form, or the standards of comparison previously used may change. This idea of changing form is consistent with the idea that the concept of QOL is "social in nature," influenced and shaped by the context within which it exists (Toulmin, 1972). The likelihood of change means that QOL will need to be examined over time both conceptually and empirically.

Sufficiency in empirical measurement of QOL from nursing and patient perspectives is unlikely to be met by a single, global item (see Chapter 8). Although a patient's response to the item may give an indication of a general perception at that moment, the response would not identify the source or domain that accounts for the change. This, then, would not provide a basis for a care intervention from nurses or other health care professionals, or a basis for not initiating an intervention. The single item would make minimal demands on the patient, but that benefit is offset by the lack of clinically useful information. Therefore, the recommendation is to avoid relying solely on a single, global item to measure QOL when the intent is to gather information that will be helpful in providing clinical care (Table 18-1).

The potential burden for patients of measuring their QOL is increased by the need to have repeated measures and by the timing of those measures. Key measurement points are those at which a change in QOL is anticipated, such as during confirmed progression of disease or nadirs. The balance between burden and the opportunity for a patient to express perceptions and values in a way that could benefit him or her or others is important to achieve. Seeking patients' QOL only at stable points may prevent health care professionals from learning essential information about QOL that may only be evident at change points, and prevent patients from sharing their views at critical times (Table 18-1).

Several psychometrically sound QOL instruments are available for use with adults. These are available in global forms and disease-specific modular forms. It is important to use these instruments consistently (rather than develop new measures) to document their ability to accurately measure QOL in different groups at varying time points (see Chapter 8). Similarly, general and disease-specific QOL instruments are now available for pediatric patients and their parents. As a result, researchers tend to use a battery of measures in an attempt to document all domains of quality of life.

Accuracy of interpreting QOL scores and capturing change in the domains of QOL also have implications for scoring QOL measures. Composite scores could obscure change in individual domains. Assigning weights to domains may also obscure the true change in intensity being obscured. Individual scores for each domain may be the more appropriate scoring method with QOL (Table 18-1).

Nursing's commitment is to support and influence in a positive manner the QOL of patients during and following care for cancer. This commitment reflects our belief that QOL is a process that changes over time and situations and that can be altered by both internal factors (e.g., cellular response to treatment) and external factors (e.g., nursing care interventions). That commitment, combined with knowledge of patients' perspectives on their QOL, will most assuredly result in care that assists patients in achieving the most positive outcomes possible in the physical, psychological, symptom-related, social, and spiritual domains.

REFERENCE

Toulmin, S. (1972). *Human understanding*. Princeton, NJ: Princeton University Press.

Descriptions/Definitions of Quality of Life by Sample (Adult or Youth) and Publication Year

Description/Definition	Dimensions	Source
ADULT		
A state of complete physical, mental, and social well-being and not merely the absence of disease and infirmity	Physical well-being Mental well-being Social well-being	World Health Organization, 1947, p. 29
The degree to which one has self-esteem, a purpose in life, and minimal anxiety		Lewis, 1982, p. 113
The degree of satisfaction with perceived present life circumstances		Young & Longman, 1983, p. 220
An individual's perceptions of well-being that stem from satisfaction or dissatisfaction with dimensions of life that are important to the individual	Health and functioning Psychological/spiritual Family Social and economic	Ferrans & Powers, 1985, p. 16
An abstract and complex form representing individual responses to the physical, mental, and social factors that contribute to "normal" living		Holmes & Dickerson, 1987, p. 16

	Social activity
	Emotional experience
	Overall current health
	Functional status
	Cognitive function
	Satisfaction
		Epstein, Hall, Tognetti,
		  Son, & Conant, 1989,
		  p. 593

Patients' appraisal of and satisfaction with their current level of functioning compared to what they perceive to be possible or ideal	Physical concerns Functional ability Family well-being Emotional well-being Spirituality Treatment satisfaction Future orientation Sexuality/intimacy Social functioning Occupational functioning	Cella & Tulsky, 1990, pp. 30–31
A personal statement of the positivity or negativity of attributes that characterize life	Psychological well-being Physical well-being Symptom control Nutritional concerns Social concerns Affective states	Grant, Padilla, Ferrell, & Rhiner, 1990, p. 261

continues

Description/Definition	Dimensions	Source
	ADULT *(continued)*	
	Physical functioning status Disease symptoms and treatment side effects Psychological status Social functioning	Aaronson, 1990, p. 62
	General health perceptions Physical suffering Self-care activities Outlook on life Meaningful activities Social relationships	Hadorn & Hays, 1991, p. 831

The perception of the impact of
the disease is both subjective
and culturally bound
	Physical function, emo-
	    tional function, or
	    psychological function
	Social function
	Symptom of disease or its
	    treatment
		Clinch & Schipper, 1993,
		    pp. 62–63

	Physical, psychological,
	    social, and spiritual
	    well-being
	Economic impact of illness
		Taylor, Jones, & Burns,
		    1995, p. 195

A multidimensional construct encompassing perceptions of both positive and negative aspects of physical, emotional, social, and cognitive functions, as well as the negative aspects of somatic discomfort and other symptoms produced by a disease or its treatment		Osoba, 1994, p. 608
The congruence or lack of congruence between actual life conditions and individuals' hopes and expectations		McDaniel & Bach, 1994, p. 19

continues

Description/Definition	Dimensions	Source
	YOUTH	
	Sensory and communication ability	Cadman, Goldsmith, Torrance, Boyle, & Furlong, 1986
	Happiness	
	Self-care ability	
	Freedom from moderate to severe chronic pain or discomfort	
	Learning and school ability	
	Physical ability	
Children's and adolescents' subjective and changeable sense of well-being that reflects how closely their desires and hopes match what is actually happening and their orientation toward the future, both their own and that of others	Hopefulness Self-esteem/self-efficacy Symptom distress Adverse physical effects of treatment	Hinds, 1990, p. 285
The impact of illness and predicament of a biologic disorder	Incidence, prevalence, physiologic dysfunction, or mortality rate	Rosenbaum, Cadman, & Kerpalani, 1990, p. 207
A term describing the total existence of an individual or group, including the more positive aspects of health	External conditions Internal conditions Personal psychological conditions	Lindstrom & Kohler, 1991, p. 121
	Mobility Physical activity Social activity	Bradlyn, Harris, Warner, Ritchey, & Zaboy, 1993, p. 250
	Physical symptoms and functionality in the areas of mobility, social activity, physical activity	Czyzewski, Mariotto, Bartholomew, LeCompte, & Sockrider, 1994, p. 966
Personal opinions reflecting satisfaction with current circumstances, participation in activities and relations, and the opportunity to have control over one's life and to make choices	Satisfaction Well-being Social belonging Empowerment/control	Keith & Schalock, 1994, p. 84
The way in which individuals view their own health and the degree to which they are satisfied with it		Vivier, Bernier, & Starfiled, 1994, p. 532

Description/Definition	Dimensions	Source
	YOUTH *(continued)*	

The degree to which a person enjoys the important possibilities of his/her life	Being
	  Physical being
	  Psychological being
	  Spiritual being
	Belonging
	  Physical belonging
	  Social belonging
	  Community belonging
	Becoming
	  Practical becoming
	  Leisure becoming
	  Growth becoming
		Raphael, Rukholm, Brown, Hill-Bailey, & Donato, 1996, p. 367

State of well-being consists of two components: 1) the ability to perform everyday activities that reflect physical, psychological, and social well-being 2) satisfaction with levels of functioning and the control of disease- or treatment-related symptoms	Physical well-being, psychological well-being, social well-being Satisfaction with functioning Control of disease- or treatment-related symptoms	Staab, Wenninger, Gebert, Rupprath, Bisson, Trettin, Paul, Keller, & Wahn, 1998, pp. 727–728

The impact of disease and treatment on an individual's physical, psychological, and social functioning, and by disease/treatment-specific symptoms	Core
	  Physical functioning
	  Psychological functioning
	  Social functioning
	Modules
	  Pain
	  Nausea
	  Procedural anxiety
	  Treatment anxiety
	  Worry
	  Cognitive problems
	  Perceived physical appearance
	  Physician/nurse communication
		Varni, Seid, & Rode, 1999, p. 128

Source: King, C. R., et al. (1997). Quality of life and the cancer experience: The state of the knowledge, *Oncology Nursing Forum, 24*(1), pp. 30–31. Used with permission.

REFERENCES

Aaronson, N. K. (1990). Quality of life research in cancer clinical trials. A need for common rules and language. *Oncology* 4(5), 59–66.

Bradlyn, A. S., Harris, C. V., Warner, J. E., Ritchey, A. K., & Zaboy, K. (1993). An investigation of the validity of the quality of well-being scale with pediatric oncology patients. *Health Psychology, 12,* 246–250.

Cadman, D., Goldsmith, C., Torrance, G. W., Boyle, M. H., & Furlong, W. (1986). Development of a health status index for Ontario children. Final report to the Ontario Ministry of Health on research grant DM 648 (00633). Hamilton, Ontario: McMaster University.

Cella, D. F., & Tulsky, D. S. (1990). Measuring quality of life today: Methodological aspects. *Oncology* 4(5), 29–38.

Clinch, J. J., & Schipper, H. (1993). Quality of life assessment in palliative care. In D. Doyle, G. Hanks, & N. MacDonald (Eds.), *Oxford textbook of palliative medicine.* New York: Oxford University Press.

Czyzewski, D. I., Mariotto, M. J., Bartholomew, L. K., LeCompte, S. H., & Sockrider, M. M. (1994). Measurement of quality of well being in a child and adolescent cystic fibrosis population. *Medical Care, 32,* 965–972.

Epstein, A. M., Hall, J. A., Tognetti, J., Son, L. H., & Conant, L. (1989). Using proxies to evaluate quality of life. *Medical Care, 27,* 591–598.

Ferrans, C., & Powers, M. (1985). Quality of life index: Development and psychometric properties. *Advances in Nursing Science, 8,* 15–24.

Grant, M. M., Padilla, G. V., Ferrell, B. R., & Rhiner, M. (1990). Assessment of quality of life with a single instrument. *Seminars in Oncology Nursing, 6,* 260–270.

Hadorn, D., & Hays, R. (1991). Multitrait-multimethod analysis of health-related quality-of-life measures. *Medical Care, 29,* 829–840.

Hinds, P. S. (1990). Quality of life in children and adolescents with cancer. *Seminars in Oncology Nursing, 6,* 285–291.

Holmes, S., & Dickerson, J. (1987). The quality of life: Design and evaluation of a self-assessment instrument for use with cancer patients. *International Journal of Nursing Studies, 24*(1), 15–24.

Keith, K., & Schalock, R. (1994). The measurement of quality of life in adolescence: The quality of student life questionnaire. *The American Journal of Family Therapy, 22*(1), 83–87.

Lewis, F. M. (1982). Experienced personal control and quality of life in late stage cancer patients. *Nursing Research, 6,* 113–119.

Lindstrom, B., & Kohler, L. (1991). Youth, disability and quality of life. *Pediatrician, 18,* 121–128.

McDaniel, R. W., & Bach, C. A. (1994). Quality of life: A concept analysis. *Rehabilitation Nursing Research 3*(1), 18–22.

Osoba, D. (1994). Lessons learned from measuring health-related quality of life in oncology. *Journal of Clinical Oncology, 12,* 608–616.

Raphael, D., Rukholm, E., Brown, I., Hill-Bailey, P., & Donato, E. (1996). The quality of life profile—adolescent version: Background, description, and initial validation. *Journal of Adolescent Health, 19,* 336–375.

Rosenbaum, P., Cadman, D., & Kerpalani, H. (1990). Pediatrics: Assessing quality of life. In B. Spilker (Ed.), *Quality of life assessments in clinical trials* (pp. 205–215). New York: Raven Press.

Staab, D., Wenninger, K., Gebert, N., Rupprath, K., Bisson, S., Trettin, M., Paul, K. D., Keller, K. M., & Wahn, U. (1998). Quality of life in patients with cystic fibrosis and their parents: What is important besides disease severity? *Thorax, 53*(9), 727–731.

Taylor, E. J., Jones, P., & Burns, M. (1995). Quality of life. In I. M. Lubkin (Ed.), *Chronic illness: Impact and intervention* (3rd ed.) (p. 195). Boston: Jones and Bartlett.

Varni, J. W., Seid, M., & Rode, C. A. (1999). The PedsQL: Measurement model for the pediatric quality of life inventory. *Med Care, 37*(2), 126–139.

Vivier, P. M., Bernier, J. A., & Starfiled, B. (1994). Current approaches to measuring health outcomes in pediatric research. *Current Opinions in Pediatrics, 6*(5), 530–537.

World Health Organization. (1947). *WHO Chronicle.* Geneva, Switzerland: Author.

Young, K. J., & Longman, A. J. (1983). Quality of life and persons with melanoma: A pilot study. *Cancer Nursing, 6,* 219–225.

Quality of Life Measurements

Selected instruments used to measure quality of life (QOL) are contained in this appendix. The instruments represent diverse approaches to quantifying QOL. These approaches include the global single item, generic measures, and cancer-specific measures.

I. EXAMPLE OF THE GLOBAL SINGLE ITEM APPROACH TO MEASURING QUALITY OF LIFE

Quality of Life
Visual Life Analogue Scale (VAS)

KATE LORIG

Contact person: Kate Lorig, RN, DrPH, Director, Stanford Patient Education Research Center, 1000 Welch Road, Suite 204, Palo Alto, CA 94304.
Source: Kate Lorig, *Outcome Measures for Health Education and other Health Care Interventions*, p. 63, copyright © 1996 by Sage Publications, Inc. Reprinted by permission of Sage Publications, Inc.

Quality of Life Visual Analogue Scale (VAS)

Take a moment and think of the best possible life and the worst possible life. Now, on the line below, place an "X" to indicate where your life is now:

Best
possible
life

Worst
possible
life

Scoring. Measure in centimeters with ruler, "10" being "Worst possible life" and "0" being "Best possible life." Enter the number where the middle of the "X" is located. Enter whole numbers, not decimals. If the "X" is between centimeters, round down if below 0.5, round up if 0.5 and above, and if exactly at 0.5, round to the nearest even number.

Note: The line must be *exactly* 10 cm long. When reproducing, make sure your printer or copy machine reproduces at exactly 100 percent. You cannot have a reliable measurement if the line is not exactly the same length each time. A small, clear, plastic ruler will make it easier to see the scoring point. Make sure all scoring is done with identical rulers.

II. EXAMPLES OF GENERIC MEASURES OF QUALITY OF LIFE

The McCorkle and Young Symptom Distress Scale

RUTH McCORKLE • KATHY YOUNG GRAHAM

Contact person: Ruth McCorkle, PhD, FAAN, Professor, The Florence S. Wald Professor of Nursing, Director, Center for Excellence in Chronic Illness Care, Chair, Doctoral Program, Yale University School of Nursing, 100 Church Street, South, PO Box 9740, New Haven, CT, 06536. Used with permission from Ruth McCorkle, PhD, FAAN.

ID# _____ DATE _____

(SDS) Each of the following sections lists 5 different statements. Think about what each statement says, then place a circle around the one statement that most closely indicates how you have been feeling during the past 7 days. Please circle one statement for each section.

1. Appetite

1	2	3	4	5
I have my normal appetite.	My appetite is usually, but not always, pretty good.	I don't really enjoy my food like I used to.	I have to force myself to eat my food.	I cannot stand the thought of food.

2. Insomnia

1	2	3	4	5
I sleep as well as I always have.	I have occasional spells of sleeplessness.	I frequently have trouble getting to sleep and staying asleep.	I have difficulty sleeping almost every night.	It is almost impossible for me to get a decent night's sleep.

3. Pain (a)

1	2	3	4	5
I almost never have pain.	I have pain once in a while.	I frequently have pain—several times a week.	I am usually in some degree of pain.	I am in some degree of pain almost constantly.

4. Pain (b)

1	2	3	4	5
When I do have pain, it is very mild.	When I do have pain, it is mildly distressing.	The pain I do have is usually fairly intense.	The pain I have is usually very intense.	The pain I have is almost unbearable.

5. Fatigue

1	2	3	4	5
I am usually not tired at all.	I am occasionally rather tired.	There are frequently periods when I am quite tired.	I am usually very tired.	Most of the time, I feel exhausted.

6. Bowel

1	2	3	4	5
I have my normal bowel pattern.	My bowel pattern occasionally causes me some discomfort.	I frequently have discomfort from my present bowel pattern.	I am usually in discomfort because of my present bowel pattern.	My present bowel pattern has changed drastically from what was normal for me.

7. Concentration

1
I have my normal ability to concentrate.

2
I occasionally have trouble concentrating.

3
I often have trouble concentrating.

4
I usually have at least some difficulty concentrating.

5
I just can't seem to concentrate at all.

8. Appearance

1
My appearance has basically not changed.

2
My appearance has gotten a little worse.

3
My appearance is definitely worse than it used to be, but I am not greatly concerned about it.

4
My appearance is definitely worse than it used to be, and I am concerned about it.

5
My appearance has changed drastically from what it was.

9. Breathing

1
I usually breathe normally.

2
I occasionally have trouble breathing.

3
I often have trouble breathing.

4
I can hardly ever breathe as easily as I want.

5
I almost always have severe trouble with my breathing.

10. Outlook

1
I am not fearful or worried.

2
I am a little worried about things.

3
I am quite worried, but unafraid.

4
I am worried and a little frightened about things.

5
I am worried and scared about things.

11. Cough

1
I seldom cough.

2
I have an occasional cough.

3
I often cough.

4
I often cough and occasionally have severe coughing spells.

5
I often have persistent and severe coughing spells.

12. Nausea (a)

1
I seldom feel any nausea at all.

2
I am nauseous once in a while.

3
I am often nauseous.

4
I am usually nauseous.

5
I suffer from nausea almost continually.

13. Nausea (b)

1
When I do have nausea, it is very mild.

2
When I do have nausea, it is mildly distressing.

3
When I have nausea, I feel pretty sick.

4
When I have nausea, I feel very sick.

5
When I have nausea, I am as sick as I could possibly be.

Demands of Illness Inventory

MEL R. HABERMAN

Contact person: Mel Haberman, PhD, RN, FAAN, Associate Dean for Research, Washington State University College of Nursing, 2917 W. Fort George Wright Drive, Spokane, WA 99224-5291. Used with permission from Dr. Mel Haberman.

Demands of Illness Inventory: Patient Version

Below is a list of events and thoughts that describe experiences some individuals have when they experience a health problem. Read each item carefully and determine the extent to which you have had the experience as the result of your health problem *during the last two weeks including today.*

Note: Please mark NA only if the item is not applicable to your particular situation, otherwise mark 0 to 4. Please do not skip any items. Thank you!

> NA = Not Applicable
> 0 = Not at All
> 1 = A Little Bit
> 2 = Moderately
> 3 = Quite a Bit
> 4 = Extremely

As the result of my illness I have experienced:

1. Headaches.	NA	0	1	2	3	4
2. Faintness or dizziness.	NA	0	1	2	3	4
3. Pains in heart or chest.	NA	0	1	2	3	4
4. Pains in lower back.	NA	0	1	2	3	4
5. Nausea or upset stomach.	NA	0	1	2	3	4
6. Soreness of muscles.	NA	0	1	2	3	4
7. Hot or cold spells.	NA	0	1	2	3	4
8. Numbness or tingling in parts of my body.	NA	0	1	2	3	4
9. Feeling weak in parts of my body.	NA	0	1	2	3	4
10. Heavy feelings in my arms or legs.	NA	0	1	2	3	4
11. Feeling rundown.	NA	0	1	2	3	4
12. Inability to stay at my usual weight.	NA	0	1	2	3	4

As the result of my illness I think about:

13. The value my life has for me.	NA	0	1	2	3	4
14. How long I might live.	NA	0	1	2	3	4
15. Not being able to achieve my goals in life.	NA	0	1	2	3	4
16. How I might reorder the priorities in my life.	NA	0	1	2	3	4
17. My own mortality.	NA	0	1	2	3	4
18. How unprepared I've been for this experience.	NA	0	1	2	3	4

Note: Patient version, Woods, Haberman, & Packard, copyright © 1984, 1987, 1993.

19. The uncertainties I face.	NA	0	1	2	3	4
20. Whether my life will ever return to normal.	NA	0	1	2	3	4
21. What will happen to my family in the future.	NA	0	1	2	3	4
22. Whether my children will face the same illness.	NA	0	1	2	3	4
23. Not having any past experience to relate this one to.	NA	0	1	2	3	4
24. How my experience compares with others having the same or a similar experience.	NA	0	1	2	3	4
25. Why is this happening to me?	NA	0	1	2	3	4
26. How unfair this experience has been.	NA	0	1	2	3	4
27. My odds of getting this illness.	NA	0	1	2	3	4
28. What has caused the illness.	NA	0	1	2	3	4

As the result of my illness our family:

29. Income has gone down.	NA	0	1	2	3	4
30. Doesn't have enough time or energy for recreational activities outside our home.	NA	0	1	2	3	4
31. Doesn't have enough money to support our usual lifestyle.	NA	0	1	2	3	4
32. Doesn't have enough time or energy to entertain friends at home.	NA	0	1	2	3	4
33. Doesn't have enough money for our health care bills.	NA	0	1	2	3	4
34. Doesn't have enough time or energy to go out with friends.	NA	0	1	2	3	4
35. Has had to change our old meal patterns.	NA	0	1	2	3	4
36. Has had to change our child care arrangements.	NA	0	1	2	3	4

As the result of my illness:

37. The children have had to take responsibility for household tasks.	NA	0	1	2	3	4
38. My partner has had to take responsibility for household tasks.	NA	0	1	2	3	4
39. The quality of my sexual activities has changed.	NA	0	1	2	3	4

40. The frequency of my sexual activities has changed.	NA	0	1	2	3	4
41. There isn't time or energy for sexual activities.	NA	0	1	2	3	4
42. I worry about how my children are reacting to my illness.	NA	0	1	2	3	4
43. The children need more emotional support.	NA	0	1	2	3	4
44. The children need more information.	NA	0	1	2	3	4
45. I need more emotional support from my family.	NA	0	1	2	3	4
46. There is a strain on my relationship with my partner.	NA	0	1	2	3	4
47. My partner has had difficulty understanding my feelings.	NA	0	1	2	3	4
48. I worry about how my partner is responding to my illness.	NA	0	1	2	3	4
49. I wish my partner were handling the illness situation better.	NA	0	1	2	3	4
50. I need to be more sensitive to my partner's moods.	NA	0	1	2	3	4
51. I need to provide more emotional support to my partner.	NA	0	1	2	3	4
52. I need to protect my partner from stress.	NA	0	1	2	3	4
53. I need my partner to be more sensitive to my moods.	NA	0	1	2	3	4
54. I need my partner to help me with my treatment.	NA	0	1	2	3	4
55. My partner has had to change his work patterns.	NA	0	1	2	3	4
56. I'm not able to work at my job.	NA	0	1	2	3	4
57. I've had to miss more time at work than usual.	NA	0	1	2	3	4
58. I'm not able to do my usual amount of work.	NA	0	1	2	3	4
59. I've had trouble finding a job.	NA	0	1	2	3	4

As the result of my illness our family has had to:

60. Make new decisions about running the house.	NA	0	1	2	3	4
61. Revise the rules for the children.	NA	0	1	2	3	4

62. Discuss things concerning the children more.	NA	0	1	2	3	4
63. Decide what is really important to us.	NA	0	1	2	3	4

As the result of my illness:

64. I go out with friends less often.	NA	0	1	2	3	4
65. My social life has decreased.	NA	0	1	2	3	4
66. I often have to help others understand my illness.	NA	0	1	2	3	4
67. It's hard to keep up with my usual pace or routine.	NA	0	1	2	3	4
68. People have been overprotective.	NA	0	1	2	3	4
69. People seem less supportive as time goes on.	NA	0	1	2	3	4
70. I find that I need to help others accept my illness.	NA	0	1	2	3	4
71. Others do not really know or understand what I am going through.	NA	0	1	2	3	4
72. Others act differently toward me.	NA	0	1	2	3	4
73. It's hard to plan social activities because I don't know how I'll feel.	NA	0	1	2	3	4

As the result of my illness I:

74. Feel self-conscious about my body.	NA	0	1	2	3	4
75. Feel less attractive.	NA	0	1	2	3	4
76. Feel dissatisfied with the way I look.	NA	0	1	2	3	4
77. Feel I cannot always rely on my body.	NA	0	1	2	3	4
78. Think more about my own sexual appeal.	NA	0	1	2	3	4
79. Think about the disfigurement caused by surgery/treatment.	NA	0	1	2	3	4
80. Think about possibly needing to undergo surgery that would result in disfigurement.	NA	0	1	2	3	4
81. Think about the possibility of undergoing surgery to improve my appearance.	NA	0	1	2	3	4
82. Think about not being able to be pregnant and have a child.	NA	0	1	2	3	4
83. Feel more susceptible to other illnesses.	NA	0	1	2	3	4
84. Concentrate on new bodily sensations that may indicate illness.	NA	0	1	2	3	4
85. Worry my illness may reoccur with its initial severity.	NA	0	1	2	3	4

86. Tend to be preoccupied with the symptoms of my illness.   NA   0   1   2   3   4
87. Think about how I'm handling my illness situation.   NA   0   1   2   3   4
88. Wonder if the illness can be controlled in the future.   NA   0   1   2   3   4
89. Wonder if the illness is spreading undetected.   NA   0   1   2   3   4
90. Wonder why I still receive treatments even though my symptoms have subsided.   NA   0   1   2   3   4
91. Think about the illness being unending.   NA   0   1   2   3   4
92. Worry my health will get progressively worse.   NA   0   1   2   3   4
93. Worry the illness will involve other parts of my body in the future.   NA   0   1   2   3   4

As the result of my medical treatment:

94. I find it difficult to continue with follow-up appointments.   NA   0   1   2   3   4
95. I find it difficult to continue the treatments.   NA   0   1   2   3   4
96. I sometimes think the adverse effects of treatment outweigh the possible benefits.   NA   0   1   2   3   4
97. I worry about the expense of treatment.   NA   0   1   2   3   4
98. I've changed my diet.   NA   0   1   2   3   4
99. I'm more regimented in the time I eat.   NA   0   1   2   3   4
100. My whole life is more regimented.   NA   0   1   2   3   4
101. I'm adjusting the way I exercise.   NA   0   1   2   3   4
102. It's difficult to find suitable clothing.   NA   0   1   2   3   4
103. I'm considering the need to undergo more treatment.   NA   0   1   2   3   4
104. I'm considering if I should try a different treatment.   NA   0   1   2   3   4
105. It's difficult waiting for the results of my medical tests.   NA   0   1   2   3   4
106. It's difficult waiting to undergo treatment or surgery.   NA   0   1   2   3   4

At times, my health care providers:

107. Are not sensitive to my preferences for treatment.   NA   0   1   2   3   4

108. Act as if my opinions are unimportant.	NA	0	1	2	3	4
109. Make decisions without my best interests in mind.	NA	0	1	2	3	4
110. Do not tell me the truth about my health status.	NA	0	1	2	3	4
111. Do not show concern for me as a person.	NA	0	1	2	3	4

As I've experienced my illness situation:

112. I do not want my health providers to tell me the truth if my health takes a turn for the worse.	NA	0	1	2	3	4
113. I want more facts about the treatments.	NA	0	1	2	3	4
114. I have questions that I want to ask but just can't.	NA	0	1	2	3	4
115. I feel rushed to make a hasty treatment decision.	NA	0	1	2	3	4
116. I want to be more assertive about expressing the direction my treatment should take.	NA	0	1	2	3	4
117. I want to be told the reason why, when asked to do something for treatment.	NA	0	1	2	3	4
118. I sometimes don't understand the treatment I'm receiving.	NA	0	1	2	3	4
119. I'm not satisfied with the progress of my treatment.	NA	0	1	2	3	4
120. I'm not satisfied with my hospital care.	NA	0	1	2	3	4
121. I feel my illness is being incorrectly managed.	NA	0	1	2	3	4
122. I'm not confident my health problems will be correctly managed in the future.	NA	0	1	2	3	4

As the result of my medical treatments:

123. I worry about the physical side effects of treatment.	NA	0	1	2	3	4
124. I worry I'll develop new physical symptoms in the future.	NA	0	1	2	3	4
125. I often feel worse rather than better after treatment.	NA	0	1	2	3	4

Demands of Illness Inventory: Scoring Procedures

Scoring: Both the frequency of demands (number or incidence of demands) and intensity of experienced demands can be computed for each item and subscale or for the total instrument.

The *frequency of occurrence score* can be calculated at several levels. At the most basic level, each item can be converted to a "Yes/No" categorical variable. As such, "item frequencies" represent the number of subjects that rated an item 1 or greater. We usually report these as percentages of the total sample. For example, if 75 out of 100 subjects rated an item 1 or greater, then 75 percent of the sample experienced that demand.

At the next level, a similar item analysis can be conducted for each subscale by summing the items rated 1 or greater within a subscale. Subscale frequencies can be reported for each subject or for the sample as a whole. The theoretical range for this score is from zero to the number of items in each subscale (or from zero to 125 for the total instrument). These scores can be expressed as whole numbers or as percentages. For example, if 2 out of a possible 4 items in a subscale are rated 1 or greater by the subject, the frequency of experienced demands for that subscale may be expressed as a 2 or as 50 percent. Similarly, if 50 out of a total of 125 items are rated 1 or greater by the subject, the frequency score for the total instrument may be expressed as a 50 or as 40 percent (50/125).

Lastly, means can be calculated from the aforementioned distributions of subscale or total instrument frequency scores. These means represent the average number of demands experienced by the sample as a whole for each subscale or for the total instrument (see Table 4, Haberman, Woods, & Packard, 1990). These means can also be rank ordered (see Table 5, Haberman, Woods, & Packard, 1990).

A variation of reporting the frequency of demands is the calculation of *incidence rates*. Incidence rates describe the percent of items in a scale marked as a demand of illness, i.e., as problematic. They represent the number of items scored a 1 or greater, divided by the number of items in the subscale (or in the total instrument) × 100. The incidence rate is insensitive to gradations in the intensity of individual items, treating ratings of "a little bit," "moderately," "quite a bit," and "extremely" identically.

For the *intensity of demands scores*, we generally use item and subscale mean scores. However, a mean intensity score also can be calculated for the total instrument. The intensity score has a theoretical range of 0 to 4 per item or per subscale. To calculate the mean intensity score for each item, sum the intensity ratings by item for the entire sample and divide by the total sample size. To calculate the mean intensity score for each subscale, sum the intensity ratings for all the items in the subscale and divide by the number of items in the subscale. Subscale intensity means for the sample as a whole can be calculated from these distributions of the individual subject's subscale intensity scores. Sample means represent the average intensity of demands experienced by the sample as a whole for each subscale dimension. The means can be reported directly or rank ordered (same format as Tables 4 and 5, Haberman, Woods, & Packard, 1990).

Demands of Illness Inventory: Patient's Version

Standardized Item Alphas

Subscale	Frequency	Intensity
Physical symptoms	.8484	.8646
Personal meaning	.8457	.9179
Family functioning	.9120	.9228
Social relationship	.8227	.8747
Self-image	.8027	.8709
Monitoring symptoms	.7835	.9104
Treatment issues	.8892	.9164
Total instrument	.9621	.9717

Sample: 96 women with breast cancer
           29 women with diabetes

Total =   125

Demands of Illness Inventory: Revision of the 1987 Version

Item change: The 1993 version has 1 item change from the 1987 version.

- 1987 Version, Item #112. *"Not thoroughly explained my health status to me."*
- 1993 Version, Item #112. *"I do not want my health providers to tell me the truth if my health takes a turn for the worse."*

Because of this item change, the Treatment Relationships Subscale lost an item and the Treatment Information Exchange Subscale gained an item (#112).

All of the remaining changes are editorial and not substantive. Minor wording changes were made to several items to improve the grammar and clarity of the items.

1. The introduction was changed, deleting an Example item and changing the Note to read: *Please mark NA only if the item is not applicable to your particular situation, otherwise mark 0 to 4. Please do not skip any items. Thank you!*

Note: Patient version, Woods, Haberman, & Packard, copyright © 1987 version.
Note: Revised version, Woods, Haberman, & Packard, copyright © 1987, 1993.

2. Not Applicable was added as a response choice. The 0 to 4 rating scale remains unchanged.
3. References to "cancer and diabetes" were removed from the tool.
4. Items #94 to 125 were changed from the past to the present tense. The present tense is more relevant especially when using the tool in a repeated measures design. The change is more consistent with the instructions which tell respondents to answer the questions *based on the last two weeks including today*.
5. Items were changed which were formally reverse scored. All the items are now scored in the same direction. The higher the item score, the greater the intensity of demand.

Demands of Illness Inventory: Patient and Partner Versions

Subscale	Total items	Item numbers
I. Physical Symptoms	12	1–12
II. Personal Meaning	16	13–28
III. Family Functioning		
A. Adaptation	8	29–36
B. Integration	13	37–49
C. Partner Caretaking	5	50–54
D. Work Situation	5	55–59
E. Decision Making	4	60–63
IV. Social Relationships	10	64–73
V. Self-Image	9	74–82
VI. Monitoring Symptoms, Self & Others	11	83–93
VII. Treatment Issues		
A. Accommodation	13	94–106
B. Relationships	5	107–111
C. Information Exchange	7	112–118
D. Evaluation	4	119–122
E. Direct Effects	3	123–125
		Total = 125

Note: Patient and partner versions, Woods, Haberman, & Packard, copyright © 1987, 1993.

REFERENCES

Haberman, M. R., Woods, N. F., & Packard, N. J. (1990). Demands of chronic illness: Reliability and validity assessment of a demands of illness inventory. *Holistic Nursing Practice, 5*(1), 25–35.

Lewis, F. M., & Hammond, M. A. (1992). Psychosocial adjustment of the family to breast cancer: A longitudinal analysis. *Journal of the American Medical Women's Association. 47*(5), 194–200.

Lewis, F. M., Hammond, M. A., & Woods, N. F. (1993). The family's functioning with newly diagnosed breast cancer in the mother: The development of an explanatory model. *Journal of Behavioral Medicine, 16*(4), 351–370.

Packard, N. J., Haberman, M. R., Woods, N. F., & Yates, B. C. (1991). Demands of illness among chronically ill women. *Western Journal of Nursing Research, 13*(4), 434–457.

Woods, N. F., Haberman, M. R., & Packard, N. J. (1990). Demands of illness inventory: Relationship to individual, dyadic and family adaptation to chronic illness. *Western Journal of Nursing Research, 15*(1), 10–30.

Quality of Life Index

GERALDINE V. PADILLA • MARCIA M. GRANT

Contact person: Geraldine Padilla, PhD, Associate Dean for Research, University of California, San Francisco, School of Nursing, Box 0604, N 339, San Francisco, CA, 94122. Used with permission from Geraldine Padilla, PhD, and Marcia Grant, RN, DNSc.

Pt. No. _____

Time given: _____

Agency: _____

1. How easy is it to adjust to your radiation treatment to date?
   not at all   very easy

2. How much fun do you have (hobbies, recreation, social activity)?
   none   a great deal

3. Do you worry about the cost of your medical care?
   not at all   extremely

4. If you have pain, how distressing is it?
   not at all   extremely

5. How useful do you feel?
   not at all   extremely

6. How much happiness do you feel?
   none at all   a great deal

7. How satisfying is your life?
   not at all   extremely

8. Is your sexual activity sufficient to meet your needs?
   not at all   extremely

9. Is your radiation treatment interfering with your sexual activity?
   not at all   a great deal

10. Are you worried (fearful or anxious) about your radiation treatment?
    not at all   constantly

11. How much can you work at your usual tasks?
    not at all   a great deal

12. How is your present ability to concentrate?
    extremely poor   excellent

13. How much strength do you have?
    none at all   a great deal

14. Do you tire easily?
    not at all   a great deal

15. Is the amount of time you sleep sufficient to meet your needs?
    not at all   completely

16. How is your quality of life?
    extremely poor   excellent

17. How is your appetite?
    extremely poor   excellent

18. Is the amount you eat sufficient to meet your needs?
    not at all   completely

19. Are you worried about your weight?
    not at all   a great deal

20. If you have nausea, how distressing is it?
    not at all   extremely

21. If you vomit, how distressing is it?
    not at all   extremely

Information on Quality of Life Index (QLI-RT)

The following information is for a Quality of Life Index which includes twenty-one linear analogue scale items.

Pelvic Radiation Sample

In the Padilla and Grant studies (Padilla, 1990 & 1992; Padilla, Grant, Lipsett et al., 1992), studies that focus on cancer patients receiving radiation treatment to the pelvic area, the QLI is measured three times: N = 186 during Radiation Treatment week one (RT Week 1); N = 174 during Radiation Treatment week three (RT Week 3); N = 146 during the first follow-up (FU) after the completion of radiation treatment (RT 1st FU).

Internal consistency thetas for the total scale are as follows: during the first week of radiation treatment = 0.86; during the third week of treatment = 0.90; during the first follow-up visit = 0.92.

Internal consistency alphas for subscales during the radiation treatment follow-up period are as follows: psychological well-being = 0.87, physical well-being = 0.87, symptoms = 0.86, sexual activity = 0.97, and worry over weight and cost of treatment = 0.42.

Source: Padilla, 1992; Padilla, 1990; Padilla, Grant, Lipsett et al., 1992.

Validity: Factor analysis is based on an N of 85 from the first week of radiation treatment. The regression analysis is based on an N of 101.

Factor analytic construct validity: Five factors (psychological, physical, symptoms, sexual activity, and worry over weight and cost of radiation treatment).

Concurrent validity: Significant *rs* of 0.58 between tension-anxiety and psychological well-being subscale; and 0.60 between fatigue and physical well-being subscale.

Head and Neck Radiation Sample

In the Padilla and Grant studies (Padilla, 1992; Padilla, Grant, Lipsett et al., 1992) that focus on cancer patients receiving radiation treatment to the head and neck area, the QLI is measured 6 times: N = 181 RT week 1; N = 176 RT week 3; N = 156 end of RT; N = 129 RT 1st FU; N = 109 3 month FU; N = 82 18 month FU.

Internal consistency theta 0.88 for the total scale (based on an N of 110 at RT week 1).

Validity: Factor analysis is based on an N of 110 at RT week 1.

Factor analytic construct validity: Six factors (psychological, physical, nutrition and pain distress, other symptom distress, sleep and worry over cost, treatment anxiety-adjustment).

REFERENCES

Padilla, G. V. (1992). Validity of health-related quality of life subscales. *Progress Cardiovascular Nursing, 7*(1), 13–20.

Padilla, G. V., Grant, M. M., Lipsett, J., Anderson, P. R., Rhiner, M., & Bogen, C. (1992). Health quality of life and colorectal cancer. *Cancer, 70*(5 Suppl.), 1450–1456.

Padilla, G. V. (1990). Gastrointestinal side effects and quality of life in patients receiving radiation therapy. *Nutrition, 6*(5), 367–370.

Padilla, G. V. , Grant, M. M., Ferrell, B. R., & Presant, C. (1996). Quality of life—cancer. In Spilker, B. (Ed.), *Quality of life and pharmacoeconomics in clinical trials* (2nd ed.), (pp. 301–308). New York: Raven Press.

III. EXAMPLES OF CANCER-SPECIFIC MEASURES OF QUALITY OF LIFE (SINGLE MEASURE APPROACH)

Quality of Life Index
Cancer Version

CAROL FERRANS

Part I. For each of the following, please choose the answer that best describes how satisfied you are with that area of your life. Please mark your answer by circling the number. There are no right or wrong answers.

How satisfied are you with:	Very dissatisfied	Moderately dissatisfied	Slightly dissatisfied	Slightly satisfied	Moderately satisfied	Very satisfied
1. Your health?	1	2	3	4	5	6
2. The health care you are receiving?	1	2	3	4	5	6
3. The amount of pain that you have?	1	2	3	4	5	6
4. The amount of energy you have for everyday activities?	1	2	3	4	5	6
5. Your physical independence?	1	2	3	4	5	6
6. The amount of control you have over your life?	1	2	3	4	5	6
7. Your potential to live a long time?	1	2	3	4	5	6
8. Your family's health?	1	2	3	4	5	6
9. Your children?	1	2	3	4	5	6
10. Your family's happiness?	1	2	3	4	5	6
11. Your relationship with your spouse/significant other?	1	2	3	4	5	6
12. Your sex life?	1	2	3	4	5	6
13. Your friends?	1	2	3	4	5	6
14. The emotional support you get from others?	1	2	3	4	5	6
15. Your ability to meet family responsibilities?	1	2	3	4	5	6
16. Your usefulness to others?	1	2	3	4	5	6
17. The amount of stress or worries in your life?	1	2	3	4	5	6
18. Your home?	1	2	3	4	5	6
19. Your neighborhood?	1	2	3	4	5	6
20. Your standard of living?	1	2	3	4	5	6
21. Your job?	1	2	3	4	5	6
22. Not having a job?	1	2	3	4	5	6
23. Your education?	1	2	3	4	5	6
24. Your financial independence?	1	2	3	4	5	6
25. Your leisure time activities?	1	2	3	4	5	6
26. Your ability to travel on vacations?	1	2	3	4	5	6
27. Your potential for a happy old age/retirement?	1	2	3	4	5	6

How satisfied are you with:	Very dissatisfied	Moderately dissatisfied	Slightly dissatisfied	Slightly satisfied	Moderately satisfied	Very satisfied
28. Your peace of mind?	1	2	3	4	5	6
29. Your personal faith in God?	1	2	3	4	5	6
30. Your achievement of personal goals?	1	2	3	4	5	6
31. Your happiness in general?	1	2	3	4	5	6
32. Your life in general?	1	2	3	4	5	6
33. Your personal appearance?	1	2	3	4	5	6
34. Yourself in general?	1	2	3	4	5	6

Part II. For each of the following, please choose the answer that best describes how important that area of life is to you. Please mark your answer by circling the number. There are no right or wrong answers.

How important to you is:	Very unimportant	Moderately unimportant	Slightly unimportant	Slightly important	Moderately important	Very important
1. Your health?	1	2	3	4	5	6
2. Health care?	1	2	3	4	5	6
3. Being completely free of pain?	1	2	3	4	5	6
4. Having enough energy for everyday activities?	1	2	3	4	5	6
5. Your physical independence?	1	2	3	4	5	6
6. Having control over your life?	1	2	3	4	5	6
7. Living a long time?	1	2	3	4	5	6
8. Your family's health?	1	2	3	4	5	6
9. Your children?	1	2	3	4	5	6
10. Your family's happiness?	1	2	3	4	5	6

How important to you is:	Very unimportant	Moderately unimportant	Slightly unimportant	Slightly important	Moderately important	Very important
11. Your relationship with your spouse/significant other?	1	2	3	4	5	6
12. Your sex life?	1	2	3	4	5	6
13. Your friends?	1	2	3	4	5	6
14. The emotional support you get from others?	1	2	3	4	5	6
15. Meeting family responsibilities?	1	2	3	4	5	6
16. Being useful to others?	1	2	3	4	5	6
17. Having a reasonable amount of stress or worries?	1	2	3	4	5	6
18. Your home?	1	2	3	4	5	6
19. Your neighborhood?	1	2	3	4	5	6
20. A good standard of living?	1	2	3	4	5	6
21. Your job?	1	2	3	4	5	6
22. To have a job?	1	2	3	4	5	6
23. Your education?	1	2	3	4	5	6
24. Your financial independence?	1	2	3	4	5	6
25. Leisure time activities?	1	2	3	4	5	6
26. The ability to travel on vacations?	1	2	3	4	5	6
27. Having a happy old age/retirement?	1	2	3	4	5	6
28. Peace of mind?	1	2	3	4	5	6
29. Your personal faith in God?	1	2	3	4	5	6
30. Achieving your personal goals?	1	2	3	4	5	6
31. Your happiness in general?	1	2	3	4	5	6
32. Being satisfied with life?	1	2	3	4	5	6
33. Your personal appearance?	1	2	3	4	5	6
34. Are you to yourself?	1	2	3	4	5	6

Quality of Life Scale

Bone Marrow Transplant

BETTY R. FERRELL • MARCIA M. GRANT

Contact person: Betty R. Ferrell, PhD, RN, FAAN, Associate Research Scientist, City of Hope National Medical Center, 1500 East Duarte Road, Duarte, CA 91010-0269. Version 1. Used with permission from Betty R. Ferrell, PhD, RN, FAAN, and Marcia Grant, DNSc, RN, FAAN.

Quality of Life in Bone Marrow Transplant Survivors

Thank you for taking the time to complete this questionnaire.

We want to ensure that your responses are anonymous and confidential. Once your completed questionnaires are received, a number will be assigned and your name will not appear on any questionnaires.

All results will go directly to the Department of Nursing Research. *Your individual responses will not be reported to your nurse, physician, or social worker.* Therefore, if you have any specific concerns, please contact your nurse, physician, or social worker directly. See the enclosed colored sheet for their telephone numbers.

Name _____ Date _____

Current address, if changes have occurred within the last year.

_____

_____

Current telephone number including area code _____

Please complete the following information.

1. Marital status prior to your bone marrow transplant (BMT).
   Single ____   Married____   Divorced____   Widowed ____   Separated____
   Marital status now.
   Single ____   Married____   Divorced____   Widowed ____   Separated____

2. Age _____

3. Height_____

4. Current weight _____

5. Are you satisfied with your current weight?
   No_____   Yes_____

6. Has a substantial weight change occurred since your BMT?
   No_____   Yes_____
   If yes, has it been an:
   Increase_____   Please identify the number of pounds _____
   Decrease _____   Please identify the number of pounds _____

7. How many colds and episodes of flu do you have per year? _____
   Is this more than_____, less than_____, or the same as_____before your BMT?

8. List all medications you are currently taking.

Medication Name and Dose	Physician's Instructions for Taking the Medication	How Are You Taking the Medication?
Example: Advil 200 mg	1 tablet 4 times a day	1 tablet 3 times a day

9. Do you have chronic graft-versus-host disease?

   No_____   Yes_____

10. Have you been able to return to work since your BMT?

   No_____   Yes (part-time) _____   Not applicable_____

   Yes (full-time) _____

11. If you have not been able to return to work, why not? _____

   _____

   _____

12. If you have returned to work, are you employed in the same occupation as before your BMT?

   No_____   Yes_____

   If no, why did you change your occupation? _____

   _____

   _____

13. Have you been able to return to school since your BMT?

    No_____   Yes (part-time) _____   Not applicable_____

    Yes (full-time) _____

14. If you have not been able to return to school, why not? _____

    _____

    _____

15. Are you using any home treatments or remedies?

    No_____   Yes_____

    If yes, please identify what you are using._____

    _____

    _____

16. Please identify any activities that you participate in such as exercise, sports, or other recreational activities._____

    _____

    _____

17. Do you currently have health insurance?

    No_____   Yes_____

18. Have you experienced any difficulty with acquiring or maintaining health insurance?

    No_____   Yes_____

    If yes, please explain._____

    _____

    _____

19. Have you experienced any problems with your employer related to your disease or treatment?

    No_____   Yes_____

    If yes, please explain._____

    _____

    _____

20. Do you belong to a support group?

    No_____   Yes_____

    If yes, to which group do you belong?_____

    _____

    _____

Directions: We are interested in knowing how your experience of having cancer and having a BMT affects your Quality of Life. Please answer all of the following questions based on *your life at this time*.

Please *circle* the number from 0–10 that best describes your experiences.
NA = not applicable to me/doesn't apply to me

Physical Well-Being

To what extent are the following a problem for you:

21. Skin changes
no problem   0   1   2   3   4   5   6   7   8   9   10   a severe problem   NA

22. Bleeding problems
no problem   0   1   2   3   4   5   6   7   8   9   10   a severe problem   NA

23. Mouth dryness
no problem   0   1   2   3   4   5   6   7   8   9   10   a severe problem   NA

24. Changes in vision
no problem   0   1   2   3   4   5   6   7   8   9   10   a severe problem   NA

25. Hearing loss
no problem   0   1   2   3   4   5   6   7   8   9   10   a severe problem   NA

26. Fatigue
no problem   0   1   2   3   4   5   6   7   8   9   10   a severe problem   NA

27. Ringing in your ears
no problem   0   1   2   3   4   5   6   7   8   9   10   a severe problem   NA

28. Appetite changes
no problem   0   1   2   3   4   5   6   7   8   9   10   a severe problem   NA

29. Physical strength
no problem   0   1   2   3   4   5   6   7   8   9   10   a severe problem   NA

30. Sleep changes
no problem   0   1   2   3   4   5   6   7   8   9   10   a severe problem   NA

31. Sexual activity
no problem   0   1   2   3   4   5   6   7   8   9   10   a severe problem   NA

32. Pain or aches
no problem   0   1   2   3   4   5   6   7   8   9   10   a severe problem   NA

33. Loss of feeling, tingling, or pain in your hands or feet
no problem   0   1   2   3   4   5   6   7   8   9   10   a severe problem   NA

34. Shortness of breath or difficulty breathing

no problem   0   1   2   3   4   5   6   7   8   9   10   a severe problem   NA

35. Constipation

no problem   0   1   2   3   4   5   6   7   8   9   10   a severe problem   NA

36. Nausea

no problem   0   1   2   3   4   5   6   7   8   9   10   a severe problem   NA

37. Fertility changes

no problem   0   1   2   3   4   5   6   7   8   9   10   a severe problem   NA

38. Rate your overall physical health

extremely poor   0   1   2   3   4   5   6   7   8   9   10   excellent   NA

Psychological Well-Being

39. Do you have any distress from visual changes?

not at all   0   1   2   3   4   5   6   7   8   9   10   a great deal   NA

40. Has it been difficult for you to adjust to your illness?

very difficult   0   1   2   3   4   5   6   7   8   9   10   not at all   NA

41. How good is your overall quality of life?

extremely poor   0   1   2   3   4   5   6   7   8   9   10   excellent   NA

42. How much enjoyment are you getting out of life?

none at all   0   1   2   3   4   5   6   7   8   9   10   a great deal   NA

43. How is your present ability to concentrate or to remember things?

extremely poor   0   1   2   3   4   5   6   7   8   9   10   excellent   NA

44. How useful do you feel?

not at all   0   1   2   3   4   5   6   7   8   9   10   extremely   NA

45. How much happiness do you feel?

none at all   0   1   2   3   4   5   6   7   8   9   10   complete   NA

46. Do you feel like you are in control of things in your life?

none at all   0   1   2   3   4   5   6   7   8   9   10   completely   NA

47. Do you enjoy the things in life now that you used to take for granted?

not at all   0   1   2   3   4   5   6   7   8   9   10   a great deal   NA

48. How satisfying is your life?

not at all   0   1   2   3   4   5   6   7   8   9   10   extremely   NA

49. How much have you been able to focus on being well again?

not at all   0   1   2   3   4   5   6   7   8   9   10   a great deal   NA

50. Has your illness or treatment caused unwanted changes in your appearance?

not at all   0   1   2   3   4   5   6   7   8   9   10   a great deal   NA

51. Are you fearful of recurrence of your cancer?

not at all   0   1   2   3   4   5   6   7   8   9   10   extremely   NA

52. How difficult is it for you to cope as a result of your disease and treatment?

not at all   0   1   2   3   4   5   6   7   8   9   10   extremely   NA

53. Has your illness or treatment decreased your self-concept (the way you see yourself)?

not at all   0   1   2   3   4   5   6   7   8   9   10   extremely   NA

54. How distressing was the initial diagnosis of your cancer?

not at all   0   1   2   3   4   5   6   7   8   9   10   extremely   NA

55. How distressing were your cancer treatments (i.e., chemotherapy, radiation, BMT, or surgery)?

not at all   0   1   2   3   4   5   6   7   8   9   10   extremely   NA

56. How distressing has the time been since your treatment ended?

not at all   0   1   2   3   4   5   6   7   8   9   10   extremely   NA

57. How much anxiety do you have?

none at all   0   1   2   3   4   5   6   7   8   9   10   severe   NA

58. How much depression do you have?

none at all   0   1   2   3   4   5   6   7   8   9   10   severe   NA

59. Are you fearful of a second cancer?

not at all   0   1   2   3   4   5   6   7   8   9   10   extremely   NA

60. Are you fearful of the spreading (metastasis) of your cancer?

not at all   0   1   2   3   4   5   6   7   8   9   10   extremely   NA

61. Rate your overall psychological well-being.

extremely poor   0   1   2   3   4   5   6   7   8   9   10   excellent   NA

Social Concerns

62. How much financial burden resulted from your illness or treatment?

none   0   1   2   3   4   5   6   7   8   9   10   extreme   NA

63. How distressing has your illness been for your family?

not at all   0   1   2   3   4   5   6   7   8   9   10   extremely   NA

64. Has your illness or treatment interfered with your personal relationships?

not at all   0   1   2   3   4   5   6   7   8   9   10   completely   NA

65. Is the amount of affection you receive sufficient to meet your needs?

not at all   0   1   2   3   4   5   6   7   8   9   10   completely   NA

66. Is the amount of affection you give sufficient to meet your needs?

not at all   0   1   2   3   4   5   6   7   8   9   10   completely   NA

67. Has your illness or treatment interfered with your sexuality?

not at all   0   1   2   3   4   5   6   7   8   9   10   completely   NA

68. Has your illness or treatment interfered with your plans to have children?

not at all   0   1   2   3   4   5   6   7   8   9   10   a great deal   NA

69. Has your illness or treatment interfered with your employment?

not at all   0   1   2   3   4   5   6   7   8   9   10   completely   NA

70. Has your illness or treatment interfered with your family goals?

not at all   0   1   2   3   4   5   6   7   8   9   10   completely   NA

71. Is the amount of support you receive from others sufficient to meet your needs?

not at all   0   1   2   3   4   5   6   7   8   9   10   completely   NA

72. Has your illness or treatment interfered with your activities at home?

not at all   0   1   2   3   4   5   6   7   8   9   10   completely   NA

73. How much isolation is caused by your illness or treatment?

none   0   1   2   3   4   5   6   7   8   9   10   complete   NA

74. Rate your overall social well-being.

extremely poor   0   1   2   3   4   5   6   7   8   9   10   excellent   NA

Spiritual Well-Being

75. How much uncertainty do you feel about your future?

none at all   0   1   2   3   4   5   6   7   8   9   10   extreme   NA

76. Do you sense a purpose/mission for your life or a reason for being alive?

not at all   0   1   2   3   4   5   6   7   8   9   10   a great deal   NA

77. Do you have a sense of inner peace?

not at all   0   1   2   3   4   5   6   7   8   9   10   completely   NA

78. How hopeful do you feel?

not at all   0   1   2   3   4   5   6   7   8   9   10   extremely   NA

79. Is the amount of support you receive from personal spiritual activities such as prayer or meditation sufficient to meet your needs?

not at all   0   1   2   3   4   5   6   7   8   9   10   completely   NA

80. Is the amount of support you receive from religious activities such as going to church or synagogue sufficient to meet your needs?

not at all   0   1   2   3   4   5   6   7   8   9   10   completely   NA

81. Has your illness made positive changes in your life?

none at all   0   1   2   3   4   5   6   7   8   9   10   extreme   NA

82. Rate your overall spiritual well-being.

extremely poor   0   1   2   3   4   5   6   7   8   9   10   excellent   NA

83. Would you recommend a bone marrow transplant to a family member or close friend with the same illness?

not at all   0   1   2   3   4   5   6   7   8   9   10   definitely yes   NA

84. Has filling out this tool been useful to you?

not at all   0   1   2   3   4   5   6   7   8   9   10   extremely   NA

REFERENCES

Grant, M., Ferrell, B., Schmidt, G. M., Fonbuena, P., Niland, J. C., & Forman, S. J. (1992). Measurement of quality of life in bone marrow transplantation survivors. *Quality of Life Research, 1*(6), 375–384.

Ferrell, B., Grant, M., Schmidt, G. M., Rhiner, M., Whitehead, C., Fonbuena, P., & Forman, S. J. (1992). The meaning of quality of life for bone marrow transplant survivors. Part 1: The impact of bone marrow transplant on quality of life. *Cancer Nursing, 15*(3), 153–160.

Ferrell, B., Grant, M., Schmidt, G. M., Rhiner, M., Whitehead, C., Fonbuena, P., & Forman, S. J. (1992). The meaning of quality of life for bone marrow transplant survivors. Part 2: Improving quality of life for bone marrow transplant survivors. *Cancer Nursing, 15*(4), 247–253.

Schmidt, G. M., Niland, J. C., Forman, S. J., Fonbuena, P., Dagis, A. C., Ferrell, B. R., Grant, M. M., Barr, T. A., Stallbaum, B. A., Chao, N. J., & Blume, K. G. Extended follow up in 201 long-term allogeneic bone marrow transplant survivors: Addressing issues of quality of life. *Transplantation,* March 1993.

Grant, M., Ferrell, B., Schmidt, G., Fonbuena, P., Niland, J., & Forman, S. Researching quality of life indicators: Their impact on the daily life of bone marrow transplant patients. In C. D. Bailey (Ed.), *Proceedings of the Seventh International Conference on Cancer Nursing* (Cancer Nursing Changing Frontiers, Vienna, August 16–21, 1992) (pp. 80–84). Oxford, UK: Rapid Communications.

IV. EXAMPLE OF CANCER-SPECIFIC MEASURE OF QUALITY OF LIFE (BATTERY APPROACH)

Quality of Life Components for Pediatric Oncology Group (POG) Protocols

ANDREW BRADLYN

Contact person: Andrew Bradlyn, PhD, Department of Behavioral Medicine and Psychiatry, Robert C. Byrd Health Sciences Center, West Virginia University, 930 Chestnut Ridge Road, Morgantown, WV 26505. Used with permission from Andrew Bradlyn, PhD.

Rand Health Status Measure (Modified) for Children Ages 0–4 Years (Day 7, Post Surgery: 1-Week Report)

Instructions

1. Read each question carefully.
2. *Circle the number* of the *one answer* that most closely fits this child.

Example:

    1. Has this child ever had a cold?
        Yes   1
        No   2

Follow any instructions next to the number you circled, which tell you to go to another question or another page.

Example:

    2. Does this child wear glasses?
        Yes   1 - Answer 2-a
        No   2 - Go to 3

  2-a. How long has this child been wearing glasses?
        Less than 1 year   1
        About 1 year   2
        About 2 years   3
        More than 2 years   4

If there are no instructions after your answer, go to the very next question.

What time is it now? _____   What is the date today? _____

During the past week (not including today):

    1. Was this child in bed for all or most of the day because of health?
        Yes   1 - Answer 1-a
        No   2 - Go to 2

  1-a. How long has this child been in bed for all or most of the day because of health?
        1 to 2 days   1
        3 to 4 days   2
        5 to 7 days   3

    2. Has this child been in a hospital or other medical facility because of health?
        Yes   1 - Answer 2-a
        No   2 - Go to 3

2-a. How long has this child been in a hospital or other medical facility because of health?

1 to 2 days	1
3 to 4 days	2
5 to 7 days	3

FL/MOB _____

3. Was this child unable to walk unless assisted by an adult or by crutches, artificial limb, or braces?

Yes, unable to walk unless assisted	1 - Answer 3-a
No, no trouble walking	2 - Go to 4
Not walking yet because of age	3 - Go to 4

3-a. How long has this child been unable to walk without assistance?

1 to 2 days	1
3 to 4 days	2
5 to 7 days	3

FL/PA_____

During the past week *(not including today)*:

4. Does this child's health limit the *kind* or *amount* of ordinary play he or she can do?

Yes	1 - Answer 4-a
No	2 - Go to 5

4-a. How long has the child's health limited the kind or amount of play he or she could do?

1 to 2 day	1
3 to 4 days	2
5 to 7 days	3

5. Does this child's health keep him from taking part in ordinary play?

Yes	1 - Answer 5-a
No	2 - Go to 6

5-a. How long has this child's health kept him or her from taking part in ordinary play?

1 to 2 days	1
3 to 4 days	2
5 to 7 days	3

FL/RA _____

6. Because of health, did this child need more help than normal for children of the same age in eating, dressing, bathing, or using the toilet?

Yes	1 - Answer 6-a
No	2 - Go to 7

6-a. How long has this child needed extra help with eating, dressing, bathing, or using the toilet?

1 to 2 days	1
3 to 4 days	2
5 to 7 days	3

FL/SC _____

During the past week (not including today):

7. Considering this child's progress in sitting up, walking, and talking, how do you feel about the way he or she is growing up or developing?

Very satisfied	1
Somewhat satisfied	2
Neither satisfied nor worried	3
Somewhat worried	4
Very worried	5

8. How do you feel about this child's eating habits?

Very satisfied	1
Somewhat satisfied	2
Neither satisfied nor worried	3
Somewhat worried	4
Very worried	5

9. How do you feel about this child's sleeping habits?

Very satisfied	1
Somewhat satisfied	2
Neither satisfied nor worried	3
Somewhat worried	4
Very worried	5

10. How do you feel about this child's bowel habits?

Very satisfied	1
Somewhat satisfied	2
Neither satisfied nor worried	3
Somewhat worried	4
Very worried	5

SAT DEV _____

11. Please read each of the following statements, and then *circle one of the numbers on each line* to indicate whether the statement is true or false for this child. There are no right or wrong answers. Some of the statements may look or seem like others, but each statement is different and should be rated by itself.

If a statement is *definitely true* for this child, circle 1.
If a statement is *mostly true* for this child, circle 2.
If you *don't know* whether it is true or false, circle 3.
If it is *mostly false* for this child, circle 4.
If it is *definitely false* for this child, circle 5.

	Definitely true	Mostly true	Don't know	Mostly false	Definitely false
A. This child's health is excellent.	1	2	3	4	5
B. This child was so sick once, I thought he or she might die.	1	2	3	4	5
C. This child seems to resist illness very well.	1	2	3	4	5
D. This child seems to be less healthy than other children I know.	1	2	3	4	5
E. This child has never been seriously ill.	1	2	3	4	5
F. When there is something going around, this child usually catches it.	1	2	3	4	5

What time is it now? _____

TOTAL HP _____   TOTAL RAND_____

Parent Satisfaction with Questionnaire

1. How much of a burden was this questionnaire for you?

1	2	3	4	5

Required
minimal effort

Required
extreme effort

2. How difficult were the questions to understand?

1	2	3	4	5

Extremely
easy

Extremely
difficult

3. How well did this questionnaire describe how your child has been doing over the past week?

1	2	3	4	5

Not well
at all

Somewhat
well

Extremely
well

Thank you for your assistance!

Parent Form

Overall health rating

1	2	3	4	5	6
Very poor	Poor	Somewhat poor	Somewhat good	Good	Very good

Using this scale (1–6), how would you rate your child's overall health during the past two weeks?

Quality of Life Rating

1	2	3	4	5	6
Very poor	Poor	Somewhat poor	Somewhat good	Good	Very good

Using this scale (1–6), how would you rate your child's quality of life during the past two weeks? By "quality of life," we mean how your child is doing overall (their physical, psychological, and social well-being).

Play-Performance Scale for Children (Parent Form)

Child's name: _____

Your name: _____

    Relationship: Mother ❏   Father ❏   Other ❏

Today's date: _____

Directions: On this form are a series of descriptions. Each description has a number beside it. Think about your child's play and activity over the past *two weeks*. Think about both good and bad days. Average out this period. Now read the descriptions and pick the one that best describes your child's play during the past *two weeks*. *Circle the number beside that one description.*

100	Fully active, normal.
90	Minor restrictions in physically strenuous activity.
80	Active, but tires more quickly.
70	Both greater restriction of, and less time spent in, active play.
60	Up and around, but minimal active play; keeps busy with quieter activities.
50	Gets dressed, but lies around much of the day; no active play; able to participate in all quiet play and activities.
40	Mostly in bed; participates in quiet activities.
30	In bed; needs assistance even for quiet play.
20	Often sleeping; play entirely limited to very passive activities.
10	No play; does not get out of bed.
0	Unresponsive.

V. EXAMPLE OF CANCER–SPECIFIC MEASURE OF QUALITY OF LIFE (MODULAR APPROACH)

The Bush Bone Marrow Transplant Symptom Inventory

NIGEL BUSH

Late Complications of BMT Module

Origin: The BMT module is an original instrument compiled following exhaustive reviews of BMT literature and from inservice discussions with staff at the Fred Hutchinson Cancer Research Center in Seattle, WA (USA). However, the BMT module is not strictly a stand-alone QOL instrument. Rather we developed it as a BMT-specific addendum or module to the European Organization for Research and Treatment of Cancer (EORTC) QLQ-C30 quality of life questionnaire (4), and as part of a battery of seven instruments encompassing four domains of QOL in BMT (physical, psychological, and social functioning, and disease/treatment symptoms).

Purpose: To complement the QLQ-C30 as a disease-specific addendum module for assessing primarily, but not exclusively, the symptomatology of long-term recovery from BMT over time in large samples of adult bone marrow and stem cell transplantation patients.

Population: Adult patients undergoing and recovering from bone marrow or stem cell transplantation. All types of transplant and treatment regimens are represented. The diseases represented in the sample may include all types of acute and chronic leukemia, preleukemia, multiple myeloma, nonHodgkins lymphoma, Hodgkins disease, aplastic anemia, and solid tumor patients receiving BMTs or stem cell transplantations.

Administration:

Rater: Has been administered and collected by mail or in person by general administrative staff or health care professionals. Questionnaire is self-assessed by patient. Scoring and assessment require relatively competent data entry and analysis person.

Time Required: Approximately 5–10 minutes. Time for self-assessed completion of entire battery of which it is a part has averaged 90 minutes.

Training: Is an integral part of a larger battery with detailed instructions. Questions are self-explanatory. Little or no guidance on the part of the patient is required.

Scoring: Follows the scoring convention of the QLQ-C30. Most of the fifty items, scaled identically to the EORTC QLQ-C30 with four-point Likert scales linearly transformed to 0–100 scales, are rated for occurrence/severity of symptoms.

Description: The module includes items which primarily index the disease/treatment symptoms domain of health-related quality of life (QOL), although the remaining three domains commonly defined (physical, psychological, and social functioning) are also represented. Multiple items are categorized by: skin, eyes, mouth/throat, joints/muscles involvement, pulmonary problems, sex/warmth/intimacy, cognitive dysfunction, infections, and fear of relapse/dying. When calculating composite scores, items from two categories, pulmonary problems and cognitive dysfunction, are combined with items from the EORTC

QLQ-C30 to form more complete BMT-specific subscales. Items already included in the EORTC QLQ-C30 are omitted from the module. Single items index physical appearance, hair and nail loss, teeth problems, abnormal sense of taste, heartburn and abdominal pain, sinusitis and runny nose, chronic GVHD, and minor symptoms/ailments.

Coverage: We have employed this instrument as a component of a much larger research assessment battery. However, we intend that a future, more refined battery will be employed by clinicians as a more comprehensive clinical outcome assessment tool.

Reliability: We recently tested the module as part of a large QOL assessment packet on 125 subjects surviving 6–18 years after BMT, and calculated alpha coefficients for the various categories. The overall Cronbach's alpha for the BMT module was 0.87 with category alphas ranging from 0.71–0.89 with four exceptions (skin = 0.55, mouth/throat = 0.69, infections = 0.32, fear of relapse/dying = 0.66). Current, ongoing use in a four-year longitudinal study of patients from pretreatment to five-year post-BMT appears, from very cursory examination, to be yielding similar figures.

Validity: Generally face-valid. Content validity for the fifty items has been derived from inservice discussions with staff at the Fred Hutchinson Cancer Research Center in Seattle, WA, and from the BMT literature.

Responsiveness: Too early to tell. Longitudinal assessment ongoing.

Strengths: Extremely comprehensive in assessing the symptomatology of long-term recovery from BMT. Easy to administer and simple enough for self-assessment. We believe the instrument complements well the QLQ-C30 as a disease/treatment specific module.

Weaknesses/Caution: The BMT module is still under development. In its present form, the BMT module does not contain rigorously psychometric scales. It includes aforementioned categories of items (e.g., eyes, skin, etc.) grouped by site or topic for convenience. We have calculated simple descriptive data such as incidences and frequencies from this instrument. At its present stage of development, we regard the module as a comprehensive *descriptive* inventory of late complications of BMT. We are currently testing it in longitudinal studies of BMT patients with yearly repeated measures at one to five years and will be using data from our QOL battery to develop new statistical methods for QOL outcome assessment. These include novel techniques (mixed effects models) for dealing with unconditional estimates of QOL trends that are not subject to attritional biases over time (missing data). We hope to develop new endpoints for BMT which will superficially resemble Q-TWIST. On completion of that study we hope to be able to shorten and refine the questionnaire.

EORTC Core Quality of Life Questionnaire (QLQ-C30) by Mail

We are interested in some things about you and your health. *Please answer all the questions yourself by circling the number that best applies to you.* There are no right or wrong answers. The information that you provide will remain strictly confidential.

Today's date (day, month, year) _____ /_____ /_____

	No	Yes
1. Do you have any trouble doing strenuous activities, like carrying a heavy shopping bag or a suitcase?	1	2
2. Do you have any trouble taking a *long* walk?	1	2
3. Do you have any trouble taking a *short* walk outside of the house?	1	2
4. Do you have to stay in a bed or a chair for most of the day?	1	2
5. Do you need help with eating, dressing, washing yourself, or using the toilet?	1	2
6. Are you limited in any way in doing either your work or doing household jobs?	1	2
7. Are you completely unable to work at a job or do household jobs?	1	2

During the past *two weeks*:

	Not at all	A little bit	Quite a bit	Very much
8. Were you short of breath?	1	2	3	4
9. Have you had pain?	1	2	3	4
10. Did you need to rest?	1	2	3	4
11. Have you had trouble sleeping?	1	2	3	4
12. Have you felt weak?	1	2	3	4
13. Have you lacked appetite?	1	2	3	4
14. Have you felt nauseated?	1	2	3	4
15. Have you vomited?	1	2	3	4
16. Have you been constipated?	1	2	3	4
17. Have you had diarrhea?	1	2	3	4
18. Were you tired?	1	2	3	4
19. Did pain interfere with your daily activities?	1	2	3	4

	Not at all	A little bit	Quite a bit	Very much
20. Have you had difficulty in concentrating on things, like reading a newspaper or watching television?	1	2	3	4
21. Did you feel tense?	1	2	3	4
22. Did you worry?	1	2	3	4
23. Did you feel irritable?	1	2	3	4
24. Did you feel depressed?	1	2	3	4
25. Have you had difficulty remembering things?	1	2	3	4
26. Has your physical condition or medical treatment interfered with your *family* life?	1	2	3	4
27. Has your physical condition or medical treatment interfered with your *social* life?	1	2	3	4
28. Has your physical condition or medical treatment caused you financial difficulties?	1	2	3	4

For the following questions please circle the number between 1 and 7 that best applies to you.

29. How would you rate your overall physical condition during the past *two weeks*?

1	2	3	4	5	6	7
Very poor						Excellent

30. How would you rate your overall quality of life during the past *two weeks*?

1	2	3	4	5	6	7
Very poor						Excellent

Former bone marrow or stem cell transplant patients sometimes report that they have the following symptoms. Please indicate the extent to which you have experienced these symptoms during the past *two weeks*.

	Not at all	A little bit	Quite a bit	Very much
31. Skin problems (overall)?	1	2	3	4
a. Rashes	1	2	3	4
b. Dryness	1	2	3	4
c. Sweating	1	2	3	4
d. Painful skin	1	2	3	4
e. Skin ulcers	1	2	3	4
32. Hair loss	1	2	3	4

	Not at all	A little bit	Quite a bit	Very much
33. Nail loss	1	2	3	4
34. Eye problems (overall)?	1	2	3	4
a. Dryness	1	2	3	4
b. Grittiness	1	2	3	4
c. Burning	1	2	3	4
d. Blurring	1	2	3	4
e. Sensitivity to light	1	2	3	4
f. Cataracts	1	2	3	4
35. Mouth/throat problems (overall)?	1	2	3	4
a. Dryness	1	2	3	4
b. Soreness	1	2	3	4
c. Burning	1	2	3	4
36. Teeth problems (dental caries, etc.)	1	2	3	4
37. Abnormal sense of taste for food or drink	1	2	3	4

During the past *two weeks*, to what extent have you experienced:

	Not at all	A little bit	Quite a bit	Very much
38. Heartburn	1	2	3	4
39. Abdominal pain	1	2	3	4
40. Weight loss	1	2	3	4
41. Sinusitis	1	2	3	4
42. Runny nose	1	2	3	4
43. Breathing problems (overall)?	1	2	3	4
a. Coughing	1	2	3	4
b. Wheezing	1	2	3	4
c. Bronchitis	1	2	3	4
d. Asthma	1	2	3	4
44. Painful joints (overall)?	1	2	3	4
a. Hip joints	1	2	3	4
b. Other joints	1	2	3	4
45. Painful muscles	1	2	3	4
46. Infections (overall)?	1	2	3	4
a. Varicella zoster (VZV)	1	2	3	4
b. Herpes simplex	1	2	3	4
c. Cytomegalovirus (CMV)	1	2	3	4
d. Pneumonia	1	2	3	4
e. Measles	1	2	3	4

	Not at all	A little bit	Quite a bit	Very much
f. Chickenpox	1	2	3	4
g. Shingles	1	2	3	4
47. Chronic graft-versus-host disease (GVHD)	1	2	3	4
48. Minor symptoms or ailments? (common cold, flu, migraine, etc.) Please describe	1	2	3	4

_____

_____

	Not at all	A little bit	Quite a bit	Very much
49. Compared with your appearance before your transplant, how satisfied are you now with your appearance?	1	2	3	4
50. Have you been satisfied with your own sexual appeal?	1	2	3	4
51. Have you been satisfied with your ability to share warmth and intimacy?	1	2	3	4
52. Have you been interested in sexual thoughts or feelings?	1	2	3	4

53. Do you have any physical problems that reduce your satisfaction with sex and intimacy?   Yes   No
Please describe (remember that your answers will be treated with the strictest confidence).

_____

_____

	Not at all	A little bit	Quite a bit	Very much
54. Have you been worried by fear of infection?	1	2	3	4
55. Have you been worried by thoughts about relapse or dying?	1	2	3	4
56. Have you had difficulty in maintaining your attention and train of thought?	1	2	3	4
57. Have you had difficulty in reasoning and thinking clearly?	1	2	3	4

58. Are there any other things that have affected the quality of your life over the past _two weeks?_

_____

_____

_____

59. Has the quality of your life over the past two weeks been typical of the past five or six months, or has it been unusual? If the past two weeks have been unusual, please describe how, in more detail.

_____

_____

_____

Please check to make sure that you have answered all of the questions.
Please use the space below for any additional comments you might have:

_____

_____

_____

REFERENCES

Aaronson, N. K., Ahmedzai, S., Bergman, B., Bullinger, M., Cull, A., Duez, N. J., Filiberti, A., Fletchtner, H., Fleishman, S. B., & de Haes, J. C. (1993). The European organization for research and treatment of cancer QLQ-C30: A quality of life instrument for use in international clinical trials in oncology. *Journal of National Cancer Institute, 85*, 356–376.

Bush, N. E., Haberman, M., Donaldson, G., & Sullivan, K. M. (1995). Quality of life of 125 adults surviving 6–18 years after bone marrow transplantation. *Social Science and Medicine, 40*, 479–490.

Haberman, M., Bush, N. E., Young, K., & Sullivan, K. M. (1993). Quality of life of adult long-term survivors of bone marrow transplantation: A qualitative analysis of narrative data. *Oncology Nursing Forum, 20*, 1545–1553.

VI. SAMPLE TOOLS FOR MEASURING QUALITY OF LIFE IN CHILDREN WITH CANCER

PedsQL™
Pediatric Quality of Life
Inventory for Young Children
(ages 5–7)

Contact person: James W. Varni, PhD, Professor and Senior Scientist, Center for Child Health Outcomes, Children's Hospital and Health Center, 3020 Children's Way, MC 5053, San Diego, CA, 92123, telephone: 858-966-4907. jvarni@chsd.org

PedsQL™
Pediatric Quality of Life Inventory

Version 4.0

PARENT REPORT for YOUNG CHILDREN (ages 5–7)

DIRECTIONS

On the following page is a list of things that might be a problem for **your child**. Please tell us **how much of a problem** each one has been for **your child** during the **past ONE month** by circling:

> 0 if it is **never** a problem
>
> 1 if it is **almost never** a problem
>
> 2 if it is **sometimes** a problem
>
> 3 if it is **often** a problem
>
> 4 if it is **almost always** a problem

There are no right or wrong answers.

If you do not understand a question, please ask for help.

In the past **ONE month**, how much of a **problem** has your child had with . . .

PHYSICAL FUNCTIONING (problems with . . .)	Never	Almost Never	Some-times	Often	Almost Always
1. Walking more than one block	0	1	2	3	4
2. Running	0	1	2	3	4
3. Participating in sports activity or exercise	0	1	2	3	4
4. Lifting something heavy	0	1	2	3	4
5. Taking a bath or shower by him or herself	0	1	2	3	4
6. Doing chores, like picking up his or her toys	0	1	2	3	4
7. Having hurts or aches	0	1	2	3	4
8. Low energy level	0	1	2	3	4

EMOTIONAL FUNCTIONING (problems with . . .)	Never	Almost Never	Some-times	Often	Almost Always
1. Feeling afraid or scared	0	1	2	3	4
2. Feeling sad or blue	0	1	2	3	4
3. Feeling angry	0	1	2	3	4
4. Trouble sleeping	0	1	2	3	4
5. Worrying about what will happen to him or her	0	1	2	3	4

SOCIAL FUNCTIONING (problems with . . .)	Never	Almost Never	Some-times	Often	Almost Always
1. Getting along with other children	0	1	2	3	4
2. Other kids not wanting to be his or her friend	0	1	2	3	4
3. Getting teased by other children	0	1	2	3	4
4. Not able to do things that other children his or her age can do	0	1	2	3	4
5. Keeping up when playing with other children	0	1	2	3	4

SCHOOL FUNCTIONING (problems with . . .)	Never	Almost Never	Some-times	Often	Almost Always
1. Paying attention in class	0	1	2	3	4
2. Forgetting things	0	1	2	3	4
3. Keeping up with school activities	0	1	2	3	4
4. Missing school because of not feeling well	0	1	2	3	4
5. Missing school to go to the doctor or hospital	0	1	2	3	4

PedsQL™
Pediatric Quality of Life Inventory

Version 4.0

YOUNG CHILD REPORT (ages 5–7)

Instructions for interviewer:

I am going to ask you some questions about things that might be a problem for some children. I want to know how much of a problem any of these things might be for you.

Show the child the template and point to the responses as you read.

If it is <u>not at all</u> a problem for you, point to the smiling face

If it is <u>sometimes</u> a problem for you, point to the middle face

If it is a problem for you <u>a lot</u>, point to the frowning face

I will read each question. Point to the pictures to show me how much of a problem it is for you. Let's try a practice one first.

	Not at all	Sometimes	A lot
Is it hard for you to snap your fingers?	😊	😐	🙁

Ask the child to demonstrate snapping his or her fingers to determine whether or not the question was answered correctly. Repeat the question if the child demonstrates a response that is different from his or her action.

Think about how you have been doing for the last few weeks. Please listen carefully to each sentence and tell me how much of a problem this is for you.

After reading the item, gesture to the template. If the child hesitates or does not seem to understand how to answer, read the response options while pointing at the faces.

PHYSICAL FUNCTIONING (problems with . . .)	Not at all	Sometimes	A lot
1. Is it hard for you to walk?	0	2	4
2. Is it hard for you to run?	0	2	4
3. Is it hard for you to play sports or exercise?	0	2	4
4. Is it hard for you to pick up big things?	0	2	4
5. Is it hard for you to take a bath or shower?	0	2	4
6. Is it hard for you to do chores (like pick up your toys)?	0	2	4
7. Do you have hurts or aches? (*Where?* _____)	0	2	4
8. Do you ever feel too tired to play?	0	2	4

Remember, tell me how much of a problem this has been for you for the last few weeks.

EMOTIONAL FUNCTIONING (problems with . . .)	Not at all	Sometimes	A lot
1. Do you feel scared?	0	2	4
2. Do you feel sad?	0	2	4
3. Do you feel mad?	0	2	4
4. Do you have trouble sleeping?	0	2	4
5. Do you worry about what will happen to you?	0	2	4

SOCIAL FUNCTIONING (problems with . . .)	Not at all	Sometimes	A lot
1. Is it hard for you to get along with other kids?	0	2	4
2. Do other kids say they do not want to play with you?	0	2	4
3. Do other kids tease you?	0	2	4
4. Can other kids do things that you cannot do?	0	2	4
5. Is it hard for you to keep up when you play with other kids?	0	2	4

SCHOOL FUNCTIONING (problems with . . .)	Not at all	Sometimes	A lot
1. Is it hard for you to pay attention in school?	0	2	4
2. Do you forget things?	0	2	4
3. Is it hard to keep up with schoolwork?	0	2	4
4. Do you miss school because of not feeling good?	0	2	4
5. Do you miss school because you have to go to the doctor's or hospital?	0	2	4

How much of a problem is this for you?

Not at all **Sometimes** **A lot**

PedsQL™
Cancer Module

Version 3.0

PARENT REPORT for YOUNG CHILDREN (ages 5–7)

DIRECTIONS

Children with cancer sometimes have special problems. On the following page is a list of things that might be a problem for **your child**. Please tell us how **much of a problem** each one has been for **your child** during the **past ONE month** by circling:

> 0 if it is **never** a problem
>
> 1 if it is **almost never** a problem
>
> 2 if it is **sometimes** a problem
>
> 3 if it is **often** a problem
>
> 4 if it is **almost always** a problem

There are no right or wrong answers.

If you do not understand a question, please ask for help.

In the past **ONE month**, how much of a **problem** has your child had with . . .

PAIN AND HURT (problems with . . .)	Never	Almost Never	Some-times	Often	Almost Always
1. Aches in joints and/or muscles	0	1	2	3	4
2. Having a lot of pain	0	1	2	3	4

NAUSEA (problems with . . .)	Never	Almost Never	Some-times	Often	Almost Always
1. Becoming nauseated during medical treatments	0	1	2	3	4
2. Food not tasting very good to him or her	0	1	2	3	4
3. Becoming nauseated while thinking about medical treatments	0	1	2	3	4
4. Not feeling hungry	0	1	2	3	4
5. Some foods and smells making him or her nauseous	0	1	2	3	4

PROCEDURAL ANXIETY (problems with . . .)	Never	Almost Never	Some-times	Often	Almost Always
1. Needle sticks (i.e., injections, blood tests, IVs) causing him or her pain	0	1	2	3	4
2. Getting anxious about having blood drawn	0	1	2	3	4
3. Getting anxious about having needle sticks (i.e., injections, blood tests, IVs)	0	1	2	3	4

TREATMENT ANXIETY (problems with . . .)	Never	Almost Never	Some-times	Often	Almost Always
1. Getting anxious when waiting to see the doctor	0	1	2	3	4
2. Getting anxious about going to the doctor	0	1	2	3	4
3. Getting anxious about going to the hospital	0	1	2	3	4

WORRY (problems with . . .)	Never	Almost Never	Some-times	Often	Almost Always
1. Worrying about side effects from medical treatments	0	1	2	3	4
2. Worrying about whether or not his or her medical treatments are working	0	1	2	3	4
3. Worrying that the cancer will reoccur or relapse	0	1	2	3	4

In the past **ONE month**, how much of a **problem** has your child had with . . .

COGNITIVE PROBLEMS (problems with . . .)	Never	Almost Never	Some-times	Often	Almost Always
1. Figuring out what to do when something bothers him or her	0	1	2	3	4
2. Solving math problems	0	1	2	3	4
3. Writing school papers	0	1	2	3	4
4. Difficulty paying attention to things	0	1	2	3	4
5. Remembering what is read to him or her	0	1	2	3	4

PERCEIVED PHYSICAL APPEARANCE (problems with . . .)	Never	Almost Never	Some-times	Often	Almost Always
1. Feeling that he/she is not good looking	0	1	2	3	4
2. Not liking other people to see his or her scars	0	1	2	3	4
3. Being embarrassed about others seeing his or her body	0	1	2	3	4

COMMUNICATION (problems with . . .)	Never	Almost Never	Some-times	Often	Almost Always
1. Telling the doctors and nurses how he or she feels	0	1	2	3	4
2. Asking the doctors or nurses questions	0	1	2	3	4
3. Explaining his or her illness to other people	0	1	2	3	4

PedsQL™
Cancer Module

Version 3.0

YOUNG CHILD REPORT (ages 5–7)

Instructions for interviewer:

I am going to ask you some questions about things that might be a problem for some children. I want to know how much of a problem any of these things might be for you.

Show the child the template and point to the responses as you read.

If it is <u>not at all</u> a problem for you, point to the smiling face

If it is <u>sometimes</u> a problem for you, point to the middle face

If it is a problem for you <u>a lot</u>, point to the frowning face

I will read each question. Point to the pictures to show me how much of a problem it is for you. Let's try a practice one first.

	Not at all	Sometimes	A lot
Is it hard for you to snap your fingers?	🙂	😐	🙁

Ask the child to demonstrate snapping his or her fingers to determine whether or not the question was answered correctly. Repeat the question if the child demonstrates a response that is different from his or her action.

Think about how you have been doing for the last few weeks. Please listen carefully to each sentence and tell me how much of a problem this is for you.

After reading the item, gesture to the template. If the child hesitates or does not seem to understand how to answer, read the response options while pointing at the faces.

PAIN AND HURT (problems with . . .)	Not at all	Sometimes	A lot
1. Do you ache or hurt in your joints and/or muscles?	0	2	4
2. Do you hurt a lot?	0	2	4

NAUSEA (problems with . . .)	Not at all	Sometimes	A lot
1. Do you get sick to your stomach when you have medical treatments?	0	2	4
2. Does food taste bad to you?	0	2	4
3. Do you get sick to your stomach when you think about medical treatments?	0	2	4
4. Do you not feel hungry?	0	2	4
5. Do some foods and smells make your stomach upset?	0	2	4

PROCEDURAL ANXIETY (problems with . . .)	Not at all	Sometimes	A lot
1. Do needle sticks (i.e., injections, blood tests, IVs) hurt you?	0	2	4
2. Do you get scared when you have to have blood tests?	0	2	4
3. Do you get scared about having needle sticks (i.e., injections, blood tests, IVs)?	0	2	4

TREATMENT ANXIETY (problems with . . .)	Not at all	Sometimes	A lot
1. Do you get scared when you are waiting to see the doctor?	0	2	4
2. Do you get scared when you have to go to the doctor?	0	2	4
3. Do you get scared when you have to go to the hospital?	0	2	4

WORRY (problems with . . .)	Not at all	Sometimes	A lot
1. Do you worry about side effects from medical treatments?	0	2	4
2. Do you worry about whether or not your medical treatments are working?	0	2	4
3. Do you worry that your cancer will come back?	0	2	4

Think about how you have been doing for the last few weeks. Please listen carefully to each sentence and tell me how much of a problem this is for you.

COGNITIVE PROBLEMS (problems with . . .)	Not at all	Sometimes	A lot
1. Is it hard for you to figure out what to do when something bothers you?	0	2	4
2. Do you have trouble solving math problems?	0	2	4
3. Do you have trouble writing school papers?	0	2	4
4. Is it hard for you to pay attention to things?	0	2	4
5. Is it hard for you to remember what is read to you?	0	2	4

PERCEIVED PHYSICAL APPEARANCE (problems with . . .)	Not at all	Sometimes	A lot
1. Do you feel you are not good looking?	0	2	4
2. Do you not like other people to see your scars?	0	2	4
3. Are you embarrassed when others see your body?	0	2	4

COMMUNICATION (problems with . . .)	Not at all	Sometimes	A lot
1. Is is hard for you to tell the doctors and nurses how you feel?	0	2	4
2. Is it hard for you to ask the doctors and nurses questions?	0	2	4
3. Is it hard for you to explain your illness to other people?	0	2	4

How much of a problem is this for you?

Not at all   **Sometimes**   **A lot**

PedsQL™
Pediatric Quality of Life
Inventory for Children
(ages 8–12)

PedsQL™
Pediatric Quality of Life Inventory

Version 4.0

PARENT REPORT for CHILDREN (ages 8–12)

DIRECTIONS

On the following page is a list of things that might be a problem for **your child**. Please tell us **how much of a problem** each one has been for **your child** during the **past ONE month** by circling:

> 0 if it is **never** a problem
>
> 1 if it is **almost never** a problem
>
> 2 if it is **sometimes** a problem
>
> 3 if it is **often** a problem
>
> 4 if it is **almost always** a problem

There are no right or wrong answers.

If you do not understand a question, please ask for help.

In the past **ONE month**, how much of a **problem** has your child had with . . .

PHYSICAL FUNCTIONING (problems with . . .)	Never	Almost Never	Some-times	Often	Almost Always
1. Walking more than one block	0	1	2	3	4
2. Running	0	1	2	3	4
3. Participating in sports activity or exercise	0	1	2	3	4
4. Lifting something heavy	0	1	2	3	4
5. Taking a bath or shower by him or herself	0	1	2	3	4
6. Doing chores around the house	0	1	2	3	4
7. Having hurts or aches	0	1	2	3	4
8. Low energy level	0	1	2	3	4

EMOTIONAL FUNCTIONING (problems with . . .)	Never	Almost Never	Some-times	Often	Almost Always
1. Feeling afraid or scared	0	1	2	3	4
2. Feeling sad or blue	0	1	2	3	4
3. Feeling angry	0	1	2	3	4
4. Trouble sleeping	0	1	2	3	4
5. Worrying about what will happen to him or her	0	1	2	3	4

SOCIAL FUNCTIONING (problems with . . .)	Never	Almost Never	Some-times	Often	Almost Always
1. Getting along with other children	0	1	2	3	4
2. Other kids not wanting to be his or her friend	0	1	2	3	4
3. Getting teased by other children	0	1	2	3	4
4. Not able to do things that other children his or her age can do	0	1	2	3	4
5. Keeping up when playing with other children	0	1	2	3	4

SCHOOL FUNCTIONING (problems with . . .)	Never	Almost Never	Some-times	Often	Almost Always
1. Paying attention in class	0	1	2	3	4
2. Forgetting things	0	1	2	3	4
3. Keeping up with schoolwork	0	1	2	3	4
4. Missing school because of not feeling well	0	1	2	3	4
5. Missing school to go to the doctor or hospital	0	1	2	3	4

PedsQL™

Pediatric Quality of Life Inventory

Version 4.0

CHILD REPORT (ages 8–12)

DIRECTIONS

On the following page is a list of things that might be a problem for you. Please tell us **how much of a problem** each one has been for you during the **past ONE month** by circling:

> 0 if it is **never** a problem
>
> 1 if it is **almost never** a problem
>
> 2 if it is **sometimes** a problem
>
> 3 if it is **often** a problem
>
> 4 if it is **almost always** a problem

There are no right or wrong answers.

If you do not understand a question, please ask for help.

In the past **ONE month**, how much of a **problem** has this been for you . . .

ABOUT MY HEALTH AND ACTIVITIES (problems with . . .)	Never	Almost Never	Some-times	Often	Almost Always
1. It is hard for me to walk more than one block	0	1	2	3	4
2. It is hard for me to run	0	1	2	3	4
3. It is hard for me to do sports activity or exercise	0	1	2	3	4
4. It is hard for me to lift something heavy	0	1	2	3	4
5. It is hard for me to take a bath or shower by myself	0	1	2	3	4
6. It is hard for me to do chores around the house	0	1	2	3	4
7. I hurt or ache	0	1	2	3	4
8. I have low energy	0	1	2	3	4

ABOUT MY FEELINGS (problems with . . .)	Never	Almost Never	Some-times	Often	Almost Always
1. I feel afraid or scared	0	1	2	3	4
2. I feel sad or blue	0	1	2	3	4
3. I feel angry	0	1	2	3	4
4. I have trouble sleeping	0	1	2	3	4
5. I worry about what will happen to me	0	1	2	3	4

HOW I GET ALONG WITH OTHERS (problems with . . .)	Never	Almost Never	Some-times	Often	Almost Always
1. I have trouble getting along with other kids	0	1	2	3	4
2. Other kids do not want to be my friend	0	1	2	3	4
3. Other kids tease me	0	1	2	3	4
4. I cannot do things that other kids my age can do	0	1	2	3	4
5. It is hard to keep up when I play with other kids	0	1	2	3	4

ABOUT SCHOOL (problems with . . .)	Never	Almost Never	Some-times	Often	Almost Always
1. It is hard to pay attention in class	0	1	2	3	4
2. I forget things	0	1	2	3	4
3. I have trouble keeping up with my schoolwork	0	1	2	3	4
4. I miss school because of not feeling well	0	1	2	3	4
5. I miss school to go to the doctor or hospital	0	1	2	3	4

PedsQL™

Cancer Module

Version 3.0

PARENT REPORT for CHILDREN (ages 8–12)

DIRECTIONS

Children with cancer sometimes have special problems. On the following page is a list of things that might be a problem for **your child**. Please tell us **how much of a problem** each one has been for **your child** during the **past ONE month** by circling:

0 if it is **never** a problem

1 if it is **almost never** a problem

2 if it is **sometimes** a problem

3 if it is **often** a problem

4 if it is **almost always** a problem

There are no right or wrong answers.

If you do not understand a question, please ask for help.

In the past **ONE month**, how much of a **problem** has your child had with . . .

PAIN AND HURT (problems with . . .)	Never	Almost Never	Some-times	Often	Almost Always
1. Aches in joints and/or muscles	0	1	2	3	4
2. Having a lot of pain	0	1	2	3	4

NAUSEA (problems with . . .)	Never	Almost Never	Some-times	Often	Almost Always
1. Becoming nauseated during medical treatments	0	1	2	3	4
2. Food not tasting very good to him or her	0	1	2	3	4
3. Becoming nauseated while thinking about medical treatments	0	1	2	3	4
4. Not feeling hungry	0	1	2	3	4
5. Some foods and smells making him or her nauseous	0	1	2	3	4

PROCEDURAL ANXIETY (problems with . . .)	Never	Almost Never	Some-times	Often	Almost Always
1. Needle sticks (i.e., injections, blood tests, IVs) causing him or her pain	0	1	2	3	4
2. Getting anxious about having blood drawn	0	1	2	3	4
3. Getting anxious about having needle sticks (i.e., injections, blood tests, IVs)	0	1	2	3	4

TREATMENT ANXIETY (problems with . . .)	Never	Almost Never	Some-times	Often	Almost Always
1. Getting anxious when waiting to see the doctor	0	1	2	3	4
2. Getting anxious about going to the doctor	0	1	2	3	4
3. Getting anxious about going to the hospital	0	1	2	3	4

WORRY (problems with . . .)	Never	Almost Never	Some-times	Often	Almost Always
1. Worrying about side effects from medical treatments	0	1	2	3	4
2. Worrying about whether or not his or her medical treatments are working	0	1	2	3	4
3. Worrying that the cancer will reoccur or relapse	0	1	2	3	4

In the past **ONE month**, how much of a **problem** has your child had with . . .

COGNITIVE PROBLEMS (problems with . . .)	Never	Almost Never	Some-times	Often	Almost Always
1. Figuring out what to do when something is bothering him or her	0	1	2	3	4
2. Solving math problems	0	1	2	3	4
3. Writing school papers or reports	0	1	2	3	4
4. Difficulty paying attention to things	0	1	2	3	4
5. Remembering what he or she reads	0	1	2	3	4

PERCEIVED PHYSICAL APPEARANCE (problems with . . .)	Never	Almost Never	Some-times	Often	Almost Always
1. Feeling that he or she is not good looking	0	1	2	3	4
2. Not liking other people to see his or her scars	0	1	2	3	4
3. Being embarrassed about others seeing his or her body	0	1	2	3	4

COMMUNICATION (problems with . . .)	Never	Almost Never	Some-times	Often	Almost Always
1. Telling the doctors and nurses how he or she feels	0	1	2	3	4
2. Asking the doctors or nurses questions	0	1	2	3	4
3. Explaining his or her illness to other people	0	1	2	3	4

PedsQL™
Cancer Module

Version 3.0

CHILD REPORT (ages 8–12)

DIRECTIONS

Children with cancer sometimes have special problems. Please tell us **how much of a problem** each one has been for you during the **past ONE month** by circling:

> 0 if it is **never** a problem
>
> 1 if it is **almost never** a problem
>
> 2 if it is **sometimes** a problem
>
> 3 if it is **often** a problem
>
> 4 if it is **almost always** a problem

There are no right or wrong answers.

If you do not understand a question, please ask for help.

In the past **ONE month**, how much of a **problem** has this been for you . . .

PAIN AND HURT (problems with . . .)	Not at all	Sometimes	A lot
1. I ache or hurt in my joints and/or muscles	0	2	4
2. I hurt a lot	0	2	4

NAUSEA (problems with . . .)	Not at all	Sometimes	A lot
1. I become sick to my stomach when I have medical treatments	0	2	4
2. Food does not taste very good to me	0	2	4
3. I become sick to my stomach when I think about medical treatments	0	2	4
4. I don't feel hungry	0	2	4
5. Some foods and smells make my stomach upset	0	2	4

PROCEDURAL ANXIETY (problems with . . .)	Not at all	Sometimes	A lot
1. Needle sticks (i.e., injections, blood tests, IVs) hurt	0	2	4
2. I get scared when I have to have blood tests	0	2	4
3. I get scared about having needle sticks (i.e., injections, blood tests, IVs)	0	2	4

TREATMENT ANXIETY (problems with . . .)	Not at all	Sometimes	A lot
1. I get scared when I am waiting to see the doctor	0	2	4
2. I get scared when I have to go to the doctor	0	2	4
3. I get scared when I have to go to the hospital	0	2	4

WORRY (problems with . . .)	Not at all	Sometimes	A lot
1. I worry about side effects from medical treatments	0	2	4
2. I worry about whether or not my medical treatments are working	0	2	4
3. I worry that my cancer will come back	0	2	4

In the past **ONE month**, how much of a **problem** has this been for you . . .

COGNITIVE PROBLEMS (problems with . . .)	Never	Almost Never	Some-times	Often	Almost Always
1. It is hard for me to figure out what to do when something bothers me	0	1	2	3	4
2. I have trouble solving math problems	0	1	2	3	4
3. I have trouble writing school papers or reports	0	1	2	3	4
4. It is hard for me to pay attention to things	0	1	2	3	4
5. It is hard for me to remember what I read	0	1	2	3	4

PERCEIVED PHYSICAL APPEARANCE (problems with . . .)	Never	Almost Never	Some-times	Often	Almost Always
1. I feel I am not good looking	0	1	2	3	4
2. I don't like other people to see my scars	0	1	2	3	4
3. I am embarrassed when others see my body	0	1	2	3	4

COMMUNICATION (problems with . . .)	Never	Almost Never	Some-times	Often	Almost Always
1. It is hard for me to tell the doctors and nurses how I feel	0	1	2	3	4
2. It is hard for me to ask the doctors and nurses questions	0	1	2	3	4
3. It is hard for me to explain my illness to other people	0	1	2	3	4

PedsQL™
Pediatric Quality of Life Inventory for Teens
(ages 13–18)

PedsQL™

Pediatric Quality of Life Inventory

Version 4.0

PARENT REPORT for TEENS (ages 13–18)

DIRECTIONS

On the following page is a list of things that might be a problem for **your teen**. Please tell us how much of a problem each one has been for **your teen** during the past ONE month by circling:

> 0 if it is **never** a problem
>
> 1 if it is **almost never** a problem
>
> 2 if it is **sometimes** a problem
>
> 3 if it is **often** a problem
>
> 4 if it is **almost always** a problem

There are no right or wrong answers.

If you do not understand a question, please ask for help.

In the past **ONE month**, how much of a **problem** has your teen had with . . .

PHYSICAL FUNCTIONING (problems with . . .)	Never	Almost Never	Some-times	Often	Almost Always
1. Walking more than one block	0	1	2	3	4
2. Running	0	1	2	3	4
3. Participating in sports activity or exercise	0	1	2	3	4
4. Lifting something heavy	0	1	2	3	4
5. Taking a bath or shower by him or herself	0	1	2	3	4
6. Doing chores around the house	0	1	2	3	4
7. Having hurts or aches	0	1	2	3	4
8. Low energy level	0	1	2	3	4

EMOTIONAL FUNCTIONING (problems with . . .)	Never	Almost Never	Some-times	Often	Almost Always
1. Feeling afraid or scared	0	1	2	3	4
2. Feeling sad or blue	0	1	2	3	4
3. Feeling angry	0	1	2	3	4
4. Trouble sleeping	0	1	2	3	4
5. Worrying about what will happen to him or her	0	1	2	3	4

SOCIAL FUNCTIONING (problems with . . .)	Never	Almost Never	Some-times	Often	Almost Always
1. Getting along with other teens	0	1	2	3	4
2. Other teens not wanting to be his or her friend	0	1	2	3	4
3. Getting teased by other teens	0	1	2	3	4
4. Not able to do things that other teens his or her age can do	0	1	2	3	4
5. Keeping up when playing with other teens	0	1	2	3	4

SCHOOL FUNCTIONING (problems with . . .)	Never	Almost Never	Some-times	Often	Almost Always
1. Paying attention in class	0	1	2	3	4
2. Forgetting things	0	1	2	3	4
3. Keeping up with schoolwork	0	1	2	3	4
4. Missing school because of not feeling well	0	1	2	3	4
5. Missing school to go to the doctor or hospital	0	1	2	3	4

PedsQL™
Pediatric Quality of Life Inventory

Version 4.0

TEEN REPORT (ages 13–18)

DIRECTIONS

On the following page is a list of things that might be a problem for you.
Please tell us **how much of a problem** each one has been for you during
the **past ONE month** by circling:

> 0 if it is **never** a problem
>
> 1 if it is **almost never** a problem
>
> 2 if it is **sometimes** a problem
>
> 3 if it is **often** a problem
>
> 4 if it is **almost always** a problem

There are no right or wrong answers.

If you do not understand a question, please ask for help.

In the past **ONE month**, how much of a **problem** has this been for you . . .

ABOUT MY HEALTH AND ACTIVITIES (problems with . . .)	Never	Almost Never	Some-times	Often	Almost Always
1. It is hard for me to walk more than one block	0	1	2	3	4
2. It is hard for me to run	0	1	2	3	4
3. It is hard for me to do sports activity or exercise	0	1	2	3	4
4. It is hard for me to lift something heavy	0	1	2	3	4
5. It is hard for me to take a bath or shower by myself	0	1	2	3	4
6. It is hard for me to do chores around the house	0	1	2	3	4
7. I hurt or ache	0	1	2	3	4
8. I have low energy	0	1	2	3	4

ABOUT MY FEELINGS (problems with . . .)	Never	Almost Never	Some-times	Often	Almost Always
1. I feel afraid or scared	0	1	2	3	4
2. I feel sad or blue	0	1	2	3	4
3. I feel angry	0	1	2	3	4
4. I have trouble sleeping	0	1	2	3	4
5. I worry about what will happen to me	0	1	2	3	4

HOW I GET ALONG WITH OTHERS (problems with . . .)	Never	Almost Never	Some-times	Often	Almost Always
1. I have trouble getting along with other teens	0	1	2	3	4
2. Other teens do not want to be my friend	0	1	2	3	4
3. Other teens tease me	0	1	2	3	4
4. I cannot do things that other teens my age can do	0	1	2	3	4
5. It is hard to keep up with my peers	0	1	2	3	4

ABOUT SCHOOL (problems with . . .)	Never	Almost Never	Some-times	Often	Almost Always
1. It is hard to pay attention in class	0	1	2	3	4
2. I forget things	0	1	2	3	4
3. I have trouble keeping up with my schoolwork	0	1	2	3	4
4. I miss school because of not feeling well	0	1	2	3	4
5. I miss school to go to the doctor or hospital	0	1	2	3	4

PedsQL™

Cancer Module

Version 3.0

PARENT REPORT for TEENS (ages 13–18)

DIRECTIONS

Teens with cancer sometimes have special problems. On the following page is a list of things that might be a problem for **your teen**. Please tell us how much of a problem each one has been for **your teen** during the **past ONE month** by circling:

> 0 if it is **never** a problem
>
> 1 if it is **almost never** a problem
>
> 2 if it is **sometimes** a problem
>
> 3 if it is **often** a problem
>
> 4 if it is **almost always** a problem

There are no right or wrong answers.

If you do not understand a question, please ask for help.

In the past **ONE month**, how much of a **problem** has your teen had with . . .

PAIN AND HURT (problems with . . .)	Never	Almost Never	Some-times	Often	Almost Always
1. Aches in joints and/or muscles	0	1	2	3	4
2. Having a lot of pain	0	1	2	3	4

NAUSEA (problems with . . .)	Never	Almost Never	Some-times	Often	Almost Always
1. Becoming nauseated during medical treatments	0	1	2	3	4
2. Food not tasting very good to him or her	0	1	2	3	4
3. Becoming nauseated while thinking about medical treatments	0	1	2	3	4
4. Not feeling hungry	0	1	2	3	4
5. Some foods and smells making him or her nauseous	0	1	2	3	4

PROCEDURAL ANXIETY (problems with . . .)	Never	Almost Never	Some-times	Often	Almost Always
1. Needle sticks (i.e., injections, blood tests, IVs) causing him or her pain	0	1	2	3	4
2. Getting anxious about having blood drawn	0	1	2	3	4
3. Getting anxious about having needle sticks (i.e., injections, blood tests, IVs)	0	1	2	3	4

TREATMENT ANXIETY (problems with . . .)	Never	Almost Never	Some-times	Often	Almost Always
1. Getting anxious when waiting to see the doctor	0	1	2	3	4
2. Getting anxious about going to the doctor	0	1	2	3	4
3. Getting anxious about going to the hospital	0	1	2	3	4

WORRY (problems with . . .)	Never	Almost Never	Some-times	Often	Almost Always
1. Worrying about side effects from medical treatments	0	1	2	3	4
2. Worrying about whether or not his or her medical treatments are working	0	1	2	3	4
3. Worrying that the cancer will reoccur or relapse	0	1	2	3	4

In the past **ONE month**, how much of a **problem** has your teen had with . . .

COGNITIVE PROBLEMS (problems with . . .)	Never	Almost Never	Some-times	Often	Almost Always
1. Figuring out what to do when something is bothering him or her	0	1	2	3	4
2. Solving math problems	0	1	2	3	4
3. Writing school papers or reports	0	1	2	3	4
4. Difficulty paying attention to things	0	1	2	3	4
5. Remembering what he or she reads	0	1	2	3	4

PERCEIVED PHYSICAL APPEARANCE (problems with . . .)	Never	Almost Never	Some-times	Often	Almost Always
1. Feeling that he or she is not good looking	0	1	2	3	4
2. Not liking other people to see his or her scars	0	1	2	3	4
3. Being embarrassed about others seeing his or her body	0	1	2	3	4

COMMUNICATION (problems with . . .)	Never	Almost Never	Some-times	Often	Almost Always
1. Telling the doctors and nurses how he or she feels	0	1	2	3	4
2. Asking the doctors or nurses questions	0	1	2	3	4
3. Explaining his or her illness to other people	0	1	2	3	4

PedsQL™

Cancer Module

Version 3.0

TEEN REPORT (ages 13–18)

DIRECTIONS

Teens with cancer sometimes have special problems. Please tell us **how much of a problem** each one has been for you during the **past ONE month** by circling:

> 0 if it is **never** a problem
>
> 1 if it is **almost never** a problem
>
> 2 if it is **sometimes** a problem
>
> 3 if it is **often** a problem
>
> 4 if it is **almost always** a problem

There are no right or wrong answers.

If you do not understand a question, please ask for help.

In the past **ONE month**, how much of a **problem** has this been for you . . .

PAIN AND HURT (problems with . . .)	Not at all	Sometimes	A lot
1. I ache or hurt in my joints and/or muscles	0	2	4
2. I hurt a lot	0	2	4

NAUSEA (problems with . . .)	Not at all	Sometimes	A lot
1. I become sick to my stomach when I have medical treatments	0	2	4
2. Food does not taste very good to me	0	2	4
3. I become sick to my stomach when I think about medical treatments	0	2	4
4. I don't feel hungry	0	2	4
5. Some foods and smells make my stomach upset	0	2	4

PROCEDURAL ANXIETY (problems with . . .)	Not at all	Sometimes	A lot
1. Needle sticks (i.e., injections, blood tests, IVs) hurt	0	2	4
2. I get scared when I have to have blood tests	0	2	4
3. I get scared about having needle sticks (i.e., injections, blood tests, IVs)	0	2	4

TREATMENT ANXIETY (problems with . . .)	Not at all	Sometimes	A lot
1. I get scared when I am waiting to see the doctor	0	2	4
2. I get scared when I have to go to the doctor	0	2	4
3. I get scared when I have to go to the hospital	0	2	4

WORRY (problems with . . .)	Not at all	Sometimes	A lot
1. I worry about side effects from medical treatments	0	2	4
2. I worry about whether or not my medical treatments are working	0	2	4
3. I worry that my cancer will come back or relapse	0	2	4

In the past **ONE month**, how much of a **problem** has this been for you . . .

COGNITIVE PROBLEMS (problems with . . .)	Never	Almost Never	Some-times	Often	Almost Always
1. It is hard for me to figure out what to do when something bothers me	0	1	2	3	4
2. I have trouble solving math problems	0	1	2	3	4
3. I have trouble writing school papers or reports	0	1	2	3	4
4. It is hard for me to pay attention to things	0	1	2	3	4
5. It is hard for me to remember what I read	0	1	2	3	4

PERCEIVED PHYSICAL APPEARANCE (problems with . . .)	Never	Almost Never	Some-times	Often	Almost Always
1. I feel I am not good looking	0	1	2	3	4
2. I don't like other people to see my scars	0	1	2	3	4
3. I am embarrassed when others see my body	0	1	2	3	4

COMMUNICATION (problems with . . .)	Never	Almost Never	Some-times	Often	Almost Always
1. It is hard for me to tell the doctors and nurses how I feel	0	1	2	3	4
2. It is hard for me to ask the doctors and nurses questions	0	1	2	3	4
3. It is hard for me to explain my illness to other people	0	1	2	3	4

Index

A

Access, 30
Accountability, 30
Acculturation, 130, 132–134
Active kinesiology, 320
Activities of Daily Living (ADL)
    cross-cultural comparisons, 128–129
    energy conservation for, 368
Adolescent Resilience Model (ARM), 153, 154
Adolescents. *See* Children/adolescents
Advisory Board, international (1992), 120
Advocacy, survivorship-related, 389–392
Affordability, 30
African Americans, 117
Age, spiritual quality of life and, 99
Agency for Health Care Policy and Research
    (AHCPR), cancer pain management
    guidelines, 207
AIDS, 117
Aistars' Organizing Framework, 352, 353, 354
Allogeneic transplants, 276
Alpha level, 188
American Cancer Society, pain management
    guidelines, 207
American Nurses' Association, Council on
    Nurse Researchers' statement, 205
AMGEN, 19–20
Anemia, cancer-related fatigue and, 264–265
Anti-cancer drug development, QOL assessment
    for, 4
Anxiety
    after stem cell transplantation, 326–327, 337
    before stem cell transplantation, 318
ARM (Adolescent Resilience Model), 153, 154
Arthritis, causal model, 58–59
Asian families, impact of stem cell transplant
    on, 334
Assessment instruments. *See* Measurement
    instruments; *specific measurement instruments*

Assessment of quality of life. *See* Measurement
    of quality of life
Assimilation, cultural, 130, 132–134
Association, of QOL variables, 189
Atheoretical approaches, to research, 81–82
Attentional fatigue, Chimprich's theory of, 352,
    353, 354
Attributes of quality of life. *See* Dimensions of
    quality of life
Audit trail, 184

B

Barriers, to nursing care, 264–265
Baseline measurements, 183–184
Bathing, energy conservation for, 367
Battery of tests
    for multidimensional assessment, 178
    vs. single instruments, 34–35
Beliefs, spiritual/religious, 97, 107–108
Benoliel, Jeanne Quint, 203
Bill of rights, for cancer survivors, 382–384
Biotherapy, fatigue from, 364
Blood product harvesting, 274–275
BMT. *See* Bone marrow transplantation
Body image changes, 248, 325, 333
Bone marrow transplantation (BMT). *See also*
        Stem cell transplantation
    definition of, 274
    harvesting stem cells for, 319
    historical aspects of, 273
    quality of life issues, 273
    stem cell sources for, 274
    as treatment, 274–275
    as unique experience, 275–278
Braden's Self-Help Model, 79–81
Breast cancer
    diagnosis, impact of
        on children, 249
        on family, 227–228

incidence, 241
interventions, QOL-related, 250
  coping skills management, 252–253
  exercise, 252
  patient education and support groups,
    251–252
mortality rates, 241
in premenopausal women, 245
research, 242–250
  future directions, 253
  physical well-being, 242–247
  psychological well-being, 247–248
  social well-being, 248–249
  spiritual well-being, 250
  tools for, 250, 251
screening, 241
survival rates, 241
symptoms
  body image changes, 248
  fatigue, 245–246
  fertility concerns and, 245
  impact of, 210
  lymphedema, 246–247
  menopausal, 243–245
  ovarian failure, chemotherapy-induced, 243
  physical, 242–247
  psychological, 247–248
  sexuality changes, 247–248
  weight gain, 246
treatment approach changes and, 242
Breast Cancer Chemotherapy Questionnaire,
  180
Buddhism, 118
Burden, 417
Bush Bone Marrow Transplant Symptom
  Inventory, 473–480
Busulfan/cyclophosphamide, 325

C

CAM (complementary and alternative
  medicine), 105
Cancer Control Research Committee of the
  Southwest Oncology Group, 70–71
Cancer experience. See also specific types of cancer
for children/adolescents, 144
meaning-making for, 106–107, 316
quality of life and. See also Perspectives, on
  quality of life

measurement and, 71
positive influences, 97
theory and, 71
spiritual needs and, 97, 98, 103
symptoms. See Symptoms; specific cancer-
  related symptoms
treatments. See Bone marrow transplantation;
  Stem cell transplantation
Cancer Rehabilitation Evaluation System
  (CARES)
applicability of, 180
coping skills, measurement of, 252
research usage, 250, 251
scoring, 35
symptom items in, 208–209
Cancer-related fatigue. See Fatigue
Cancer-related pain. See Pain
Cancer-specific assessment instruments, 180, 181
Cancer survivors. See Survivorship
Cardiovascular disease, ovarian failure and, 244
Care coordinator, after stem cell transplantation,
  336–337
Caregivers
of children in pain, 211
family as, 224, 226
  categories of, 226
  primary strains from, 222–223
  secondary strains from, 222, 223
optimism, 227
personal perspective of, 406
strain/burden, after death of family member,
  230
stress/coping, 222–224, 225
CARES. See Cancer Rehabilitation Evaluation
  System
Caring, as spiritual support, 108–109
Causal modeling, 190
Chemotherapy
ovarian failure from, 243
personal stories, 397–401
Childbirth Fatigue Framework, 352, 353–354
Childhood cancer survivor, personal story,
  397–401
Children/adolescents
with cancer, quality of life and
  conceptualization of, 145, 160–162
  definition of, 143–149, 145–147
  meaning/importance of, 144

Children/adolescents (*continued*)
measurement, 156–160. *See also*
Measurement instruments,
children/adolescents
pain experiences of, 211
recommendations for future, 161–162
refusal to eat/drink, 333
research, 149, 161–162
significance of, 148–149
of parents with cancer, 221, 249
Chinese Americans, 117
Christianity, 118
Chronic illness, theoretical model of QOL for,
56, 57
CINAHL (*Cumulative Index of Nursing and
Allied Health Literature*), 10
Circular causality, 220
City of Hope Model (Ferrell & colleagues)
for bone marrow transplant survivors,
279–280
for cancer survivors, 7, 8
definition of HRQOL and, 123–124, 127
development of, 53
dimensions of, 53
nurse's perceptions and, 261–263
research usage of, 49
Clarity, conceptual. *See* Concept of quality of
life, clarification
Clinically obscure research-based QOL
information, definition of, 267
Clinical sensitivity, of measurements, 158
Clinical significance, of measurements, 159
Clinical staff. *See* Health care providers
Clinical trials
design characteristics, 188
endpoints, 172–174
enrollment, encouragement of, 191
premature closure of, 156–157
for stem cell transplantation, 317
Clowns, pediatric patients and, 333
Coding schemes, for cross-cultural research, 134
Colony stimulating factors, 364
Community, cancer-related advocacy and,
391–392
Complementary and alternative medicine
(CAM), 105
Concept of quality of life
analysis, 77
in assessment, 81–82

broad, 415
changes in, 416
for children/adolescents, 145, 160–162
clarification, 30–31, 416
guidelines for, 70–82
for pediatric oncology, 143–148
variable specification for, 77
definitional/descriptive issues. *See* Definition,
of quality of life
dimensions of. *See* Dimensions of quality of
life
fatigue and, 352
for healthy persons, 348
inadequacy of, 81
indicators *vs.* related concepts, 66
measurement issues and, 66–70
Medical Outcomes Study's framework for,
59–60
models. *See* Models, conceptual
multidimensional, 45, 46, 59
for nurse *vs.* patient, 413–415
for pediatric oncology patients, 144
specifying for assessment, 76–81
spiritual, 94–96
subjective, 59
Conceptual equivalence, of health-related
quality of life, 129–130, 131
Conceptual-theoretical-empirical structure, of
quality of life
critique of, 49–51
description of, 47–48
Confounding, 79
Consensus Statement on Adjuvent Therapy for
Breast Cancer, 242
Consumers
health care, 30
model of survivorship for, 385–386
Coping strategies
for breast cancer survivors, 252–253
for caregivers, 222–224
definition of, 222
to lessen stress symptoms, 224
to manage meaning, 224
nursing role in, 336
for situational management, 223–224
spiritual/religious, 93, 105
Core plus module approach, for measurement,
35–36
Cost-effectiveness analysis, 190–191

Criterion equivalence, HRQOL, 130
Cross-cultural comparisons, of health-related
 quality of life, 128
Cross-national studies, of health-related quality
 of life, 117–118
Culture
 assimilation/acculturation, 130, 132–134
 disease prevalence/epidemiology and, 134–135
 functions of, 118, 119, 135
 quality of life and
  for children/adolescents, 144–145, 159
  definition of, 119–121, 135–136
  health-related quality of life definition and,
   119–128, 135–136
  measurement issues, 37, 159
 universal needs, fulfillment of, 118
 vs. ethnicity, 119
 vs. race, 118–119
*Cumulative Index of Nursing and Allied Health
 Literature* (CINAHL), 10
Cure, sustained, 388–389
Cyclophosphamide
 premature ovarian failure and, 243
 in stem cell transplant conditioning regimen,
  325

D
Dance, similarity to quality of life, 261, 262
Databases, national, 134–135
Data collection
 multiple methods, 190
 standardized procedures, 184
Death
 of family member, 230, 233
 fear of, children and, 331
 preparation for, 98, 233
Definition
 of fatigue, 351–352
 of health-related quality of life, cultural
  aspects and, 122–128
 of quality of life, 413
  for adults, 421–422
  in arthritis causal model, 59
  broad/global, 415
  in cancer context, 348–349
  cancer survivor's bill of rights, 382–384
  for children/adolescents, 145–147,
   423–424

clarification of, 65
conceptual, 55
 in conceptual models. *See* Models,
  conceptual
consistency/consensus, lack of, 46, 279, 317
controversial issues in, 30–31, 66
cultural aspects of, 119–121, 135–136
for families, 226
individual perspectives, 382
lack of specific measurement and, 171–172
multidimensionality of, 6–8, 55, 160
for pediatric oncology, 143–148
by publication year, 421–424
for research studies, 20
subjectivity of, 55
theoretical, 50–51
universally accepted, 59
vs. health-related quality of life, 122
by World Health Organization, 7, 119–120,
 122
 of response shift, 75
 of spirituality, 94
 of symptom management, 202–204
Demands of Illness Inventory, 180, 435–445
Dependency, 80, 329
Depression
 after stem cell transplant, 327, 337
 interventions for, 369
 optimism and, 227
Descriptive statistics, 189
Determinants, vs. dimensions, 122–126
Development, child
 quality of life and, 144–145
 sensitivity of measurement instruments and,
  158
 stages of, 221
 stem cell transplantation and, 333
Developmental theory, families and, 219–222
Diagnostic impact of cancer
 on children, 249
 on family, 221, 227–228
Dimensions of quality of life
 atheoretical, 78
 for children/adolescents, 145–147
 controversial issues, 31–32
 functional domains. *See* Domains, functional;
  specific functional domains
 in health-related quality of life, 122–126

Dimensions of quality of life (*continued*)
  measurement issues, 66–68, 317, 415–416
    comparisons between domains, 67
    endpoints, 172, 173
    scoring, 35
    unidimensional assessment, 177–178
  multiple. *See* Multidimensionality, of quality
    of life
  nursing process and, 49, 52–53
  vs. determinants or predictors, 122–126
  vs. related concepts, 66–67, 78
Discrimination, QOL measures for, 33
Disease
  incidence, ethnic differences in, 130, 132–133
  phases, 76
  prevalence, cultural/ethnic diversity and,
    134–135
  progressive relationship with QOL domains,
    123
  specific groups of, assessment of, 74
  symptoms from. *See* Symptoms
Disease-related domain, 66
Domains, functional
  in cancer *vs.* noncancer-based theories, 50–51
  for children/adolescent measures, 160
  in City of Hope Model, 53
  comparisons between, 67
  disease-related, 66
  emotional, in Ferrans and Powers' Model,
    54–55
  existential, 94, 95, 121, 370
  in Ferrans and Powers' Model, 54–55
  hierarchical relationship of, 54–55
  impact of symptoms on, 201–202
  measurement issues, 66–68, 415–416
  in Padilla and Grant model, 49, 52–53
  physical. *See* Physical well-being
  progressive relationship with disease and, 123
  psychological. *See* Psychological well-being
  social. *See* Social well-being
  spiritual. *See* Spiritual well-being
Drawings, in communicating with children, 332
Dressing, energy conservation for, 367
Drug development, quality of life assessment for,
  4
Drug therapy, for osteoporosis prevention, 244
Dying process, 76
Dyspnea, 205

E
EBMT (European Group for Blood and Marrow
  Transplantation), 315, 318
Economic/financial factors
  in combating fatigue, 370
  impact of cancer on family, 228–229
  in measurement/assessment, 317
  stem cell transplant recipients and, 323, 330
Edwards' Theory of Neuromuscular Fatigue, 352,
  353
Effect size, 188
Emotional domain, in Ferrans and Powers'
  Model, 54–55
Employment, caregivers and, 223
Empowerment, survivorship and, 386
Enabling skills, 80
End-of-life
  care
    conceptual models for children/adolescents,
      155–156
    family experiences during, 229–230
  as developmental phase, 76
  preparation for death, 98, 233
Endpoints, QOL, 75, 78, 172–174
Energy conservation, for cancer-related fatigue,
  367–368
Environmental characteristics
  definition of, 267
  impact on quality of life, 152–153
EORTC (European Organization for Research
  and Treatment of Cancer), QOL Core
  Questionnaire, 5, 35–36, 250
EORTC Quality of Life Questionnaire, 176
Epidemiology, cultural/ethnic diversity and,
  134–135
Epoetin alpha, 362
Equation, QOL, 349–350
Ergonomics, 352, 353
Estrogen replacement therapy (ERT), 244
Ethical issues
  principles of quality cancer care, 392–393
  purpose identification and, 73
Ethnicity
  coding schemes, 134
  differences in disease incidence/mortality and,
    130, 132–133
  disease prevalence/epidemiology and,
    134–135

health care disparities and, 117
vs. culture, 119
Ethnography, 176–177
European Group for Blood and Marrow Transplantation (EBMT), 315, 318
European Organization for Research and Treatment of Cancer (EORTC), QOL Core Questionnaire, 5, 35–36, 250
Exclusion criteria, for research sample, 187–188
Exercise interventions
  for breast cancer, 252
  for fatigue, 365
  for stem cell transplant patients, 321, 325
Existential domain
  in combating fatigue, 370
  cultural aspects of, 121
  spiritual quality of life and, 94, 95
Existential well-being subscale, of Spiritual Well-Being Scale, 112
Exploratory factor analyses, 67

F

FACIT-Sp (Functional Assessment of Chronic Illness Therapy-Spiritual Well-Being), 101–102, 111
FACT. *See* Functional Assessment of Cancer Therapy
FACT-B (Function Assessment of Cancer Treatment-breast), 250, 251, 252
FACT-G (Functional Assessment of Cancer Therapy-general scale), 180, 208–209
Faith, 96
Family
  assessment, 231–232
  cancer experience
    future directions for, 234
  as caregiver. *See* Caregivers, family as
  of children in pain, experiences of, 211
  defining quality of life for, 226
  financial/economic impact of cancer on, 228–229
  functioning, 220
  impact
    of diagnosis on, 221, 227–228
    of end stage of cancer on, 229–230
    of follow-up care on, 229
    of recurrence on, 229
    of rehabilitation on, 229
    of treatment on, 227–229

as information source QOL assessment, 298
nursing interventions for, 230–233
perspective in assessing child's QOL, 144
relationship issues, 69, 222, 329
research on quality of life, 227–230
spouses, 249, 409–410
structure, 220
theoretical perspectives, 219–226
  caregiver stress and coping, 222–224, 225, 231
  comparison of, 225
  developmental, 219–220, 221–222, 225, 231
  systems, 219, 220, 225, 231
Fatigue
  after stem cell transplantation, 327
  in breast cancer survivors, 245–246
  as clinical symptom, 363–370
  during data collection, 185–186
  definitions of, 351–352, 359
  epidemiology, 361
  etiology of, 347
  factors related to, 346
  impact on quality of life, 346–348
  interventions for, 363–365
  measurement
    in children/adolescents, 158
    physiologic, 360
  as multidimensional/multifactorial construct, 345, 359
  patient description of, 200–201, 359
  prophylactic entiemetics for, 361
  quality of life equation and, 349–350
  research, 345, 358–362
  subjective nature of, 359
  teaching sheets, 367–368
  theories, 350–358
FDA (Food and Drug Administration), 4
Feedback loop, in Winningham's Psychobiological Entropy Hypothesis, 357
Female cancer survivors, spiritual well-being and, 99
Ferrans and Powers' QOL Model. *See* Quality of Life Index
Ferrell and colleagues' model. *See* City of Hope Model
Fertility issues
  after stem cell transplantation, 326
  breast cancer and, 245

Financial factors. *See* Economic/financial factors
Finland, stem cell transplant support groups, 330
FLIC (Functional Living Index-Cancer), 35, 208–209, 253
Follow-up care, impact on family, 229
Food and Drug Administration (FDA), 4
Food restrictions, during isolation, 332
Friendships, 328, 369
Functional Assessment of Cancer Therapy (FACT)
    breast scale, 251, 252
    general scale, 180, 208–209
    as quantitative measure, 176
    scoring, 35
    symptom items in, 208–209
Functional Assessment of Chronic Illness Therapy-Spiritual Well-Being (FACIT-Sp), 101–102, 111
Functional domains. *See* Domains, functional; *specific functional domains*
Functional Living Index-Cancer (FLIC), 35, 208–209, 253

G

Gender differences, in caregiver strain/burden, 228
Generic assessment instruments, 179–180, 181
Genetic differences, of population groups, 118–119
Genitourinary symptoms, menopausal, 244
Genuineness, of caring, 109
Global health status scales, 179
Glorification of recovery, 389
God, 96, 97
GOG (Gynecologic Oncology Group), 11
Graft-versus-host disease (GVHD)
    allogeneic stem cell transplants and, 276–277
    sexuality and, 325
    stem cell transplants and, 317, 324–325
Grandjean's General State of Fatigue Theory, 352–353
Gratitude, 97
Grooming, energy conservation for, 367
Grounded theory, 77, 176–177
GVHD. *See* Graft-versus-host disease
Gynecologic Oncology Group (GOG), 11

H

Happiness, client, 55
Health, definition of, 122, 381–382
Health care costs
    inadequate insurance and, 30
    symptom management and, 206–207
Health care providers. *See also* Nurses
    as information source for assessments, 298
    perspective in assessing child's QOL, 144
    responder burden of, 185–186
Health care system, problems with, 30
Health insurance, lack of, 30
Health paradigm, fatigue theories in, 352
Health profiles, 34
Health-related outcomes, QOL research outcomes and, 174
Health-related quality of life (HRQOL)
    clinical evaluation, 124, 126
    conceptual models, 122–128
    core dimensions/domains, 66–67, 93
    cross-cultural comparisons, 128
        conceptual equivalence, 128–129
        operational equivalence, 128–129
        relevance/usefulness of, 128
    cross-national studies, 117–118
    cultural diversity and, 120
    cultural universality and, 120
    definition, cultural aspects of, 122–128
    determinant-dimension relationship and, 122–126
    integration/assessment, 124, 126
    outcomes, 124–125, 174
    relevant characteristics of, 122
    spiritual well-being and, 93, 99–104
Helplessness, feelings of, 228
Hematopoietic stem cell transplantation. *See* Stem cell transplantation
Herbal remedies, for menopausal symptoms, 244
Hermeneutics, 176–177
HIV, 117
HLA (human leukocyte antigen), 274
Home care, for symptom management, 206
Hope, 95–97
Hormonal therapies, weight gain from, 246
Hospice, 230
Hospice Quality of Life Index, 111
Hospitalization costs, 206–207
HRQOL. *See* Health-related quality of life

Human leukocyte antigen (HLA), 274

I

Illness, meaning-based models and, 150
Illness paradigm, fatigue theories in, 352,
   353–358
Inclusion criteria, for research sample, 187–188
Indicators of QOL. *See* Dimensions of quality of
   life
Inductive research, approaches for, 77
Infection, fear of, 329
Information sources, survivors as, 298–303
Insurance, lack of, 30
Interest, in quality of life, 3–5
Interferon alpha, fatigue and, 200–201
Interleukin-2, 364
International quality of life activities, 4–6
International Society for Chemo-
   Immunotherapy, 5
International Society for Quality of Life
   Research (ISQOL), 4–5
Interpersonal well-being, 68
Irritability, during data collection, 185–186
Isolation procedure, for stem cell transplant
   patients, 321
ISQOL (International Society for Quality of Life
   Research), 4–5

J

Japanese language, quality of life in, 120, 121

K

Karnofsky Performance Scale (KPS), 69,
   177–178, 179
Kitchen activities, energy conservation for,
   367–368
KPS (Karnofsky Performance Scale), 69,
   177–178

L

LAD (lymph node dissection), 248
Language, in distinguishing QOL for children,
   145
Leukemia survivor, personal story of, 397–401
Levels, of quality of life. *See* Dimensions of
   quality of life
Life-Span Development Framework, 149–150,
   151–152
Linear causality, 220

Long-term monitoring, of cancer survivors, 190
Loss, family, 222–223, 233
Lymphedema, 246–247
Lymph node dissection (LAD), 248
Lymphoma survivor, personal story of, 401–406

M

Management. *See* Treatment
Marital relationship, breast cancer and, 249
McCorkle and Young Symptom Distress Scale,
   208–209, 431–433
McGill Quality of Life Questionnaire, 99, 100
Mead Model, 319
Meaning
   of cancer experience/treatment, 67–68
   finding purpose and, 98
   positive, ascribing to cancer experience,
      106–107
   of situation, coping strategies and, 224
   spiritual quality of life and, 96
Meaning-based model, 67–68, 69
Measurement, 66–70
   across domains, 67
   applications, 33
   children/adolescents, 156–160
      after HSCT, 294–295
      clinical sensitivity, 158
      cultural sensitivity, 159
      developmental sensitivity, 158
      guidelines for, 159–160
      purpose of, 159
      standards of comparison, 158
   clarification for, 65, 70–81
   in clinical trials, 33
   conceptual issues, 171–174
      clarity, guidelines for, 70–81
      lack of specific definition, 171–172
      multidimensionality, 171–173
      QOL research outcomes, 172–174
   conceptual/theoretical framework, 72, 76–81
      relationship specification, 78–81
      variable specification, 77
   controversial issues, 33–37
   core plus module approach for, 35–36
   criteria, 72, 81
   dimensions of, 7, 32. *See also* Dimensions of
      quality of life
   domains and, 32, 415–416. *See also* Domains,
      functional

Measurement (*continued*)
  family, 231–232
  future research directions, 190–191
  health-related quality of life
    cross-cultural comparisons, 129
    cross-cultural strategies, 129–130, 131
    cross-cultural translation validation, 130,
      131
  importance of, 3–4
  interest in, 3–4
  meaning-based *vs.* function-based, 75
  in nursing research studies, 11
  patient's perceptions and, 265
  perspective, outcome focus and, 75–76
  population of interest, 73–75
  process or outcome focus, 75–76
  by proxy, 31
  purpose of, 33, 72, 73–76
  qualitative, 176–177
  of quality cancer care, 392–393
  quantitative, 176
  reliability of, 180, 182
  research design issues. *See* Research, design
    issues
  sensitivity/responsiveness, 69–70
  spiritual, 107–108
  stem cell transplant, 293–295
  of symptoms management, 208–211
  theoretical basis of, 49, 50–51
  time points for, 37
  timing of, 75–76
  utility, 4
  validity, 180, 182
Measurement instruments. *See also specific*
    measurement instruments
  for breast cancer research, 250, 251
  cancer-specific, 180, 181
  children/adolescents, 156–160
    clinical sensitivity, 158
    cultural sensitivity, 159
    developmental sensitivity, 158
    disease-specific, 160
    generic, 160
    premature closure of clinical trials, 156–157
    self-reports, 157
    standards of comparison, 158
  cultural adaptation of, 5–6
  culturally sensitive, 37
  dimension *vs.* total scores, 35

  interpretation, 417
  modular, 250
  psychometric inadequacy of, 81
  quantitative *vs.* qualitative, 36
  questionnaires. *See* Questionnaires
  recommendations on, 35–36
  reliability/reproducibility of, 33
  responsiveness of, 33
  selection of, 20, 182
    for children/adolescents, 159–160
    for stem cell transplantation, 295
  self-report *vs.* proxies, 36
  single *vs.* battery of tests, 34–35
  specific *vs.* generic, 34
  for stem cell transplantation QOL, 281–293
  symptom items in, 208–209
  for symptoms/symptom distress, 207
  validity of, 33
Medical model of survivorship, 385
Medical Outcomes Study (MOS)
  conceptual framework, 59–60
  Short Form-36, 34
  Short Form General Health Survey, 180
Medical treatment, 73, 124, 126. *See also specific*
    medical treatments
Menopausal symptoms, in breast cancer,
    243–245
Methodological triangulation, 177
Metric equivalence, HRQOL, 130
Mind-body relationship, 336
Miscel's uncertainty in illness theory, 77
Models, conceptual, 47, 416. *See also* City of
    Hope Model; Quality of Life Index
  function-based, 68–69, 150
  in future research, 60–61
  health-related quality of life, 122–128
  Life-Span Development Framework, 149–150,
    151–152
  meaning-based, 67–68, 150–151
  measures of HRQOL and, 123
  of nurses' relationship-based perception of
    patients, 265–267
  for pediatric oncology, 149–156
  in research, 49, 52–53
  of subjectively perceived QOL, 55–56
  substantive, 152–156
  vs. theory, 47–48
  Zhan's, 55–57
Modular assessment approach, 179, 473–480

Morbidity, cultural/ethnic diversity and, 134–135
Mortality rates
  breast cancer, 241
  cultural/ethnic diversity and, 134–135
Mortality rates (*continued*)
  ethnic differences in, 130, 132–133
MOS. *See* Medical Outcomes Study
Multidimensionality
  of definition for quality of life, 7, 8
  of measurement/assessment, 76–77, 178
    battery approach, 178
    questionnaires, 178
  of quality of life, 31, 67, 171–172
  of symptoms, 205–206
Multidimensional Model of Fatigue, 352, 353
Multidimensional QOL questionnaire, 69

N

National Cancer Institute (NCI), 11, 172
National Coalition for Cancer Survivorship (NCCS), 384
National Comprehensive Cancer Network, cancer pain management guidelines, 207
National health care policy, 29–30
National Institutes of Health (NIH), 242
National Surgical Adjuvant Project for Breast and Bowel Cancer (NSABP), 11
Nausea, 203
NCCS (National Coalition for Cancer Survivorship), 384
NCI (National Cancer Institute), 11, 172
Needs
  spiritual, 97, 98, 103
  universal, culture and, 118
Netherlands, stem cell transplant support groups, 330
NIH (National Institutes of Health), 242
Noncancer QOL models, 55–59
Nottingham Health Profile, 34
Nurse administrators, QOL issues for, 149
Nurse-patient relationship, definition of, 267
Nurses. *See also* Nursing interventions
  educational issues, 148–149
  impact on stem cell transplantation QOL, 335–337
  implications of SCT QOL assessment, 301–303

interest in QOL, 10–11
  perceptions of patient's QOL, 261, 263–267
    definition of, 267
    vs. patient's perceptions, 263–264
  quality of life perspectives
    future research and, 413–414
    patients' perspectives and, 413–418
  spiritual support from, 104–105
  symptom management and, 199
Nursing interventions, 417–418
  for anemia, 364–365
  assessment of illness response, 261
  barriers, 208, 264–265
  for QOL improvement
    clinical practice methods for, 268–270
    patient's perceptions of, 268
  relevance of quality of life for, 21–22
  settings, for symptom management, 206
  spiritual care, 104–106
Nursing process. *See also* Nursing interventions
  dimensions of quality of life and, 49, 52–53
  practice scope, quality of life and, 9–10
  quality of life outcomes and, 124–125
Nursing strategies, definition of, 267
Nutritional status, 320

O

Oncology Nursing Foundation (ONF)
  major grants program, 16–17
  small grants program, 12–16
Oncology Nursing Society (ONS)
  Annual Quality of Life Award, 17–19
  Quality of Life Lectureships, 17, 19
  research activities, 12–20
  research priorities, 20
  State-of-the Knowledge Conference, 20, 264–265
Oncology Nursing Society Congress, 264
ONF. *See* Oncology Nursing Foundation
ONS. *See* Oncology Nursing Society
Operational equivalence, 129–130, 131
Osteoporosis, 244
Outcomes
  of cancer treatment, in QOL assessment, 3, 4, 75–76, 191
  in clinical trials, 191
  health-related quality of life, 124–125, 174
Outpatient care, symptom management and, 206

Ovarian cancer
   fatigue and, 369
   HRQOL domains and, 98
   spiritual quality of life and, 96–97
Ovarian failure, 243, 244

P

Padilla and Grant model. *See* Quality of Life
      Index, Padilla & Grant adaptation
Pain
   children's experiences with, 211
   impact
      on family, 228
      on quality of life, 203
   management guidelines, 207
   multidimensional view of, 205–206
   quality of life dimensions and, 123–124
Palliative care, 4, 74–75
Paradigm, quality of life, 66
Parents
   of children in pain, experiences of, 211
   of children receiving SCT, 331
   perspective, congruence with child's
         perspective, 144
   of stem cell transplant patients, 334
Passive kinesiology, 320
Patient education, breast cancer, 251–252
Patient-focused approach, 67
Patient-nurse relationship, 335
Patient's perceptions
   as best QOL measure, 265
   differences in, 76
   future research and, 413–414
   of nursing ability to improve QOL, 268
   personal stories
      childhood cancer survivor, 397–401
      nurses' perceptions from, 266–267
   of quality of life, 266–267
      fatigue and, 200–201
      nurses' perceptions and, 266–267
      nurses' relationship-based perception of,
         265–266
   vs. health provider's perceptions, 263–264
Pediatric Oncology Group (POG), 150, 465–471
Pediatric oncology patients
   definition of QOL for, 143–148
   significance of QOL for, 148–149
Pediatric Quality of Life Inventory for Young
      Children (PedQL™)

   for ages 5-7, 482–493
   for ages 8-12, 496–505
   for ages 13-18, 508–517
Perceived quality of life, 55–56, 58
Peripheral stem cell transplantation. *See* Stem
      cell transplantation
Perspectives, on quality of life
   assessments, 75–76
   parent-child congruence of, 144
   personal, 407–409
   spiritual support and, 104–105
   of spouse, 409–410
Phenomenology, 77, 176–177
Physical care interventions, for fatigue, 364–365
Physical well-being (domain)
   in adult clinical trials, 66
   after stem cell transplant discharge, 317,
      324–326
   of breast cancer survivors, 242–247
   cancer pain and, 123–124
   for children/adolescents, 145–147
   in City of Hope Model, 53, 68
   description of, 32, 173
   in Ferrans and Powers' Model, 54–55
   importance to cancer patients, 98
   research on, 242–247
   symptom control and, 199
   variables, 80
Physicians' Desk Reference, 4
Physiological domain, 46
Pilot testing, 186
Piper Fatigue Scale, 200–201, 362
Piper's Integrated Fatigue Model, 353,
      354–355
Pluripotent stem cells, 274
POG (Pediatric Oncology Group), 465–471
POMS (Profile of Mood States), 253
Population of interest
   defining, 73–75
   demographics, 74
Positive outlook, 97
Predictors, of quality of life. *See also* Domains,
      functional; specific functional domains
   measurement of, 33
   theoretical aspects, 68, 77
   vs. dimensions or attributes, 122–123
Pregnancy, breast cancer survivors and, 245
Premature ovarian failure, cyclophosphamide
      and, 243

Pretesting, 186
Process focus, of assessment, 75–76
Profile of Mood States (POMS), 253
Prostate cancer, African Americans and, 117
Proxies, *vs.* self-reports, 36
Psychiatric interventions, 320–321
Psychobiological Entropy Hypothesis, 352, 353, 355–358
Psychological well-being (domain)
  in adult clinical trials, 66, 317
  after stem cell transplant
    adults, 326–328
    children, 333
  breast cancer survivors, 247–248
  cancer pain and, 123–124
  for children/adolescents, 145–147
  in City of Hope Model, 53
  description of, 32, 173
  importance to cancer patients, 98
  interventions for fatigue, 365, 368–369
  spiritual quality of life and, 94, 95
  during stem cell transplantation
    adults, 320–322
    children, 332–333
  theoretical aspects, 46, 68
Psychometric inadequacy, 81
Psychometric instruments, 417
Psychosocial theories, 78–79
Psychosocial well-being, pre-stem cell transplant
  adult, 318–319
  children and, 331–332
Publications, QOL, 6
Purpose, for assessing QOL, 72, 73–76

Q
QALY (quality adjusted life year), 73
QOL Core Questionnaire, 5, 35–36, 250
Qualitative research
  instruments for, 36
  measurement, 176–177
  model of survivorship, 385–386
  spiritual quality of life, 109–110
  stem cell transplant survivors, 295
  symptom management, 210
Quality adjusted life year (QALY), 73
Quality cancer care, 392–393
Quality of life. *See specific aspects of*
Quality of Life Index
  bone marrow transplant version, 208–209

breast version, 208–209, 250, 251
Ferrans & Powers version, 187
  cancer version, 362
  definition of quality of life for, 54
  development of, 49
  domains in, 46, 54–55
  faith in God and, 96
Padilla & Grant adaptation, 447–450
  cancer-related pain and, 123–124, 125, 127
  cancer version, 451–454
  development of, 6, 49, 52–53
  psychological/spiritual domain, 112
Quality of Life Lectureships, 17, 19
Quality of Life Scale, 455–463
Quantitative research
  measurement, 36, 176
  model of survivorship, 385
  spiritual quality of life, 110–112
Questionnaires
  development of, 71
  lack of gold standard for, 175–176
  modular-type, 179
  multidimensional, 180
  scoring, 186–187
Questions, open-ended, 176, 177

R
Race
  coding schemes, 134
  vs. culture, 118–119
Rand Health Status Measure for Children, 466–471
RBI (Religious Belief Index), 100
Recurrence of cancer, impact on family, 229
Rehabilitation, impact on family, 229
Relationship specification, for assessment, 78–81
Reliability
  of assessment instruments, 33
  of cultural/racial/ethnic coding schemes, 134
  of measurement, 180, 182
Religion
  after stem cell transplantation, 330
  coping strategies and, 93
  needs from, 98
Religiosity, *vs.* spirituality, 95
Religious Belief Index (RBI), 100
Religious well-being subscale, of Spiritual Well-Being Scale, 112
Remission, 76, 388–389

Repeated-measures design, 182–183
Reproducibility, of assessment instruments, 33
Rescue, bone marrow, 274
Research
    Annual Quality of Life Award, 17–19
    breast cancer. *See* Breast cancer, research
    children/adolescents, 149, 161–162
    conceptual models in, 49
    cross-cultural
        on acculturation, 130, 133–134
        coding schemes for, 134
    descriptive symptomatic, 207
    design issues, 174–190
        baseline data, 183–184
        cancer-specific instruments, 180, 181
        entry criteria, 187–188
        generic instruments, 179–180, 181
        lack of gold standard, 175–176
        modular assessment, 179
        multidimensional assessment, 177–178
        pilot testing, 186
        pretesting, 186
        quantitative *vs.* qualitative approaches,
            176–177
        responder burden, 185–186
        scoring of questionnaires, 186–187
        self-report data, 184–185
        single- *vs.* repeated-measures, 182–183
        standardized data collection procedures,
            184
        statistical analysis plan, 188–190
        statistical power, 188–190
        treatment effectiveness designs, 188
        unidimensional assessment, 177–178
    EBMT nurses group, 318
    ethnic, limitations of national databases,
        134–135
    family, 227–230
    on fatigue and quality of life, 358–362
    future directions
        children/adolescents, 161–162
        conceptual models in, 60–61
        in measurement, 190–191
        nursing perspectives and, 413–414
        patient perspectives and, 413–414
        stem cell transplantation, 295–297
    interdisciplinary approaches, 11
    interest in, 4
    interpretation of, 21

    missing data in, 21
    Oncology Nursing Foundation projects, 12–17
    outcome, QOL as, 172–174
    participants, responder burden, 185–186
    priorities, for Oncology Nursing Society, 20
    as priority, 11
    psychological well-being, 247–248
    qualitative. *See* Qualitative research
    quality of life issues, 20–21
    quality of life theory and, 47–49
    quantitative. *See* Quantitative research
    questions, cancer *vs.* noncancer-based, 50–51
    recommendations for, 37–38
    spiritual quality of life, 96–104, 109–112
    stem cell transplantation, 280–293
    on symptoms management
        as focus of, 205
        interventional, 207
        lack of, 207
        measurement issues in, 208–211
    theory-generating, 46
    theory-testing, 46
        examples of, 46–47
        lack of explicit theories and, 47
Resources
    allocation, QOL assessment for, 73
    for family, 233
Responder burden, 185–186
Response shift
    definition of, 75
    health-related quality of life and, 125, 127,
        128
Responsiveness, of assessment instruments, 33
Roy's Adaptation Model, 205

S

Sample size
    statistical power and, 189
    test batteries and, 35
Satisfaction, client, 55
Scalar equivalence, 130
School return, after stem cell transplant, 333
SCT. *See* Stem cell transplantation
SDS (Symptom Distress Scale), 208–209,
    431–433
Self-advocacy, 389–390
Self-awareness, 107
Self-care agency, 227–228
Self-help, definition of, 79–80

Self-Help Model, 79–81
Self-reports
  children/adolescents, 157
  data from, 70, 184–185
  limitations of, 185
  vs. proxies, 36
Self-Sustaining Model, 153–155
Self-transcendence, 96
Semantic equivalence, 129
Sensitivity, of measurement tools, 157
Sequelae of disease/treatment, 73
Serial measurement, 182–183
Sexuality
  after stem cell transplantation, 325–326,
    328–329
  assessment, 336
  breast cancer survivors and, 247–248
Showering, energy conservation for, 367
Siblings, of children undergoing SCT, 276, 332,
  334
Sickness Impact Profile (SIP), 34, 180
Side effects, 80. *See also* Symptoms
Simultaneous concept analysis, 77
SIP (Sickness Impact Profile), 34, 180
Social role performance, 69
Social support, for stem cell transplant
  recipients, 322–323
Social well-being (domain)
  in adult clinical trials, 66
  of breast cancer survivors, 248–249
  cancer pain and, 123–124
  for children/adolescents, 145–147
  in City of Hope Model, 53
  description of, 32, 173
  in Ferrans and Powers' Model, 54–55
  importance to cancer patients, 98
  interaction, 317
    after stem cell transplantation, 328–330
    interventions to combat fatigue, 369–370
    during stem cell transplantation, 322–323
  theoretical aspects, 46, 68–69, 77
Somatic dimension, 32
Southwest Oncology Group (SWOG), 11
Spilker model, 124, 126, 127
Spirituality
  definition of, 94
  different manifestations of, 103
  HRQOL and, 96–97

  importance of, 409–410
  as QOL domain, 67
  vs. religiosity, 95
Spiritual practices, support for, 107–108
Spiritual quality of life (SpQOL)
  clinical implications, 104–109
  conceptualization, 94–96
  degree of, 98–99
  elements of, 94, 95
  empirical research, 96–104
    qualitative, 109–110
    quantitative, 110–112
  factors related to, 99–104
  indicators of, 96–98
  promotion, nursing approaches for, 105–106
  spiritual needs and, 97–98
Spiritual well-being (domain), 46
  of breast cancer survivors, 97, 250
  cancer pain and, 123–124
  for children/adolescents, 145–147
  in City of Hope Model, 53
  in combating fatigue, 370
  cultural aspects of, 121
  description of, 32
  health-related quality of life and, 93, 99–104
  HRQOL and, 93
  importance to cancer patients, 98
  of stem cell transplant recipients, 323–324,
    330
Spiritual Well-Being Scale (SWBS), 100, 101,
  110–112
Spouses
  of breast cancer survivors, 249
  personal perspective of, 409–410
SpQOL. *See* Spiritual quality of life
Sprangers and Schwartz model, 125, 127, 128
Statistical analysis plan, 189–190
Statistical power, 188–190
Statistical significance, 159
Stem cell transplantation (SCT), 274–275,
  315–316
  adult care during, 319–324
    economic status, 323
    physical status, 320
    psychological status, 320
    social interaction, 323–323
    spiritual aspects, 323–324
  adult psychosocial care prior to, 318–319

Stem cell transplantation (*continued*)
  allogeneic, 276
    graft-versus-host disease and, 276–277
    outpatient, 337
  autologous, 276, 337
  candidates, 275
    risks for, 275–276
    underlying diseases of, 276
  conditioning regimen, 321, 325
  cost of, 277
  cytotoxic protocols, 277
  definition of, 274
  discharge, care after, 324–330
  disclosure of risks/side effects, 318–319
  European Group for Blood and Marrow
      Transplantation, 315
  harvesting of stem cells for, 319
  measurement of QOL, 293–295
  nursing, 335–337
  parents of patients, 334
  patient independence and, 316
  potential recipients, 276
  psychosocial aspects, pre-transplant
      for children, 331–332
  QOL assessment, 303–304
    challenges, 299–300
    comparison groups, 300–301
    concerns for, 299
    information sources, 298–303
    nursing practice implications, 301–303
    pretransplant, 299–300
  research, 280–293
    future directions, 295–297
  siblings of pediatric patients, 334
  sources of stem cells, 274
  survivors
    global quality of life, 294
    modular approach, 473–480
    personal story of, 401–406
    quality of life for, 9–10, 277–278, 278–280
    Quality of Life Scale, 455–463
    as volunteers, 321–322
  syngeneic, 276
  theoretical approach to QOL, 278–279
  as treatment, 274–275
  types of, 276–277
  as unique experience, 275–278
Stress, caregiver, 222–224
Structural analysis, 77

Subjectively perceived quality of life, model of,
    55, 56
Subscales, summing scores from, 186–187
Suffering, transcending, 106–107
Support groups
  for breast cancer, 251–252
  for hematologic malignancies, 323
  for stem cell transplant patients, 330
Survivorship
  bill of rights for, 382–384
  breast cancer, 241
  defining, 385–386
  historical perspective, 381–382
  personal story of, 397–401
  shift toward, 384–385
  spiritual well-being and, 99
  SpQOL and, 103
  stages, 387–389
  stem cell transplant. *See* Stem cell
      transplantation, survivors
SWBS (Spiritual Well-Being Scale), 100, 101,
    110–112
SWOG QOL questionnaire, 35, 36
Symptom Distress Scale (SDS), 208–209,
    431–433
Symptoms. *See also specific symptoms*
  in breast cancer. *See* Breast cancer, symptoms
  disease-related, 173
  distress, 203–204, 208
  fatigue. *See* Fatigue
  impact on quality of life, 201–202, 210
  intensity/severity of, 205, 208
  management, 199
    barriers to, 207–208
    clinical issues in, 204–207
    definition of, 202–204
    future research on interventions for, 211
    goal of, 204–205
    health care costs and, 206–207
    interventions, future research on, 211
    lack of research on, 207
    qualitative research, 210
    research issues, 208–211
  menopausal, 243–245
  multidimensionality of, 205–206
  in oncology literature, 204
  relationship specification, 78–81
  treatment-related, 173
Syngeneic transplants, 276

Systems theory, families and, 219, 220

T

Tamoxifen™, 242, 246
Technical equivalence, of health-related quality
of life, 130
Terminal illness
family experiences during, 229–230
preparation for death, 98, 233
Theories, quality of life
cancer-related fatigue, 350–358
cancer *vs.* noncancer-based, 49, 50–51
dimensions of. *See* Dimensions of quality of
life
explicit, lack of, 47
implications of, 47–49
models. *See* Models, conceptual
specifying for assessment, 76–81
for stem cell transplant, 278–280
vs. conceptual model, 47–48
Timing
of assessment, 75–76
of symptoms management assessment, 208
Total scores, for assessment instruments, 35
Transcendence, 96
Treatment
advances, 417
changes, in breast cancer, 242
disputes, resolution of, 73
effectiveness studies. *See* Clinical trials
impact on family, 227–229
medical
HRQOL and, 124, 126
justification, 73
refuting, 73
phases, 76
quality of life data collection during, 186
selection, 73
strategies, for family coping, 223–224
of symptoms. *See* Symptoms, management
symptoms from, 173. *See also* Symptoms
transplantation. *See* Bone marrow
transplantation; Stem cell
transplantation

Treatment-related symptoms domain, 66
Tumor necrosis factor, 364

U

Uncertainty in illness model, 79, 80
Unidimensional assessment, 177–178
Upjohn Corporation, Annual Quality of Life
Award, 17–19
U.S. Food and Drug Administration, 4
Utility measures, 34

V

Vaginal dryness, 325, 326
Validity
of assessment instruments, 33
of cultural/racial/ethnic coding schemes, 134
exploratory factor analyses and, 67
of measurement, 180, 182
Variable specification, for assessment, 77
VAS (Visual Analogue Scale), 429–430
Vasomotor symptoms, in breast cancer, 243–244
Veteran-rookie connection, 390
Visual Analogue Scale (VAS), 429–430
Volunteers, stem cell transplant survivors as,
321–322

W

Ware model, 123, 127
Watchful waiting, 387–388
Weight gain, from hormonal therapies, 246
WHO. *See* World Health Organization
"Windows of time" concept, 232
Winningham's Psychobiological Entropy
Hypothesis, 352, 353, 355–358
Workshop on Quality of Life Research in
Cancer Clinical Trials, 7
Work simplification, for cancer-related fatigue,
366
World Health Organization (WHO)
definition
of health, 381–382
of quality of life, 7, 119–120, 122
global cancer control program, 4
Tokyo QOL conference of 1984, 121